MULTI-BILLION-DOLLAR PET FOOD FRAUD

Other books by the author

Raw Meaty Bones: Promote Health 2001
Work Wonders: Feed Your Dog Raw Meaty Bones 2005

MULTI-BILLION-DOLLAR

PET FOOD FRAUD

HIDING IN PLAIN SIGHT

DR TOM LONSDALE

RIVETCO PTY LTD

First published in 2023 by:
Rivetco Pty Ltd
PO Box 6096
Windsor Delivery Centre
NSW 2756
Australia

Email: info@rivetco.com.au
Phone: +61 2 4577 6236
Website: www.thepetfoodcon.com | www.rawmeatybones.com

National Library of Australia Cataloguing-in-publication entry:

Lonsdale, Tom, 1949–
Multi-billion-dollar pet food fraud: hiding in plain sight

Includes index

ISBN 978-0-6457265-0-3
ISBN 978-0-6457265-1-0 (ebook)
ISBN 978-0-6457265-2-7 (audiobook)

NATIONAL LIBRARY OF AUSTRALIA

A catalogue record for this book is available from the National Library of Australia

This book has been written and published in good faith. However, when dealing with biological systems, for instance the health of animals, problems can occur. The publisher is therefore unable to guarantee that, in every circumstance, the information presented here will be of benefit, and neither does the information constitute professional advice upon which you should rely.

The author and publisher have made extensive efforts to trace the copyright holders for borrowed material. If they have inadvertently overlooked any, they will be pleased to rectify matters at the first opportunity.

If you find errors of fact or interpretation contained within these pages, please contact the publisher.

ABBREVIATIONS

AAFCO	Association of American Feed Control Officials
ABC	Australian Broadcasting Commission (Corporation since 1983)
ACVS	Australian College of Veterinary Scientists
AVA	Australian Veterinary Association
BVS	Board of Veterinary Surgeons
CDC	Centers for Disease Control and Prevention (US)
CT	computerised tomography
CVE	Centre for Veterinary Education
EDM	early day motion (UK Parliament)
FDA	Food and Drug Administration (US)
FLUTD	feline lower urinary tract disease
FOI	Freedom of Information
MRI	magnetic resonance imaging
NSW	New South Wales (Australia)
PFIAA	Pet Food Industry Association of Australia
PFMA	Pet Food Manufacturers Association (UK)
RCVS	Royal College of Veterinary Surgeons
RMB	raw meaty bones
RSPCA	Royal Society for the Prevention of Cruelty to Animals
RVC	Royal Veterinary College (University of London)
SASH	Small Animal Specialist Hospital (Sydney)
UK	United Kingdom
US	United States (of America)
VOHC	Veterinary Oral Health Council
VPB	Veterinary Practitioners Board of New South Wales
VSIC	Veterinary Surgeons Investigating Committee

CONTENTS

INTRODUCTION

Why the need for this book now? Why the provocative title?

The year was 2011. Not one person venturing up the path, entering the reception room and then the consulting room in my newly opened vet practice, had ever been given sound, healthy dietary advice for their pet. No matter whether they nursed a baby kitten, a puppy or a geriatric cat, or coaxed a dog on a lead, the situation was (and still is) the same. All new clients grew up in a world programmed to accept commercial pet food as normal. All had been following the advice of qualified vets, and all were unwittingly harming their pets—multi-level failings on a tragic scale.

Now 10 years later, after ministering to the needs of thousands of pets and their owners, I felt it was time to rise in defiance, to again blow the whistle on the multi-billion-dollar pet food fraud hiding in plain sight.

Back in 1991, vet Breck Muir and I first blew the whistle on the alliance between the junk pet food industries, vets and fake animal welfare groups. We explained in simple terms how junk pet foods, similar to or worse than human junk foods, were devastating the health of carnivorous pets. We objected to vets knowingly harming the pets under their care. We condemned the cruelty of subjecting pets to a lifetime of dental suffering. We deplored the overservicing by vets when a simple diet change would, in many cases, obviate the need for pet owners to consult the vet.

Breck complained: 'Here we have the perfectly engineered commercial circle—a problem doesn't exist, so we create one, and then come up with all the remedial treatments.'

Overservicing by the vet profession was bad in 1991. It's way worse now. Vets in tandem with fake animal welfare organisations proclaim the alleged superiority of the junk pet food offerings. Bought and paid for by giant companies, vet professional bodies and welfare organisations provide a protective cordon—innocence by association—for the companies. The community of pet owners and the community more generally is accustomed to believe in the integrity of the vet profession and welfare groups when, in fact, the vets and welfare groups abuse the trust.

Imagine if all the auto mechanics in a town had a deal with oil companies. Imagine if they knowingly sold defective fuel and worked on the fuel-related engine problems without first draining the fuel tank. Imagine if every petrol (gasoline) station in the town sold adulterated fuel, that the government regulators knew about and condoned the scam. Unthinkable, do I hear you say? Unfortunately, not just in an imaginary town, but the whole world over, pets are 'fuelled' by junk food and the pet mechanics, the vets, dream up all manner of tests and treatments without either acknowledging or dealing with the fundamentals of the pandemic induced by junk pet food.

Government regulators know, or should know, about the problem. It's the same for journalists, scientists, administrators and anyone with a role providing checks and balances against the pet food fraud. Basic biological and nutritional definitions tell us that carnivores with anatomy, physiology and behaviour fashioned by nature over aeons should not now be forced to dwell in solitary confinement forced to consume industrial grain-based junk.

When new materials, technology or methods are introduced, their manufacturers and promoters need to demonstrate suitability and safety as compared with the systems they are replacing. The onus of proof is on the manufacturers to show that, for instance, cars are superior to horses for carrying passengers and goods. Regulators review the company data, conduct further tests and provide certificates of compliance. However, with industrial pet foods, the system has been upended, with the result that artificial, harmful junk is nowadays considered to be the gold-star standard. Vets, pet welfare organisations and government regulators disparage the natural evolutionary standard—whole carcasses or the pragmatic option, raw meaty bones.

Evidence of the pet food hoax goes well beyond basic definitions. In 1992 I gave a presentation to Sydney general practitioner vets entitled 'Pandemic of periodontal disease: a malodorous condition'. I urged the audience, including six academic vets, to take up the challenge and research the aetiology, prevention and treatment of the mouth rot pandemic. Laughter was their response. At that moment, I resolved that if they would not address the issues, then I would. Over the ensuing years I researched, wrote and campaigned against the junk pet food monster hiding in plain sight.

The resultant documents and books fill archives, nowadays mostly obscured from view by relentless junk pet food propaganda. Consequently, I've placed some key articles and representative historical data in Part II of this book, 'Pet health matters'. The realisation that raw meaty bones exert miracle preventative and therapeutic benefits for pets has filled me with awe at the majesty of nature's grand design. It's a tiny realisation with immense implications for pets, people and the planet.

Part III, 'Confronting reality', describes how vet schools and associations are variously compromised and corrupted. There's a chapter on the 'alternative' raw feeding movements that misappropriated aspects of the straightforward 'raw meaty bones' solution for their own advancement and suppressed the rest. The media and politicians have mostly failed a dependent public. The public deserves to know. Part IV recommends that we 'press on regardless' spreading the vital good health message by any and all available means—including legal actions against pet food companies, vets and animal welfare groups.

Disclaimer

Printed words on the page are our medium of communication. And words have a depressing habit of meaning different things to different people. Indeed: 'One man's meat is another man's poison'. The supermarket aisle carries the signs 'Dog food' and 'Cat food'. The cans bear labels describing the contents as 'pet food'. With endless, regular use the concepts stick. The signs and labels seem to provide a reasonable description.

To my mind, it would be closer to the truth to hang signs 'Dog poison' and 'Cat poison' over the supermarket aisle. The contents of the can or packet should not bear the benign label 'pet food' but

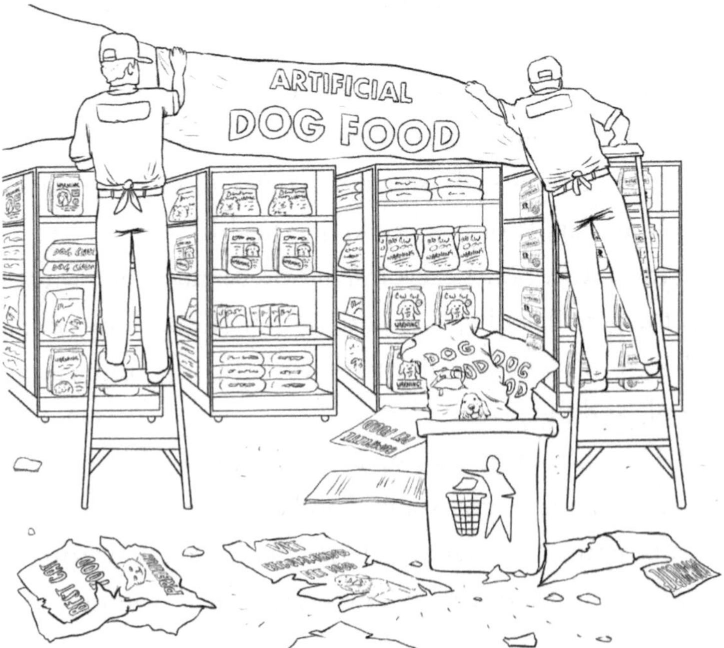

warn the purchaser that the contents are at best 'artificial' or 'industrial' or 'fake'. However, I don't wish to be obtuse, and I don't have another term to replace the ubiquitous 'pet food'. So, for the rest of the book, I use the term, but always use it in a 'manner of speaking'. If the substance being described is in some way manufactured, then you can be sure it does not deserve the unqualified label 'pet food'.

I have similar reservations about the use of the word 'carnivore' meaning 'meat eater'. People easily get lulled into the idea that a meat diet is sufficient for lions, wolves, domestic cats and dogs. But meat alone is *not* sufficient. 'Carnivores' need both meat and bone to stay healthy. 'Carcassivores' would be a more apt term.

However, putting pedantry aside, throughout the book I use the terms 'pet food' and 'carnivore' and hope that you will make the necessary mental adjustments.

Getting started

Much of the information in the book challenges established beliefs. No matter your starting point, I request that you suspend disbelief until you're more familiar with the material. This is especially the case if you're a vet or other pet professional invested in the current system. And for all people, I recommend watching the television segments and videos at the Tom Lonsdale YouTube channel.

Regarding vet reluctance to switch sides, Dr Mei Yam provides a vivid example. Most young vets took around six months working in my practice before gaining an understanding and becoming proficient in raw meaty bones theory. Mei Yam was an exception. She took 18 long months before her illusions fell away, before she rejected her vet school indoctrination and became a raw meaty bones champion. It took time for Mei to tease apart the extensive, interwoven strands that bind the junk pet food culture. It took time for her to see and connect the dots giving her a clear picture of the industrial scale, pet food cultural conditioning. But when she did, she bought the veterinary practice, enabling me to retire from clinical work and write this book. Mei, I salute you.

If you are a pet owner, you may like to start with three inspiring pet owner testimonials submitted to the 2018 Australian Parliament Inquiry into the pet food industry located at Appendixes A, B and C. Three pet owners describe the dramatic health improvements of their pet dogs and cats upon switching diets from processed junk to a diet of predominantly raw meaty bones. Also, before your next visit to the vet, I suggest that you read the 'Preventative dentistry' article at Appendix D. The article sets out precautionary principles and basic standards, standards most vets are unaware of and do not follow. Yes, until vets turn through 180 degrees and drop their slavish adherence to junk pet food dogma, pet owners must rely on their own research.

Regardless of your entry point into the book, I hope you enjoy the onward journey. There's lots of ground to cover—best to start slowly.

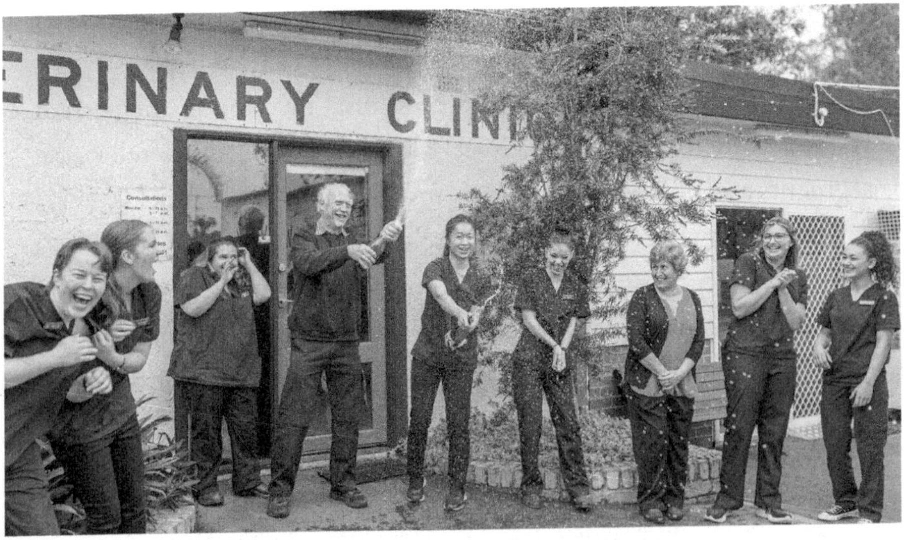

Dr Mei Yam becomes the new owner of Bligh Park Pet Health Centre—27 October 2020.

PART I

1

SOME BACKGROUND, SOME CONTEXT

London veterinary school

Fifty-five years ago, in September 1967 to be precise, I commenced my studies at the Royal Veterinary College (RVC), University of London. Wide-eyed, perhaps not innocent, I was an English country kid heading out on a fabulous adventure in the big city. It was the Summer of Love. The Beatles, Jimi Hendrix and the Rolling Stones topped the charts. A restlessness and sense of excitement filled the air. The price of inclusion, for me, entailed passing exams. So long as I passed the annual exams, I could spend another year soaking up the delights life had in store.

At the end of the first academic year, during the summer holidays, I took a cheap student flight to New York, then a standby flight to San Francisco and a Greyhound bus to San Jose. Through July and August, I worked 10-hour shifts, six nights a week in the Del Monte pickle works. At weekends I mingled with university students from Stanford and Berkeley and the hippie crowd in San Francisco. In September I travelled on a Greyhound bus pass throughout North America before catching the flight back to London for the new university year. The English country kid had grown up fast.

Foundation work in veterinary science involves studies in anatomy, physiology and biochemistry. Memorising vast amounts of information by rote was the accepted way of learning. Most lecturers presented information as incontrovertible fact that in some unspoken way was supposed to provide us with a foundation for later studies in animal husbandry, pathology, medicine and surgery. Frankly, I was amazed at the seeming ease with which our teachers poured forth reams of information. But how did all that information come into being in the first place? To me it seemed that diligent super brains, greatly exceeding my intellectual capacity, had assembled a formidable body of information in the service of humans and the animals under our care.

So, my life roughly divided into two halves. At the university I was intent on learning the nuts and bolts of how to be a vet. Proficiency involved knowing lots of facts, good hand–eye coordination skills, and an ability to find practical solutions to practical problems. Outside university there was no ready-made formula for the other half of my life. Economic necessity always constrained my choices. No lavish lunches, holidays or expensive clothes. However, I did travel widely. I simply hitchhiked wherever I wanted to go—Europe, Turkey, Morocco, the USA and Canada. Along the way political, philosophical and spiritual questions phased in and out of focus. What was the meaning of life? I had no idea, but the 1960s and 70s were a great time to be alive.

Quest for meaning

Looking to the future, I was not entirely content with the prospect of being a vet. Sure, I liked animals, and practical endeavour is always satisfying. But for me the question increasingly arose: How does the veterinary profession fit into and serve the wider community? I gained the feeling that veterinary science was conducted in a vacuum and that that it did not have a sound connection with the society it was supposed to serve. Consequently, that being a vet felt more like being an animal technician.

In the quest for answers, I made long-term plans. I enlisted as a volunteer with Voluntary Service Overseas so that soon after graduating as a vet I took off for Nairobi as lecturer at the Animal Health and Industry Training Institute. Then I hitchhiked through Kenya, Tanzania and Zambia before returning to London. I had a place lined up at the London School of Economics (LSE) where, I thought, I would gain critical insight into politics, philosophy and economics and thus understand how veterinary endeavours fitted into the needs of society.

You likely can spot this as the naive delusions of youth. The LSE was uninterested in answering questions about the place of veterinary science in the world, just as the RVC was not the least interested in going beyond the immediate bounds of mechanistic 'science' within a veterinary culture. Chastened by the experience, I dropped out and set off for Africa again, this time as traveller with a casual commission as a photographer for two children's books on Egypt and Kenya.

First full-time vet job

Lesley my girlfriend and the gravitational pull of London drew me back to the UK. And by lucky chance I secured a job with Tony Todd as a vet working at a frantically busy small animal clinic close to the Angel, Islington. Fortunately, Tony my boss and work colleague Malcolm Corner gave me support during the first few weeks and soon I was reasonably proficient at the technical aspects of diagnosis and medical and surgical management of cases. We worked for a fee. Clients asked our opinion; we provided advice. We dealt with the superficial and obvious presenting signs.

Looking back almost 50 years I can honestly say the matter of diet seldom arose and, if it did, only in passing. If clients fed their animals out of a can or dry kibble out of a bag, that was OK by me.

All animals—100 per cent—must be fed. But at the vet school little or no time was devoted to the subject. The common assumption was that so long as animals ate *enough* food—of almost any diet or combination—that was all that mattered.

Then as now, dental disease was running at pandemic proportions. It probably affected all pets to some degree, but was clinically obvious as stinky breath and sore and bleeding gums in around 85 per cent of the pet population. Seldom did we initiate discussion about the dental disease. When owners showed an interest or concern, we would respond by offering to scrape the accumulated calculus off the teeth and maybe remove obviously loose, diseased teeth. As dirty work, by which I mean not sterile surgery, this work was usually performed last in the day's schedule and done in a hurry.

Second full-time vet job

My last proper vet job in the UK took me to Bedford and the practice of Alex Scott and Brian Cox. Farm animals, horses, dogs and cats were our regular patients. However, it was the exotic patients that held special fascination for me. From A for aardvark to Z for zebra and a host of species in between, we had responsibility for the animals at a wild animal quarantine station and the Woburn Safari Park. Luckily for me, I got to make regular visits to Woburn and struck up a wonderful friendship with head ranger Peter Litchfield and his team.

Cats and dogs never speak about their pain and discomfort. Indeed, for their ancestors in the wild, obscuring health issues was a vital survival mechanism. Prey, predators and competitors would all be sure to take advantage of an obviously weakened individual. Of course, wild animals in the zoo hide their problems. They also flee the vet and resent being handled. The challenge then is to look more carefully and think more deeply about the animals' presenting signs, their biology, ethology, nutrition and environment. All our discussions about our zoo patients referred to their place in nature. Put simply, nature knows and knows best.

Australian adventure

My next stop was Manjimup, Western Australia, where I caught up with old school friend John Lumley. John had graduated from Glasgow vet school and migrated to Australia soon afterwards. Beside the welcome hospitality, I gained a gentle introduction to Australian vet life in John's mixed veterinary practice. Then, in January 1981, I took a job as a locum pet vet flying into and out of mining towns in the arid Pilbara region—all good experience for starting my own practice.

The next phase in the adventure was about to begin. Lesley flew in from London. We bought an old caravan, hitched it to the Holden van and set off across the Nullarbor Plain in the direction of Adelaide, Melbourne and ultimately Sydney. Filled with immigrant vigour, curious and entranced by the delights, the size and scope of Australia—Godzone, the Lucky Country—we pushed forward.

Adam Smith, the famed Scottish economist, in his book the *Wealth of Nations*,[1] identified three necessary components of human economic endeavours—land, capital and labour. When time came to start a practice, I found an empty shop in Riverstone, an outer western suburb of Sydney. That was the 'land' component. Regarding capital I had meagre savings and needed extra funds in order to equip and stock the new vet practice. Bank number one rejected my application outright. Bank number two offered me a $500 loan. I declined the derisory offering but did open an account at that branch. With insufficient capital, the solution was to contribute more 'labour'. And so it was, working from dawn until late at night seven days a week—initially painting and decorating and renovating old desks, sinks and office furniture—that I opened my new practice.

Half a world away from family and friends it was no problem to immerse myself in work. In those days an epidemic of heartworm disease afflicted the canine population. With the appearance of angel hair spaghetti, the adult worms clog the right side of the heart and pulmonary arteries. Apparently, so the story goes, Captain Scott stopped off in Sydney on his way to the Antarctic. His dogs, acquired in Siberia, were said to harbour heartworm and so infected the Sydney dogs. Due to the lack of veterinary care over many years the heartworm disease pandemic took hold. Fortunately, after a couple of misdiagnoses, I wised up and started testing dogs and treating the positive cases.

Heartworm testing and treatment became the mainstay of the practice. At the end of the first full year the two vet nurses, Merry and Marilyn, baked a heart-shaped cake sprouting jelly worms. We were proud of our successes and as you can tell, as yet oblivious to the more sinister, ubiquitous afflictions affecting our patients: junk diet, dental disease and obesity.

I cannot be sure when the blinkers started to fall off and when I finally twigged that all, yes all, of my small animal patients were suffering the consequences of a processed 'food' diet. I do, however, remember being conscience stricken when I realised how my contributory negligence had ensured the end-stage ill health and disease of Duchess the Maltese terrier.

Waking up in a blur

You know how it is waking up blinking in the first light of day. Slowly your eyes focus through the blur. Ears start to tune out a vivid dream and tune in to real sounds in the real world. That's what if felt like as I came to terms with the reality facing Duchess, a long-time patient of the practice. I'd known her since she was a little ball of white fluff barely eight weeks old. I'd administered the obligatory vaccines and supplied intestinal worm pills, heartworm pills and flea treatments. Duchess was cute and charming and her elderly owners genial and trusting. A bond was struck, and a ritual established that carried us through the next decade.

On each anniversary of a patient's first visit, we sent out a vaccination 'booster' reminder notice in the mail. And dutifully without fail the owners would appear at the practice with Duchess sporting a neat ribbon in her topknot. Following a cursory clinical examination, the 'booster shot'—against mostly non-existent diseases—was administered and worm pills were supplied against the either non-existent or relatively insignificant intestinal worms. After the usual amiable banter, the owners would make their way to reception to pay the bill. Duchess had no say in the matter, but the humans were happy enough.

To the best of my recollection we never spoke about Duchess's lineage direct from her wolf forebears. Neither did we speak about her junk food diet, whether out of the can or packet, or human left-overs. The tartar on her teeth, receding gums and stinky breath were standard, normal and not worth discussion. Errors of omission are some of the hardest errors to first identify and then secondly to remedy. We don't know that which we don't know.

We, Duchess's owners and I, settled into a pattern where fundamental errors of omission were our standard *modus operandi*—the effect of which was catastrophic. Eventually after some years I took account of the murmur of the failing heart, noticed the accumulation of ascitic fluid in the abdomen and the sparse dull coat. The dental ill health started to elicit my attention and the owners told me Duchess was getting slower in her advancing years.

For many years I had followed the conventional veterinary path, thinking I was providing the best of veterinary care. A subtle arrogance and hubris supported my ego—and little Duchess was the innocent victim of my wretched incompetence. When I recovered from the jumble of misplaced, confusing thoughts I was, to say the least, conscience stricken. I realised that it was not so much that Duchess was getting older, but rather that her junk food diet led to signs of premature aging. As I recall from over 30 years ago, the owners were understanding and forgiving when I told them this.

Veterinary frame of reference

Vets, through the ages, have put about the notion that they are the best placed, best informed and most conscientious people who can be relied upon to do the right thing for pets, people and the planet. It is the myth that sustains the belief that the veterinary profession must be provided with 'self-regulatory' status. Vets, the argument goes, need to spend many years learning the essentials of their profession. Only *they* know when things are out of kilter and needing diagnosis and treatment. Only *they* can be relied upon to employ scientific thinking on behalf of the wider community.

Unfortunately, I must tell you, this 'self-regulatory' status confers immense privileges and little by way of responsibility on the self-serving 'profession'. There is a widespread and erroneous belief that scientific thinking imbues the profession; that 'evidence-based medicine' is something tangible and that which all vets strive for. Unfortunately, passing fashion, more than high-minded cerebral function, is the determinant of what passes for acceptable veterinary practice.

The 'influencers' of veterinary fashion are the trade advertisers with their packaged, gift-wrapped concepts about veterinary drugs, diets and equipment designed to catch the attention and speak to the self-interest of the vets. The advertisements—in vet newsletters, drug catalogues and electronic media—pay lip-service to the needs of pets and their owners. But it's the opportunity to make a buck that motivates the merchants and their target audience of general practitioner vets.

Here in Australia, in the late 1980s and early 1990s the dominant new fashion was the promotion and sale of expensive mobile dental workstations. These workstations on wheels, similar to your dentist's chair-side compressed air-driven hand tools, were hailed as the new profit centre for vets. A rich seam of untapped wealth was accessible, the ads suggested, when justifying the many thousands of dollars needed to buy the machines. The ready population of dogs and cats with stinky breath and tartar-encrusted teeth could be treated on a six-monthly basis. 'Dental prophy' (a shortened form of 'prophylaxis') was the euphemism emanating from the USA and used to describe the scale and polish of a dog's 42 teeth and a cat's 32 teeth.

Visiting salesmen and speakers at vet dental seminars encouraged practitioner vets to send out six-monthly client reminders after pet 'prophies'—earn a fee this month and again six months later. It was the guaranteed way to polish the smile on the practice accounts manager's face. These days, over 30 years later, the same cynical marketing continues apace, only more so. There are doggy toothbrushes, dental chews, mouth washes, dental diets and a panoply of products and plans designed to exploit to the maximum the pandemic of dental disease affecting our furry friends. In the USA, UK and Australia the organised vet 'profession' promotes 'dental health month' where owners are encouraged to present their pets for a dental assessment.

It's a systematic con designed to part owners from their hard-earned cash—relentlessly and regularly throughout the life of the pet.

Back in the 1980s and 90s some vets began to question the need for such active intervention disguised as prophylaxis or prevention. What did dogs and cats do prior to the advent of dental workstations? More to the point, what did and what do wild carnivores do to prevent dental disease?

After my experience working in zoos, and on safari in Kenya in the 1970s, it did not take much effort to figure out that wild animals have zero access to a dentist and nonetheless do just fine. In fact, their fangs are kept immaculate by scything through meat, tendon and bone of their prey—not once every six months but at every meal.[2] Observe the feeding frenzy, the ripping and tearing at the carcass, and you'll understand what I mean. It's that vigorous activity that serves to scrape and polish the teeth while massaging the gums.

Contrasting nature's way with that of the dental workstation merchants, we needed to know how to harness the power of nature in the domestic setting. In nature every meal is tough and chewy. Was there a compromise whereby a raw bone could be provided once a week but otherwise the diet could consist of industrial 'food' in the can or packet?

Unfortunately, this was not a question that could be simply put and simply answered. Clients present their animals for treatment or for conventional vaccinations. They don't want or expect the vet to launch off on some experimental journey—especially when that journey is replete with potential hazards. Raw bones are known to break teeth, get stuck in the digestive tract, carry a multitude of bacteria and give rise to dog fights or aggressive behaviour directed at children. There's a belief raw bones carry parasites affecting pets and people. Raw bones attract flies and maggots, become stinky and messy, especially after your dog retrieves the bone from the hidey-hole in the garden bed.

Other considerations weighing with us were the ever-present threat of Veterinary Board attention. Vet regulators don't like vets to stray too far from conventionally approved thinking that dogs and cats are supposed to be fed cooked concoctions in the can and packet. Vets, competing with each other, could be relied upon to capitalise on any mishaps and to pour scorn wherever scorn could be poured. That was then and it's still the same today. Yes, it just shows you the durability of the veterinary mind locked shut against anything that challenges its preferred position of power and control.

We were right to be wary of the ruthless vets, then and now. As mentioned in the introduction not one of my new clients in the decade 2011 to 2021 came to me equipped with the understanding that raw meaty bones are an essential, indeed the main, component of a carnivore's diet. This notwithstanding that locally in this part of Australia we have been popularising the feeding of raw meaty bones since the late 1980s. Even though the local press, radio and television have carried plenty of stories on the fundamental requirements of carnivores, local vets have not and do not promote the health benefits of a natural diet.

Back in the 1980s and 90s we knew things were bad, but nevertheless we pressed on in hope of better days to come.

Environmental protection

A third motivating factor—additional to the awareness of the widespread dental disease and the cynical exploitation of said disease by the vets—was the increasing awareness of environmental degradation and the concomitant need for change.

Rachel Carson is credited with kickstarting the environmental revolution with her seminal 1962 work *Silent Spring*.

> Despite condemnation in the press and heavy-handed attempts by the chemical industry to ban the book, Rachel Carson succeeded in creating a new public awareness of the environment which led to changes in government and inspired the ecological movement.[3]

Gradually over the succeeding decades awareness and alarm intensified such that Margaret Thatcher, the Iron Lady, said at the 1990 Second World Climate Conference:

> The danger of global warming is as yet unseen, but real enough for us to make changes and sacrifices, so that we do not live at the expense of future generations.
>
> Our ability to come together to stop or limit damage to the world's environment will be perhaps the greatest test of how far we can act as a world community. No-one should under-estimate the imagination that will be required, nor the scientific effort, nor the unprecedented co-operation we shall have to show. We shall need statesmanship of a rare order. It's because we know that, that we are here today.
>
> [**Man and nature: out of balance**]
>
> For two centuries, since the Age of the Enlightenment, we assumed that whatever the advance of science, whatever the economic development, whatever the increase in human numbers, the world would go on much the same. That was progress. And that was what we wanted.
>
> Now we know that this is no longer true.
>
> We have become more and more aware of the growing imbalance between our species and other species, between population and resources, between humankind and the natural order of which we are part.
>
> In recent years, we have been playing with the conditions of the life we know on the surface of our planet. We have cared too little for our seas, our forests and our land. We have treated the air and the oceans like a dustbin. We have come to realise that man's activities and numbers

> threaten to upset the biological balance which we have taken for granted and on which human life depends.
>
> We must remember our duty to Nature before it is too late. That duty is constant. It is never completed. It lives on as we breathe. It endures as we eat and sleep, work and rest, as we are born and as we pass away. The duty to Nature will remain long after our own endeavours have brought peace to the Middle East. It will weigh on our shoulders for as long as we wish to dwell on a living and thriving planet, and hand it on to our children and theirs.[4]

Well said, Lady Thatcher. Her well-chosen words ring in the ears to this day and henceforth. We must, absolutely must, be cognisant

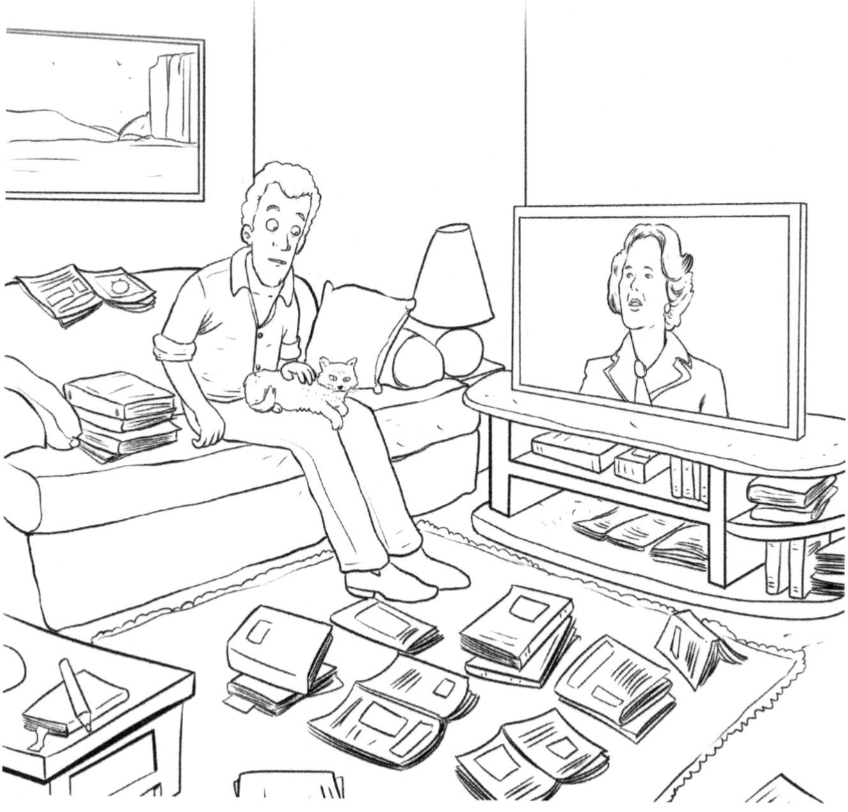

of the wonderful world and the all-supplying environment that we inhabit.

In 1990 I asked the President of the Sydney branch of the Australian Veterinary Association (AVA) if he would allow me to present a short paper echoing the Thatcher sentiments at an upcoming scientific and social meeting. On the appointed evening I was gratified to see Bob Kibble, the AVA National President, sitting in the front row. Things moved rapidly from there. And very soon it was announced that the 1991 joint Australia–New Zealand veterinary conference would be entitled Veterinarians and the Environment.

Back then I was 41 years old and brimful of zeal and enthusiasm. I leapt at the chance to join the organising committee and then to present a paper at the conference describing veterinary environmental impacts and what could be done to ameliorate those impacts. Brainstorming those subjects, ideas soon started to billow like large cumulous clouds overlapping and augmenting each other. Drawing on my education and life experience, thinking about vets and their place in the world, I realised the importance of the veterinary environmental footprint. Vets in the 1990s mostly treated pets—pets afflicted with periodontal disease. And by 1990 I had finally worked out that pets suffered from periodontal disease as a result of the junk pet food diet.

'Follow the money trail' is recurring good advice for anyone seeking to understand the motivators within any given system. The impacts of vets on the environment could easily be seen as intrinsic to the whole pet/vet and then the pet food economy. Veterinary pharmaceuticals depend on toxic chemicals and antibiotics that enter the environment. Processing, packaging and transportation place huge burdens on the environment, not least the processing, packaging and transportation of industrial pet foods.

Bingo, that was it, all roads, all money trails led to the industrial pet food industry. The vet profession was integral to the entire pet ownership promotion, pet resultant ill health and pet food industry protective cordon. I saw the junk pet food bubble economy in stark relief. However, for vets, as long as they kept their heads down, concentrated on fixing diseases and not questioning where those diseases came from then the gravy train would keep on delivering—regardless of the environmental consequences.

At the conference I seem to recall the handful of delegates who attended my talk provided polite acceptance but without enthusiasm. There was no exchange of telephone numbers (it was before the advent of email), no commitment to discussing things further. In the interests of piety, a gesture had been made. 'That surely was enough' seemed to be their message.

Myself, I was more moved by Margaret Thatcher's entreaties; to do our duty by Mother Nature. Besides I had spent the better part of the previous 40 years wondering about the meaning of life. I had been a rebel without a cause. Now suddenly numerous disparate threads coalesced making sense of a disorderly jumble. I had stumbled upon a purpose; I had discovered a cause.

PART II

PET HEALTH MATTERS

2

ERUPTION OF DISSENT

Life wasn't meant to be easy.

Malcolm Fraser
Australian Prime Minister 1975–1983

Laying foundations

The Australian Veterinary Association (AVA) May 1991 Vets and the Environment Conference came and went—a feel-good marketing blip with no lasting benefit.

I continued to fret and then became affronted. The AVA announced that they would host a series of 'educational' evenings sponsored by the Mars Corporation and featuring two speakers from the Royal Veterinary College, University of London, and also two speakers from Mars's Waltham Research Institute in the UK. The Sydney evening meeting was full to overflowing with small animal practitioners lapping up the conventional junk pet food inspired propaganda delivered by vet establishment spruikers.

Variously exasperated, enraged, despondent, I decided something needed to be done about the blatant junk pet food brainwashing. As I saw it, the veterinary profession was engaged in a vast confidence trick with widespread animal cruelty and consumer fraud implications. If I were to blow the whistle would anyone hear? Would anyone care?

I submitted a piece (see below) to the Sydney University Post Graduate Committee in Veterinary Science newsletter *Control & Therapy*.[1] Dr Douglas Bryden, the editor, was known to be fair-minded and straight-talking. Before becoming a vet, he had been a schoolteacher and rugby football referee.

Oral disease in cats and dogs

The stench of stale blood, dung and pus emanating from the mouths of so many of my patients has finally provoked this eruption of dissent.

The sheer numbers passing through the practice, when extrapolated to the world situation, tells me that oral disease is the source of the greatest intractable pain and discomfort experienced by our companion animals.

This is a great and mindless cruelty we visit upon our animals from the whelping box to the grave. Just imagine having a mouth ulcer or toothache for a lifetime.

The internal factors are these:

Puppies and kittens cut their deciduous teeth between 2 and 6 weeks of age. An inevitable consequence of this is gingivitis. A diet of processed food ensures lack of gum massage and the gingivitis persists. The growing animal develops grooming behaviour and adds hair and faecal materials to the accumulated food scraps clogging the interdental spaces.

Between four and six months of age the permanent teeth erupt into a soup of blood, pus and saliva. The gingivitis is now well established and not infrequently one finds a young kitten or puppy with a complete set of deciduous teeth hanging from inflamed gingival shreds.

Even on a diet of processed food the deciduous teeth must eventually fall out. The permanent teeth come to occupy a diseased mouth and by this time the animal has learned not to chew on anything because of the pain involved.

The exquisite mechanism of teeth and gums, designed by nature to be cleaned, massaged and stressed daily, is left to rot. Compare mining machinery properly maintained which can excavate a mountain but by disuse can be rendered useless.

A lifetime of inescapable pain is bad enough. The sequelae of endocarditis, iliac thrombosis, nephritis and all those other entities attributable to a permanent septic focus finally condemn this situation as being intolerable.

The external factors are these:

Foremost are the pet foods which are promoted as 'complete diets, only water needed'. Along with petroleum and coffee, pet food is one of the biggest industries worldwide.

Reacting to the now universal dental needs of our animals the dental instrument, the dental machine and even the imitation bone industries have flourished.

I believe many veterinary practitioners have reacted passively, perhaps providing some dental care as an afterthought and virtually no advice. Since cats and dogs don't complain, owners don't realize and don't seek advice. Many vets just don't seem to be pro-active in this vital area.

As vets we need to provide more than palliative care.

Brushing teeth and regular prophys [dental scaling under anaesthetic] are not enough when advice on diet and food to massage the gums is so vitally important.

What's to be done?

a. The internal system

Help pets control their two bouts of physiological gingivitis before it becomes pathological. Older larger dogs need raw bones and cats need raw meat on the bone.

b. The external system

The external commerce driven system did not exist before the 50's and now it seems such an inescapable part of life. It may take a while to alter course.

The profession can do much to re-educate itself and in turn the public. A few practice surveys and university-based research projects would set the tone.

The pet food manufacturers will need advice on the problems caused by processed food. One pet food company gives bi-annual 'prophys' to its research animals (personal communication).

However, they may be persuaded to voluntarily print cautionary advice on their packaging. **Failing that a few class actions by aggrieved pet owners would probably work wonders.**

What benefits can we expect?

Innumerable. Pets will be fed on cheap unprocessed bi-products some of the time. The environment will benefit, clients will be an average $1000 per animal/per lifetime better off. Certainly, the pets can be expected to live longer as they enjoy their lives seeking to 'steal bones out of the freezer'.

As vets we will be happy to see more pain free, healthier pets and grateful owners.

In December 1991, four months after I first submitted the draft, the article appeared in print. Apart from fixing my atrocious spelling and punctuation, Dr Bryden's main editorial change was removal of the line: 'Failing that, a few class actions by aggrieved pet owners would probably work wonders'.

It was a change I could live with. The overall tone and content were clear enough. Vets needed to do more than pay lip-service to their scientific, moral, ethical, legal and social obligations.

That same month, December 1991, the *AVA News* carried a letter from my old mate Breck Muir. For as long as I had known him, Breck railed against the junk pet foods. He now put pen to paper, providing the wider profession with some home truths.

Canned pet food not the healthiest

The pet food situation has concerned me for some years, my feelings brought to this by the current competitive marketing of various dental work stations for veterinary use.

The scene as I see it goes like this: 'Here is the best food ever made for your dog Mrs Jones' handing her a can of commercial dog food or dry food, 'but he may develop problems with his teeth, so here is a special toothbrush and paste for you to use to clean his teeth regularly, and then if that doesn't keep the periodontal disease at bay then we have the very latest in dental equipment just like our own dentist has, and we can give Fido that perfectly enamelled ivory grin'—that he would have had had you not fed him the commercial food in the first place.

Here we have the perfectly engineered commercial circle —a problem doesn't exist, so we create one, and then come up with all the remedial treatments.

Infiltration

The infiltration of the commercial pet foods into our lives is one of the great success stories of the business world. Gross sales figures for a single product type is probably only bettered by petroleum products worldwide.

We as a profession have been led by the nose by vested interests into a current situation where most younger vets actually recommend commercial pet foods as the best available way of feeding domestic pets—because they have never known of any other way. Before they had their first pet, they were bombarded with constant mass media advertising instilling into them that the various commercial foods were the only way to go, and when they graduated and went to postgraduate nutrition courses again they had this idea reinforced by visiting lecturers who actually mentioned brand names in their notes.

My experience with commercial canned and dry pet foods is that they:

- are a prime cause of periodontal disease in all breeds of dogs and cats
- are associated with an increased incidence of gastric dilation and/or torsion
- are a cause of diarrhoea in a substantial number of dogs

> - cause intestinal 'allergies' with associated dermal pruritus and behavioural changes in a significant number of cases
> - are a prime cause of flatulence and offensive odour in dogs—some brands more than others.
>
> We are objectively educated, of above average intelligence, trained to observe and reason as undergraduates. We should develop the ability to assess products for what they are in spite of extremely effective advertising claiming otherwise. This is a mammoth and ongoing task for all of us and certainly not just with pet foods.
>
> In this case we should be giving clients advice to correct their pets' diet towards more natural one and not justify the financial outlay on the latest dental equipment available by advocating the wholesale feeding of commercial pet foods.[2]

We were seeing Breck's wise words in print for the first time. Matters of scientific, moral, ethical, legal and social obligations take time to evolve—requiring free, uncensored debate. Ordinarily the *AVA News* letters page was reserved for AVA members who would first see the printed version and then could send in their thoughts for publication in the *next* edition of the newsletter. On this occasion, however, the AVA had provided John Wingate, president of the Pet Food Manufacturers Association of Australia, with special advance notice of Breck's letter. Wingate, although neither a vet nor member of the AVA, was provided with space to launch a pre-emptive counter-attack in the *same* edition of *AVA News* designed to quell any upheaval. His statement published alongside Breck's letter stated:

> We are surprised by the content of Dr Muir's letter, which is an attack on the integrity of the pet-food manufacturers of this country.[3]

Fifteen spin- and platitude-filled paragraphs later he concluded:

> With the economic strife Australia now faces, we would have thought it more appropriate to encourage ever increasing standards of excellence in a successful export industry such as the prepared pet food industry. Instead, this letter attempts to cut the 'tall poppy' down.

And so began the back and forth of a partially truncated debate in the monthly *AVA News*. Two members of the Australian Veterinary Dental Society jumped in on the side of the AVA and pet food manufacturers. Mars Corporation vet Duncan Hall claimed: 'The relationship between nutrition and periodontal disease is not clear', but then incriminated Mars, his employers and owners of the Waltham Centre:

> The pet-food industry currently commits considerable financial resources towards researching pet nutrition and product development. An example of this research is the work of the Waltham Centre for Pet Nutrition where a technique for staining and objectively grading plaque development in dogs is now being used to examine the effect of different food textures on canine dental health. The ultimate aim of such research is to develop products which can assist in preventing the development of this complex and sometimes distressing disease.[4]

OK! Mars Corporation, biggest junk pet food maker on planet Earth, speaking to you. You know food *texture* counts. You know that periodontal disease is to say the least, 'distressing', and you surely know that Mars canned and dry concoctions are the scourge of pet dogs and cats the world over.

Of course, the vet dentists and pet food makers' arguments were off beam. They were based on spin and make-believe with the ever-present danger, for them, that they would make self-incriminating statements likely to come back to haunt them. Avoiding engagement, saying nothing, is generally their best strategy. We cannot be sure to what extent the vet dentists and manufacturers pressured the AVA to ban further letters page discussion. We do know that in March 1993 the *AVA News* carried the following abrupt notice:

> *AVA News* believes that this issue has been aired fully over the last year and does not intend to run further correspondence.[5]

Dr Bryden to the rescue

Fortunately, over at the Sydney University Postgraduate Foundation we still had an ally. Dr Bryden had been following the *AVA News* letters page discussions and agreed to visit my practice to see the evidence for himself. On arrival at 7 am on the appointed day I asked how long he expected to stay. 'Half an hour', came the curt reply. Five hours later he departed the practice a changed man. Douglas Bryden saw for himself the impressive results when animals are switched from junk food diets to a diet based on raw meaty bones. He saw how puppies and kittens thrive when fed appropriately.

Some days later the telephone rang. Douglas Bryden was on the line. Could I write down the things I had told him and have the manuscript to him inside two weeks? He planned to publish the work as an extra chapter entitled 'Preventative dentistry' in the course proceedings for the upcoming five-day course on veterinary dentistry. I could not refuse but noted many constraints. The very next day I was due to take my two young sons on a two-week beachside holiday. In the event things turned out OK. The three of us had fun times at the beach by day and at night I sat out on the balcony under the streetlights writing the manuscript.[6]

Unfortunately, though, most vets have not read the chapter and consequently neither know nor apply the principles. Better if pet owners fill the void, focusing on ensuring their pets have healthy mouths and encouraging their vets to adopt the same focus (see Appendix D). It's the single most important thing you can do to ensure a healthy pet.

Brief history of manufactured pet food

It is said that behind every great fortune lies a great crime.[7] As we chronicle the junk pet food devastation and the struggle to expose and overcome it, it is helpful to know that it was not always a fact of life. It is useful to know where the modern concept of 'pet food' came from and that ultimately we can revert to healthier options from bygone times.

As early as 1841, the *Quarterly Journal of Agriculture* warned against unnatural foods and recommended the need for bones.

> Barley-meal, indeed, is an unnatural food, unless it be varied with bones, for a dog delights to gnaw, and thus to exercise those potent teeth with which nature has furnished him; his stomach, too, is designed to digest the hard and tough integument of animal substance; hence, barleymeal, as a principal portion of his subsistence, is by

> no means to be desired. In small private families it is not always possible to obtain a sufficiency of meat and bones for the sustenance of a dog, and recourse is too frequently had to a coarse and filthy aliment, which is highly objectionable, especially if the creature be debarred from taking daily exercise, fettered by a chain ...[8]

How clear-eyed, how prescient that writer was back in 1841. Imagine if he were to reappear 180 years later to see the pet food aisles full of 'filthy aliment' intended for pets kept in solitary confinement in millions of homes worldwide.

Jack Spratt, dry biscuits

Jack Spratt is the man credited with inventing industrialised processed pet food. Sometime in the 1860s Spratt left his native Cincinnati, Ohio, and arrived in London by ship. Noticing the stray dogs scavenging for ship's biscuits on the quayside, he hit on the idea to manufacture his Wheat Fibrine Dog Cakes, a concoction of wheat, beetroot and beef blood.

Within a few years, Spratt teamed up with the young Charles Cruft (of Cruft's Dog Show fame) and together they launched pedigree dog shows. Business boomed and in the 1870s Spratt's pet food venture expanded to the USA.

> Spratt's became a relentless advertiser, convincing Americans who usually fed their dogs table scraps to buy a product they didn't need. The company employed snob appeal to hook the public, targeting participants and spectators at dog shows, and, in 1876, focusing on the centennial exhibition with free food for exhibitors. The

> company bought the entire front cover of the first journal of the American Kennel Club in January 1889 to broadcast its involvement with American and European kennel clubs, and to trumpet the company's 'Special Appointment' to Queen Victoria.[9]

From the get-go 'Spratt's was one of the most heavily marketed brands in the early 20th century, with product recognition developed through logo display, lifestyle advertising, and support through devices such as cigarette cards'.[9] Always at the forefront with distortion and confidence trickery, Spratt's advertised their wares with the first coloured billboard erected in London, England—depicting a *Native American buffalo hunt*!

Objectively speaking, buffalo in their natural state were an appropriate source of food and medicine for packs of American wolves. However, peeling the metaphorical labels 'food' and 'medicine' from the flanks of a buffalo and affixing them to grain-based, packaged junk food required a huge leap of imagination—which sadly too many pet owners were and are prepared to make.

Chappel Brothers, canned products

In the 1920s, after World War I, there was a vast population of unwanted army horses that entrepreneur Philip Chappel decided to seal in cans and sell as dog food. Very soon he had a booming business based in Chicago, Illinois.

> One of the advertisements for Ken-L-Ration was a jingle that became the favorite of children across the nation—'My dog's bigger than your dog, my dogs faster than yours. My dogs better 'cause he eats Ken-L-Ration, my dog's bet-

> ter than yours'. The alliance of pet food and advertising got its start when Philip Chappel incorporated the famous canine radio and cinema star, Rin Tin Tin, into his efforts to sell Ken-L-Ration to American dog owners. One week in July was declared 'Ken-L-Ration Week' and more than four million dogs were being fed horse meat via 150,000 stores across the nation. Chappel's network expanded rapidly into a wide-open market and Ken-L-Ration became an international power in the dog food business.[10]

Some people were opposed to the canning of horsemeat. Frank Litts, for instance, tried to take the law into his own hands and attempted to dynamite the Chappel packing plant. He was caught in the act, shot several times and carted off to jail where he later died. Other critics were upset with the treatment of the horses shipped in by rail:

> The railroad, seeing how the horses were destined for slaughter, did not go out of their way to provide any food, water or medical care for the animals. The starving animals would chew the tails off of other horses and if any would fall during transport, they were trampled. Several cases were brought up against Chappel but all were overturned as the Chappel Brothers were making everyone rich.

Purina, kibble

In the 1950s breakfast cereal producer Purina experimented with extruding kibble. Ingredients were pushed through a tube, cooked under high pressure and puffed up with air. The result: 'Purina Dog Chow was introduced in 1957 and in two years became the leading brand of dog food in the US'.[11]

Such technological wizardry would have seemed like alchemy, turning base metals into gold. For pets it was a case of turning cheap grain and assorted chemicals into a substitute for the gold star standard—a deer racing through the woods, a bird flying in the air or a fish darting in a stream. With the pets unable to complain and the public, vets, regulators and politicians hoodwinked, the same basic industrial process produces most of the junk dry pet 'food' sold today.

Nowadays

Nowadays, after amalgamations the pet food industry is headed by the ultra-secretive Mars family.[12,13] Nestlé, the world's largest packaged food and confectionery company, comes in second and Colgate the toothpaste maker is third. The three giant companies compete in the cooked packaged junk food market, a market that they create from the ground up in countries around the globe.

In past times it was European countries that were the colonisers, Great Britain, Spain, France and others. Now it's the turn of the giant corporations to act as economic colonisers, to alter the thought processes of consumers whether in first or third world countries across the globe.

On their website Purina commit to 'helping make pets' lives better worldwide'. And their reach is indeed worldwide: the website lists 15 countries and regions in Asia/Oceania/Africa, 24 countries in Europe and 21 in Central and South America as having Purina sites.[14]

Purina International Sites

North America	Asia/Oceania/Africa	Europe	South America
United States	Australia	Austria	Argentina
Canada	Hong Kong SAR, Greater China	Bulgaria	Bolivia
	Israel	Croatia	Brazil
	Japan	Czech Republic	Caribe
	Korea	Denmark	Chile
	Mainland China, Greater China	Estonia	Colombia
	Malaysia	Finland	Costa Rica
	Middle East & North Africa	France	Ecuador
	New Zealand	Germany	El Salvador
	Philippines	Greece	Guatemala
	Singapore	Holland	Honduras
	South Africa	Hungary	Jamaica
	Taiwan, Greater China	Italy	Mexico
	Thailand	Latvia	Nicaragua
	Turkey	Lithuania	Panama
		Norway	Paraguay
		Portugal	Peru
		Russia	Rep. Dominicana
		Serbia	Trinidad and Tobago
		Slovakia	Uruguay
		Spain	Venezuela
		Sweden	
		Switzerland	
		United Kingdom	

With the sheer size and reach of the giant companies, there are plenty of nooks, cracks and crannies. Niche marketers follow close behind the giant companies, actively seeking out gaps, duping the public and pushing their version of:

> ultrapremium, natural, raw, organic, grain free, human-quality ingredients and protein-focused diets. There are also niche products for skin health, gut health, dental health, urinary tract health, hairball prevention, pets with allergies and many more.[15]

This dizzying array of 'alternative' packaged food jostles for attention using false concepts and tricky advertising similar to that of the multinational conglomerates—with nary a legislator or regulator in sight. We come back to this issue in Chapter 10.

3

FOOD AND MEDICINE

In the decades since Douglas Bryden commissioned my preventative dentistry article, things have turned from bad to worse. The pet food behemoths have done their utmost to tighten their grip on the veterinary mind. Decades of brainwashing veterinary student innocents until they all talk in tongues—they talk in the confected language of a bizarre cult divorced from dietary good health fundamentals.

At vet schools the world over, they sit listening to the slick presentations by junk pet food industry 'nutritional experts'. Students wear shirts emblazoned with the logos of Hill's—the Colgate-Palmolive brand—and take notes with pens and paper supplied by Royal Canin—the flagship of Mars Inc. They are drilled to the point of paranoia on the extreme dangers allegedly posed by the feeding of bones, coupled with which they are filled with dread of the teeming death-delivering bacteria in every morsel of real food.

Insofar as they think—and they don't think much, with minds brimful with assumptions inspired by the junk pet food industry—they believe that only commercial products can deliver the 'complete and balanced' formula. Programmed to believe the relentless propaganda, their lecturers do nothing to offset the company lies. In fact, lecturers pile on the scaremongering so that insecure, inexperienced future vets are desperate to stay safe.

Young vets are told how the US Food and Drug Administration published the 2010 consumer health information sheet on the nasty impacts of bones whether cooked or raw.[1]

The idea that it's natural for dogs to chew on bones is a popular one. However, it's a dangerous practice and can cause serious injury to your pet.

mouth injuries

rectal bleeding

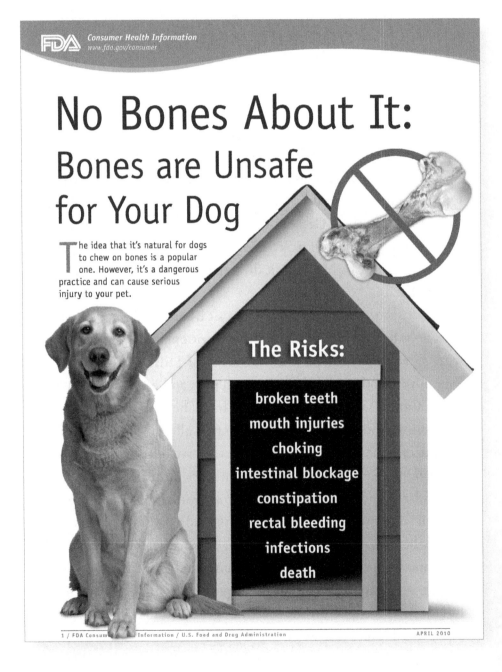

FDA Consumer Health Information
www.fda.gov/consumer

"Make sure you throw out bones from your own meals in a way that your dog can't get to them."

"Some people think it's safe to give dogs large bones, like those from a ham or a roast," says Carmela Stamper, D.V.M., a veterinarian in the Center for Veterinary Medicine at the Food and Drug Administration. "Bones are unsafe no matter what their size. Giving your dog a bone may make your pet a candidate for a trip to your veterinarian's office later, possible emergency surgery, or even death."

"Make sure you throw out bones from your own meals in a way that your dog can't get to them," adds Stamper, who suggests taking the trash out right away or putting the bones up high and out of your dog's reach until you have a chance to dispose of them. "And pay attention to where your dog's nose is when you walk him around the neighborhood—steer him away from any objects lying in the grass."

Here are 10 reasons why it's a bad idea to give your dog a bone:

1. **Broken teeth.**
   This may call for expensive veterinary dentistry.

2. **Mouth or tongue injuries.**
   These can be very bloody and messy and may require a trip to see your veterinarian.

3. **Bone gets looped around your dog's lower jaw.**
   This can be frightening or painful for your dog and potentially costly to you, as it usually means a trip to see your veterinarian.

4. **Bone gets stuck in esophagus, the tube that food travels through to reach the stomach.**
   Your dog may gag, trying to bring the bone back up, and will need to see your veterinarian.

5. **Bone gets stuck in windpipe.**
   This may happen if your dog accidentally inhales a small enough piece of bone. This is an emergency because your dog will have trouble breathing. Get your pet to your veterinarian immediately!

6. **Bone gets stuck in stomach.**
   It went down just fine, but the bone may be too big to pass out of the stomach and into the intestines. Depending on the bone's size, your dog may need surgery or upper gastrointestinal endoscopy, a procedure in which your veterinarian uses a long tube with a built-in camera and grabbing tools to try to remove the stuck bone from the stomach.

7. **Bone gets stuck in intestines and causes a blockage.**
   It may be time for surgery.

8. **Constipation due to bone fragments.**
   Your dog may have a hard time passing the bone fragments because they're very sharp and they scrape the inside of the large intestine or rectum as they move along. This causes severe pain and may require a visit to your veterinarian.

9. **Severe bleeding from the rectum.**
   This is very messy and can be dangerous. It's time for a trip to see your veterinarian.

10. **Peritonitis.**
    This nasty, difficult-to-treat bacterial infection of the abdomen is caused when bone fragments poke holes in your dog's stomach or intestines. Your dog needs an emergency visit to your veterinarian because peritonitis can kill your dog.

"Talk with your veterinarian about alternatives to giving bones to your dog," says Stamper. "There are many bone-like products made with materials that are safe for dogs to chew on."

"Always supervise your dog with any chew product, especially one your dog hasn't had before," adds Stamper. "And always, if your dog 'just isn't acting right,' call your veterinarian right away!" FDA

Find this and other Consumer Updates at *www.fda.gov/ForConsumers/ConsumerUpdates*

Sign up for free e-mail subscriptions at *www.fda.gov/consumer/consumerenews.html*

With only propaganda to rely on, what do the young vets do when first out in the real world of vet practice? Yes, you guessed it: they double down on the propaganda.

Young vets mostly work for bosses, frequently in corporate vet chains, who stock their waiting areas with the so-called high-end pet food products and prescription 'foods'. Even before starting in the vet course it is often the case that students are given a 'goody bag' by the giant pet food company at the new student orientation day. Five years later they emerge as qualified vets clutching an indexed handbook advising which packaged 'foods' to recommend when treating each particular malady. It's all there in neatly tabulated form—no thinking, only reading required.

Often the 'boss' is the Mars Corporation.[2] The junk pet food makers boast that they employ 50,000 veterinary professionals[3] in hundreds of vet practices in the USA[2], UK[4] and Europe.[3] In Australia hundreds of vets work for a corporate chain with close ties to the junk pet food makers.[5]

Theory, practice, experience

From every angle the young vets are cornered and don't realise it. Feeding pets involves opening a can or packet, as far as they are concerned.

1. The theory underlying their practice derives from the junk pet food industry.
2. The practical know-how, insofar as they have any, derives from opening a can or packet.
3. The only experience they gain derives from 1 and 2 above. They become highly practised and expert at doing the *wrong* thing.

Alas they have no idea that the ingesta of carnivores should fulfil both *nutritional* and *medicinal* needs. New vets, almost all vets, have no clue that:

a. The theory of feeding pet carnivores should depend on evolutionary concepts and the teachings of nature.

b. Their practical know-how should be substantially a matter of reaching into the refrigerator or freezer and tossing a carcass or large piece of raw meaty bones to the hungry pet.
c. By combining a and b they would become experienced in doing the *right*, the *healthful* thing for their carnivore patients.

Setting the record straight

Vet school academic and journal editor Dr Richard Malik is the exception that proves the rule. Back in 1992, as a young University of Sydney academic, he attended my lecture, 'Pandemic of periodontal disease a malodorous condition',[6] which he told me 'struck a chord'. Richard became known for openly espousing the need for a more natural diet—despite the risks to his academic career.

In 2018, as editor of the Centre for Veterinary Education's *Control & Therapy* journal, he published a paper detailing how a fragment of lamb bone got stuck in a dog's oesophagus. The paper's author concluded: 'That's just one of the reasons why I don't recommend bones.'

Richard knew that there are powerful reasons vets *should recommend bones.* He reached out to me:

> Could you provide a comment on what is the most suitable RMB to feed a Staffordshire Bull terrier? I am surprised that the lamb shank [in the article] caused a problem
>
> I would be happy to publish a comment by you, or a separate article, about choosing the right bone for each dog or cat. I know it's in your book [*Raw Meaty Bones: Promote Health*], but we have a new generation of vets.

I replied:

> For sure I'd like to comment ... the recommended 'throwing the baby out with the bathwater' is a major issue. They simply don't recognise the baby. Oh dear!

And that is how the 'Raw meaty bones essentials' article came to be written.

> **Raw meaty bones essentials**
>
> Raw meaty bones are easily the strongest, safest, most gentle, most effective medicine for all domestic carnivores. Raw meaty bones are the key that unlocks the carnivore code. Catching, killing and consuming raw meaty bones is for carnivores the *sine qua non*, the motivation for living. It's their job. They take it seriously and building on genetic determinants and with practice become highly skilled at devouring the food/medicine combined.
>
> Ideally raw meaty bones come covered with fur, feathers and fins. But even in the butchered form, providing the bones are of a suitable size, then the medicinal benefits are adequate for most practical purposes.
>
> Medicinal modes of action include:
>
> 1. Feeding frenzy—release of endorphins/immune stimulation—therapeutic.
> 2. Physical exercise—release of endorphins/immune stimulation—therapeutic.
> 3. Tooth cleaning—preventative medicine—therapeutic.
> 4. Stimulate gut enzymes/motility—therapeutic.
> 5. Natural food contains intracellular enzymes and is thus pancreas sparing—therapeutic.

6. Probiotics, maintenance of the microbiome—therapeutic.
7. Substrate conditioning of the colon environment leading to healthy balance of bacteria—therapeutic.
8. Behavioural conditioning (avoidance of stress/neurosis)—therapeutic.
9. Natural array of biochemicals—nutrition in the commonly used sense and providing all the essential macro and micro nutrients in the appropriate balance for optimal cellular growth, function and repair.

Clearly then, the medicine man, the vet, needs to have a good grasp of the biology, ecology, ethology, physiology and *pharmacology* of this most important carnivore medicine. And as with all medicines it's essential to be up to speed with procurement, storage, handling and administration.

Therapeutic risk management

All medicines come with inherent risks. Raw meaty bones are no exception—although happily if one keeps as close as possible to Nature's way of delivering the medicine then benefits are optimal and adverse effects minimal.

Eighteen years ago, when writing *Raw Meaty Bones: Promote Health*, I asked my contacts in two UK zoos to tell how captive wild carnivores deal with their food/medicine. See below.

Once one begins to think biologically it's easy to see that dry, virtually meatless bones are not a suitable medicine. A bored dog locked in solitary confinement may choose to chomp down on a lamb shank producing a potential foreign body. Or as is the case with femurs and bones cut lengthwise to expose the marrow, teeth, especially carnassials, get broken. And of course, cutting up the bones into small pieces only serves to increase the hazards and reduce the essential medicinal benefits of ripping and tearing.

In summary raw meaty bones are not an adjunct—they are the essential food and medicine for all carnivores from the time they cut their first teeth at three weeks of age. Nature does not apply labels; Nature does not differentiate between food and medicine. It's past time that the veterinary profession got up to speed.

For the future

Please go to: www.rawmeatybones.com. Check out the articles and view the TV segments and videos. Please feel free to visit us. Take a tour of our shipping container freezer plant/medicine chest; meet our wonderfully enthusiastic staff and clients; ask any questions. Back in 1993 Dr Douglas Bryden, Director of the CVE, made a short courtesy call. We satisfied his most searching questions, whereupon he commissioned the raw meaty bones preventative dentistry chapter: www.rawmeatybones.com/PrevDent.html

If, as a profession, we pull together we can revitalise vet medicine; we can create an innovative Australian petfood/medicine industry providing health and wellbeing for pets, pet owners and the wider community. Most certainly we should try.

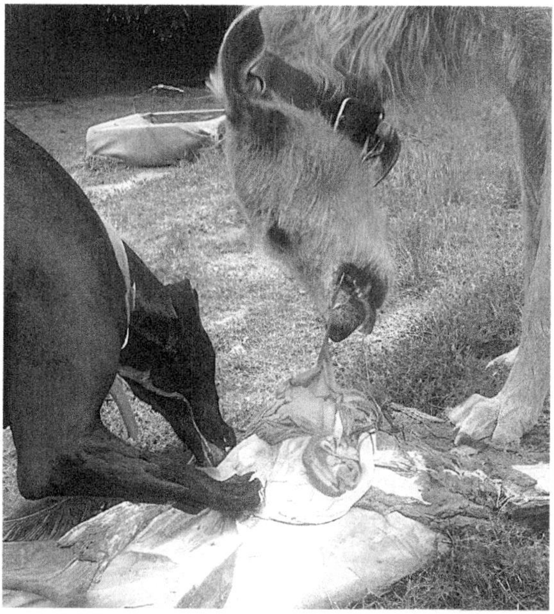

Figure 1. *Sam, 12-year-old staghound, and Needle, two-year-old whippet, floss their teeth and get a natural high*

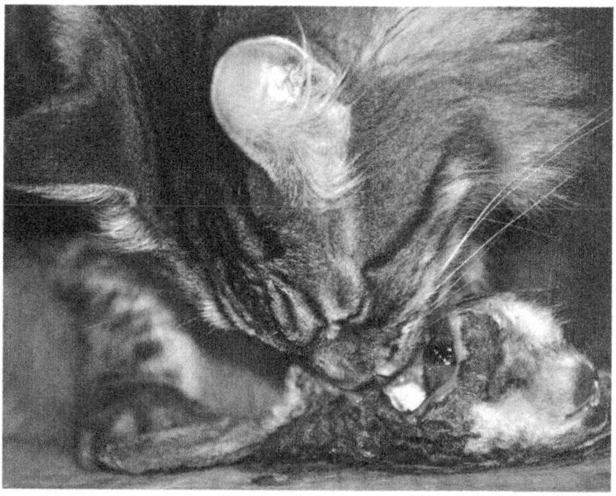

Figure 2. *George, 11-year-old, chows down on a rabbit head. Presented in September 2012 with severe diabetic polyuria/polydipsia and periodontal disease. Treated with quail and rabbit heads. Now in 2018, raw meaty bones are his sole 'medicine'—correct weight, no gum disease, no polyuria/ polydipsia. (See testimonial in Chap. 5, pp 72-6.)*

Diets of zoo species of similar weight to domestic cats and dogs

Rusty-spotted Cat (India, Sri Lanka—2 kg)

Mouse: Eaten completely. Very occasionally stomach left.

Rat: Stomach, colon and tail not eaten. Occasionally the liver is also left.

Day-old chick: Wing tips and feet uneaten. Gizzard occasionally left.

They have not been observed eating faeces, either theirs or that of other animals. Grass is regularly eaten. Some animals are known to do this daily. (Evidence in faeces samples and grass vomit.)

Desert Cat (Pakistan, India—4 kg)

Fish: Everything eaten except sperm sac and roe. Occasionally heads left.

Day-old chick: Gizzard, wing tips and feet are occasionally uneaten.

Mouse: Eaten completely.

Rat: Stomach, colon and tail not eaten. Occasionally the liver is also left.

Pigeon: All internal organs, feet and wing tips left. Plucked before eaten.

Quail: Eaten completely after first being plucked. Caecum sometimes left.

Guinea pig: Plucked. Colon left. Occasionally the pelt is turned inside out and left.

They have not been observed eating faeces, either theirs or that of other animals. Grass is occasionally eaten.

Timber Wolf (Canada, USA—33 kg)

Calf, horse, deer, goat

Carcass opened at groin, liver and heart eaten, lungs often left. The rumen is usually dragged across the enclosure; when this ruptures the contents are left where they lie. The colon, once dragged from the carcass, is usually left. The contents of the rumen are frequently rolled on by all members of the pack. The hide is turned inside out and left. Fur is not eaten. Horns are left although antlers are chewed and partially eaten. Hooves are eaten but only if from the carcass of a young animal. Bones from a young animal are mostly eaten, the exception being the larger bones. Bones from a larger animal are generally chewed on the ends. Particularly strong-smelling male goats are avoided by most animals.

Rabbit: Sometimes eaten completely, at other times the pelt is left.

Fish: Eaten completely. Often rolled on.

Chicken: Preferred when feathers removed.

Carcass turned inside out to get at flesh. They have not been observed eating grass or faeces, either theirs or that of another animal.

Bush Dog (South America—6 kg)

Chicken: Eaten completely. Gizzard and colon occasionally left.

Rabbit: Eaten completely.

Quail: Eaten completely.

Rats: Eaten completely.

Fish: Eaten completely.

Pigeon: Eaten completely. Wing tips, gizzard and colon occasionally left.

Fruit: Bananas, pears and grapes offered. Small amounts eaten.

Antlers: Antlers in velvet (during the annual growth phase) mostly eaten, hardened antlers partially eaten.

Grass often eaten.[7]

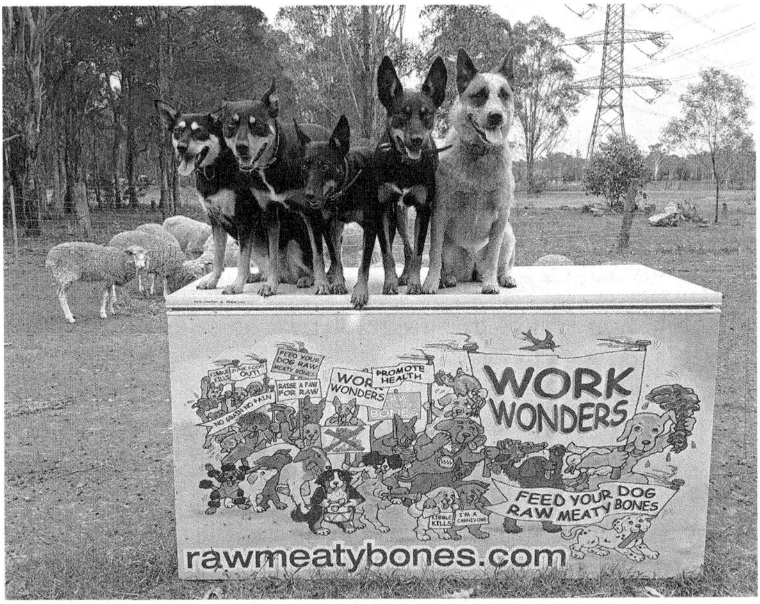

Fig 3. Five working dogs on a raw-meaty-bones tucker box/medicine chest. Note the glossy coats and sunny smiles. The owners, Australian Working Dog Rescue, know a thing or two about feeding working dogs. They rescue around 1500 dogs a year from Australia's pounds. workingdogrescue.com.au

Did the *Control & Therapy* subscribers consume, digest and assimilate the vital information? Did they incorporate any of the information into their practice? I very much doubt they did. No-one spoke with me about the subject and as far as I know there were no follow-up comments in the journal. Subject closed.

Clearly that's not good enough. What can we, the sincere and the well-informed, do until the revolution comes and sweeps away the bogus vet teaching? I suggest that at the least we should memorise the points '1. Feeding frenzy' down to '9. Natural array of biochemicals' (see pages 50-1).

We need this information first to help us overcome our own cultural conditioning. Thereafter it's the nine-point shield and weapon of attack against the junk pet food makers and their allies in the vet profession and fake animal welfare organisations. It's also fundamental information to help combat the madness of the BARFers, prey-modellers and other raw feeding cults with their emphasis on madcap recipes and percentages of fruit, vegetables and bizarre supplements.

By contrast the sad reality

OK, so we've had a detour via the 'Raw meaty bones essentials'. Whole carcasses or raw meaty bones provide essential nutritional and medicinal benefits. Raw meaty bones are the key that unlocks the carnivore code. Everyone should gain awareness. Every pet should derive the benefit on a regular basis.

Alas in reality, as important as the information is, for the most part it remains in the realms of theory. The majority of vets and pet owners did not see the article, and for the Centre for Veterinary Education it was a mere token gesture in 2018. Their refresher courses for vets continue as before. For example, an advertisement for a CVE online professional development course in 2021 entitled 'Small Animal Nutrition' included the claim that 'commercial foods, formulated to meet the known nutrient requirements of dogs and cats, have ensured good nutritional health'—and was accompanied by a photograph of six cute puppies eating from a tray of kibble.[8]

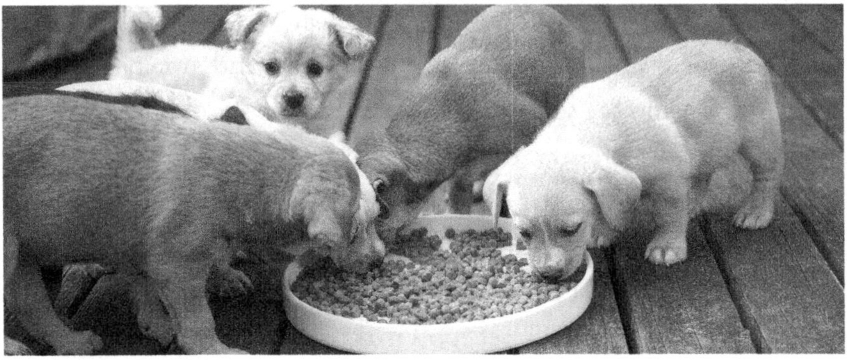

Breck Muir and I were outraged. A picture is worth a thousand words—conveying the CVE belief that compacted grain-based pellets ensure 'good nutritional health'?! Although the CVE had commissioned and published the 'Raw meaty bones essentials' article, and although they had seen videos and photos of dogs and cats consuming their proper food, they nonetheless reverted to teaching vets that desiccated junk was 'food' fit for young puppies.

We wrote to the new director of the CVE and when that failed, we sent an open letter to the chancellor of the university and the state minister of education:

> Dear Chancellor, Dear Minister,
>
> Please find correspondence below regarding the Centre for Veterinary Education (CVE) continued involvement with industrial junk food— involvement that the founding Director of the CVE, in 2001, labelled as 'foolish' and 'brain-dead'.
>
> Previously, in 1993, Director of the CVE Dr Douglas Bryden commissioned and published a chapter in *Veterinary Dentistry, Proceedings 212*: Preventative Dentistry

which chapter included a legal opinion regarding potential actions against veterinarians:

> Potential claims by pet owners under various pieces of consumer legislation throughout the States and Territories of Australia.
>
> In the Federal sphere potential Trade Practices Act claims for false or misleading claims may be made either in relation to advertising or promotional material or labels.
>
> The new Truth in Labelling activities instituted by the Federal Government.
>
> Potential problems or claims under the recently introduced Product Liability provisions in Part V of the Trade Practices Act.
>
> The, as yet, unknown effect of class actions which have been lawful in Australia since the 5th day of March 1992 which may tend to overcome the existing drawbacks to actions brought by individual pet owners, namely the high cost of litigation and claims which may amount to only several hundreds of dollars in relation to an individual pet.
>
> The foregoing relates to potential claims against manufacturers, distributors and possibly even retailers of processed pet food. Query what may be the legal problems of veterinarians who fail to consider the issues in this paper or fail to address those issues in advising pet owners who make known to the veterinarian that they rely wholly and solely on

> **processed pet food to supply their pets' diet. Is it too much to suggest that, as pet owners, in common with everyone else in the community become more litigious, veterinarians may some day share top billing on a Writ?'**
>
> Now 28 years later, we believe that the *Prevention of Cruelty to Animals Act*, and *Education for Overseas Students Act* may also apply.
>
> It's our confirmed opinion that Directors Hungerford and Bryden were right to condemn the teaching and promotion of junk pet-food feeding.
>
> If the CVE continues on its current course, please advise what legal opinions the University of Sydney and the Federal Department of Education rely on in support of such conduct.
>
> In the event that legal opinions obtained by the University and the Government oppose the CVE conduct, please advise.

Within days a terse reply arrived.

> Dear Dr Lonsdale,
>
> I refer to your email to the Chancellor, Ms Belinda Hutchinson AC, forwarding your earlier correspondence with the Director of the Centre for Veterinary Education, Dr Simone Maher.
>
> Dr Maher has detailed the content and aim of the CVE's Small Animal Nutrition TimeOnline course, which is to

> enhance a veterinarian's understanding of a dog or cat's nutritional needs. We reject your assertions regarding the CVE's approach to small animal nutrition, and request that you cease making disparaging claims about its courses and, by implication, its tutors.
>
> Please be advised that the University will not respond to any further correspondence from you on this matter.
>
> Kind Regards,
>
> Paul.
>
> Professor Paul Sheehy | Acting Head of School & Dean
> THE UNIVERSITY OF SYDNEY
> Faculty of Science | Sydney School of Veterinary Science

Nature sets the standard for pet nutrition. All other alternatives must be *better* than, the *same* as, or *inferior* to the natural standard. For dogs with 42 sharp teeth and cats with 32 sharp teeth designed to rip and tear at whole carcasses, plainly desiccated pebbles of compacted grain are inferior, but by what margin are they inferior?

In previous chapters we've looked at some of the dental and related health impacts. Now I'd like to mention other aspects arising out of a junk diet:

- Failing to provide appropriate food is to deprive an animal of its birthright and all the health-giving properties of that diet.
- Simultaneously pets tend to become used to what their owners feed them, even addicted to it.
- Which in turn depends on the owners developing habits that are hard to break.
- The worldwide fashion for feeding kibble, as in the CVE illustration (p. 58), has immediate and interminable bad effects on the unfortunate animals.

Over the years I've seen dry kibble pass all the way through cats and dogs and come out the rear end barely changed from when it went in the front end. Cats and dogs often vomit up kibble with outward appearance much the same as when ingested. Two dramatic cases brought home to me the cruel reality facing most pets that are fed kibble.

Ruby

When Ruby the five-month-old toy poodle ate some Easter chocolate, her owner was anxious that Ruby should not suffer from the toxic elements in chocolate. As a precaution we administered an emetic and eagerly waited to see the resultant vomit. The verdict: little or no chocolate but instead three piles of Nestlé Purina Supercoat kibble. It was slimy and moist, but otherwise the nuggets were about the same size and shape as when ingested—*12 hours previously*.

Seeing the evidence in context, we reasoned that it would have been several more hours before the junk was softened enough to travel on down through the intestinal tract. More than likely, without our intervention, in those hours Ruby would have eaten more of the dry

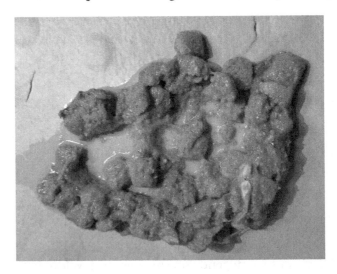

junk. But for the chance encounter with chocolate, the owner was primed to feed Ruby on doom nuggets for the rest of her life. Twenty-four hours a day, seven days a week Ruby would have been in the company of millions of animals, chock-a-block with indigestible junk.

A little further reflection tells us what it means to have a stomach full of factory-made pebbles. Dogs don't chew their food; they don't grind dry pebbles with saliva. They hear the rattle as the pebbles cascade into a bowl. They come running, quickly wolfing down the addictive junk in seconds without so much as a sip of water. Softening of the pebbles inevitably takes hours and is dependent on moisture from the stomach wall, which in turn dehydrates the pet. Sometimes the pebbles don't absorb sufficient moisture, triggering further problems.

I posted on YouTube the Supercoat ad featuring television celebrity vet Harry Cooper where he claims: 'No matter what stage of life your dog's at, there's a Supercoat meal providing natural nutrition to keep him happy and healthy'.[9] Alongside I posted two videos demonstrating the *un*natural, *un*happy and *un*healthy Nestlé Assault on Pets Part I[10] and Part II.[11]

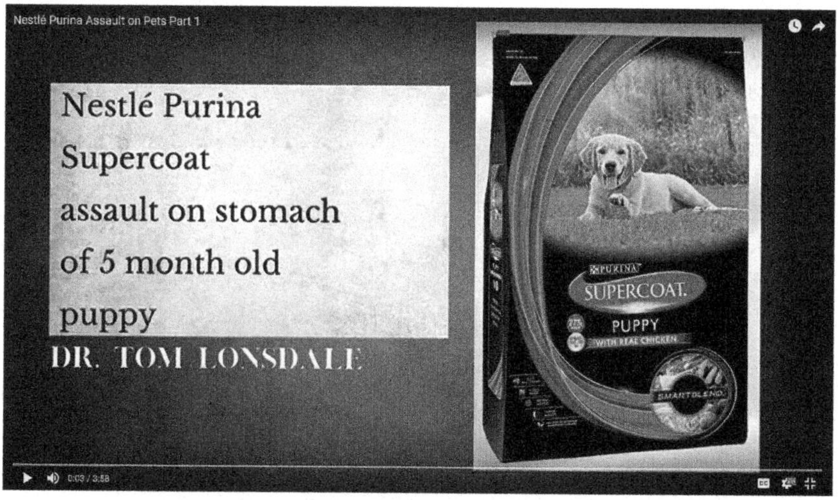

YouTube video: Nestlé Purina Supercoat assault on puppy

Jack

Jack, a handsome cross-breed dog, had been off his food and vomiting for two days. He had a reputation for chewing brushes and shoes and the clinical signs suggested that he was suffering from a bowel obstruction. We took radiographs and monitored the passage of barium contrast material down his bowel. After due discussion with Jack's owner, we agreed to perform exploratory surgery to confirm the diagnosis and, hopefully, allow us to effect a cure. Even after all these years as a general practitioner vet, I was staggered to see not one obstruction, but several. The junk dry pebbles had exited the stomach and were distributed down the small intestine, slowly, painfully making their way out of the patient.

Millions of pets suffer from intermittent vomiting. Quite a few are subject to expensive investigations, even to the point of exploratory surgery. These are some of the junk pebble issues hiding in plain sight. Imagine how much more we will learn when those in universities, government and other positions of power and responsibility change their attitude. At the very least, they should permit, even welcome, discussion!

4

PROTECTING YOUR PETS

Everyday reality in the consulting room

So that we can better protect your pet, please allow me to welcome you into the consulting room and follow the progress of some real-life patients.

First some context. After 14 years writing articles and books and touring the world on the raw meaty bones campaign, I ran out of money. The trouble was made worse by my longstanding veterinary tenant moving out of the Bligh Park vet clinic, taking his equipment and clients with him. I was trying not to worry when Sandra Sultana, a vet nurse who had worked for me years earlier, arrived at the critical time. Together we refurbished and restocked the empty premises, hung out an 'Open' sign and waited for clients to come.

In previous practices I had supplied clients with a list of butchers and pet shops where they could obtain raw meaty bones and offal. In the new practice I resolved to make things easier, more economical and efficient in the hope more people would respond to the raw meaty bones message. We sourced second-hand chest freezers which we stocked with a range of raw meaty bones and offal—chicken frames (the bony leftover after most of the meat has been removed for human consumption), quail frames, kangaroo tails, abattoir offal, sheep heads, rabbit heads and whole wild rabbits.

On the consulting room walls we arranged photos of healthy

dogs and cats ripping at raw meaty bones. A large drug company poster helped pet owners understand the significance of gum disease.

> **Get a dental checkup for your dog**
>
> **Before his breath gets worse than his bite.**
>
> Your dog's bad breath can be more than annoying. It can signal serious dental problems that threaten the animal's health as well.
>
> **More than 8 out of 10 adult dogs have periodontal disease.**
>
> Recent veterinary surveys reveal that 85 percent of adult dogs suffer from some form of periodontal disease.
>
> **Neglected teeth can lead to serious health problems.**
>
> Periodontal disease or gum disease can result in infected gums, abscesses, loose teeth, even destruction of bone tissue around the teeth.[1]

We highlighted the Mars Corporation advertising feature from a UK vet magazine promoting their milk and rice dental chew. Mars didn't tell vets that their junk products trigger the gum disease pandemic, but they did acknowledge in heavy bold type the magnitude of the resultant problem.

> **Major health problems can start with gum disease**
>
> Dental problems are known to increase with age and are increasingly being linked to vital organ disease—most notably kidney and liver. This is of particular concern

> when you consider that in many small animal practices, periodontal disease is the most common reason for anaesthesia. It is unnecessary to alarm dog owners but such scientific findings do have a role to play in stressing the need for daily oral care. Perhaps then it may be given a higher priority in the everyday care of animals.[2]

A 2004 *Time* magazine cover, enlarged and laminated, grabbed attention emphasising the effects of inflammation on human health and thus by extension the effects on the health of all animals.

> **THE SECRET KILLER**
> The surprising link between INFLAMMATION and HEART ATTACKS, CANCER, ALZHEIMER'S and other diseases.[3]

Sad to say, none of the clients venturing in to see the new (old) vet in town had any prior knowledge of the diet + gum disease + inflammation nexus. Neither did they know that junk food chemicals, while only taking minutes to consume, remain in the body 24 hours a day, seven days a week, posing another serious challenge to the overtaxed immune system. And for the owners of fat dogs and cats, the recent scientific findings that obesity is associated with inflammation throughout the body was indeed 'secret' and 'surprising' information.

It is no surprise that pet owners steeped in false and misleading propaganda in favour of junk pet food might be somewhat ignorant. One might suppose, however, that those who have consulted vets may have received at least partial enlightenment. Not so. No-one had any idea. Instead, they had been denied true, accurate useful information and simultaneously exposed to a welter of false and misleading information and massive overservicing that passes for modern-day veterinary 'care'.

Given this level of cultural conditioning you can begin to understand why no-one ever thought to consult us about diet, gum disease, obesity or inflammation, the main determinants of health, life and death for pet dogs and cats—and also ferrets, which are common pets in the US. It was mostly by chance that clients visited us, whether about minor concerns through to serious end-stage disease. Vaccinations—against mostly controlled or non-existent diseases—was another reason clients visited the practice. In each instance, clients expected us to address the presenting complaint. However, more in line with the pet's long-term interests, it was our opportunity to address the distress and suffering induced by junk food and affecting the pet 24 hours every day.

The permanent vile stench wafting from the animals' mouths, I advised, were poisonous gases escaping into the atmosphere—and if we were temporarily unlucky, up our noses. For the pets, however, there could be no escape. As animals they would be abundantly aware of their fetid breath. Significantly, the capillary beds and lymphatics in the gums would be transporting the poisonous juices away from the diseased gums and into the general circulation 24 hours a day. Once in the circulation the heart, liver, kidneys and immune system need to be constantly at work detoxifying the septic sludge.

Diagnosing the triple assault on the pets—junk food ingredients, gum disease and obesity—I pointed out, requires no fancy instrumentation, no thermometers, stethoscopes, X-ray machines, pathology tests or referral to specialists. Four senses, excluding taste, are all that we need.

What's before our eyes

Dull, lifeless, moth-eaten coat

Saggy belly, or obesity or rake-like thinness

Dull of eye, constant licking of lips

What's up our nose

Stinking mouth odours

Greasy dog skin odour

What's in our ears

Client's description of junk food diet and copious, offensive faecal output

What's at our fingertips

Dry lifeless brittle coat or greasy coat or sparse coat

Body flaccid to the touch or flabby—as opposed to the taut, trim and terrific form of the canine or feline athlete

Then as now I cannot say that all clients listen with rapt attention. If, however, time permits and the client is somewhat receptive, I press on, mindful that this is an opportunity to act as the animal's advocate. The pets cannot speak. I must speak for them.

I attempt to demonstrate how vet practice has gone a long way down the dead end of techno-medicine. I explain some of the deficiencies.

The fact that most vets' waiting areas are stocked with plastic bags of junk labelled as 'food' is an affront to common sense and in breach of 'truth in labelling' laws. Catch a rabbit in the woods and affix 'pet food' and 'pet medicine' labels and you would be truthful. However, those same labels cannot be peeled off the rabbit and truthfully affixed to the side of a can or packet of artificial grain-based recipes.

I gesture to the dog and cat skulls and the model of human teeth. Note the difference in number and shape of the teeth, I say. Note how the dentition of a 15 kg (33 pound) dog is, relatively speaking, eight to 10 times as large as that of a 75 kg (165 pound) human. Coupled with this disparity in size and shape, dogs and cats live on average 15 years compared with a human average of 75 years.

Consequently, the impacts of dental disease are speedier and proportionately much greater for pets so afflicted.

As for the vets who book animals for six-monthly 'prophies'—teeth scaling and polishing under general anaesthetic—I cast doubt. Dental plaque forms constantly and, if left undisturbed, begins to calcify within 24 hours. Dogs and cats need *daily* vigorous cleaning of the working parts. Many vets delegate the 'prophy' task to their vet nurses and technicians who take immense pride in polishing the ivories—and *pride in not removing* teeth. Just as polishing the ivories of an antique piano puts on a shine but fails to help the long-dead elephant, so it is with pets' diseased teeth. Teeth may gleam, but if they're only loosely attached in diseased jaws, those teeth must be extracted. Often pets have recently undergone 'prophies' at other clinics and when presented at our clinic need multiple teeth extractions.

Thermometers, stethoscopes, elaborate diagnostic machines and instrumentation and the ubiquitous blood tests only measure when reserve capacity and compensatory mechanisms have failed. Only imperfectly do they tell us about the end stage when something has gone wrong. At some level the need for diagnosis and treatment bespeaks a failure of prevention. And in every case the biggest failure constitutes the continued poisoning of the pets with artificial concoctions neither suitable nor safe for ingestion by living carnivores.

What do I mean by reserve capacity and compensatory mechanisms? Imagine you're at the foot of the stairs, your heart beats steadily at a resting rate, but as you climb the stairs your heart rate increases to *compensate* for the needed extra effort. If you are unfit your heart rate soon approaches or reaches its maximum rate. However, if you are physically fit your *reserve capacity*, the potential extra output of your heart, will be greater, but nevertheless your heart will still need to compensate, to beat faster. Apply the same reasoning for pets' body systems—heart, liver, kidneys, immune system—stressed by *constant need* to deal with junk food toxins, periodontal disease and obesity and you can see how compensatory mechanisms and reserve capacities are constantly stressed and, in many instances, reach their limits.

If you put the wrong fuel in your car it will likely blow smoke and probably won't get you home. You'll need to call a mechanic who will straight away drain the fuel tank and make necessary repairs. If you put the wrong 'fuel' in your pet, unfortunately its onboard mechanics—the compensatory mechanisms—will attempt to make necessary repairs to keep things functional 24 hours a day, seven days a week. When dogs and cats are diagnosed with a failing heart, liver, kidneys or immune system I say it's generally not so much that systems have failed, but that they have been toiling valiantly before finally collapsing under the constant load.

Speaking about blood tests, I tell clients there's a massive inbuilt fallibility. The tests are expensive and frequently misleading or wrong. So many of my patients have been rotting alive from the mouth and its consequences, but nevertheless blood test results frequently fall within the so-called 'normal' range. For vets overly dependent on 'reading the tea-leaves' of the blood test 'snapshot' it's akin to an airline pilot relying on his faulty altimeter as he and his passengers plunge to earth.

It sounds a bit extreme, but that's the reality for millions of pets the world over. The measurers and recorders (the vets), fixated on their instruments, order more and more tests, employ more and more failed treatments until the poor animals are in end-stage decline.

Owners are fleeced by the massive overservicing when simply stopping the junk food and feeding the animals appropriately is all that's needed.

Returning to a discussion of the pet's coat, I point out that the coat provides an outward manifestation of inner health. The skin represents 12 per cent of body weight and can only be as healthy as the underlying internal organs, circulatory and immune systems. Hair follicles can only be as healthy as the skin in which they're located, and the resultant hair growth will be affected accordingly. These days I show a video of Milo the 12-month-old Maine Coon cat with a dull, moth-eaten coat contrasted with George the 12-*year*-old Maine Coon with a rich lustrous coat and confident demeanour.[4]

Testimonials—the before and after of junk diets

George the Maine Coon cat

For George it was not always thus. When first presented at our clinic as a six-year-old cat, he was a physical wreck. Six years later his owner wrote to the Australian Government Senate Standing Committees of Rural and Regional Affairs and Transport.

> Dear Sir/Madam
>
> **RE: Regulatory approaches to ensure the safety of pet food**
>
> **Summary**
>
> We believe our cat's life-threatening diabetes was caused by the high-grain content of the vet-recommended, dry pet food that we innocently fed him, due to the prevailing misinformation available to pet owners. Since his diagnosis in 2012, after changing his diet to a more natural, traditional diet of raw meaty bones he is disease-free, medication-free, and far healthier than previously.
>
> We recommend a complete overhaul of the pet-food industry, or at the very least, an independent body is required to regulate and oversee pet food standards.

Background

In October 2010 we adopted our gorgeous cat, 'George,' from Katoomba RSPCA, and before leaving the store we purchased the food they recommended—Hill's Science Diet dry and tinned cat food. Because it was an expensive, 'reputable' name brand highly recommended by vets, we didn't think twice about checking the ingredients or doing some research on it. It was also extremely convenient, and we thought we were feeding him one of the best products available. We included some tinned wet foods in our cat's diet, but found he didn't do very well on it, often vomiting it back up again, so we dropped it out almost altogether, and he was fed practically exclusively on Hill's Science Diet dry food.

Our cat seemed to be in relatively good health, except for a mucus-like discharge from one or both eyes, which would never seem to clear up. We were a little surprised by how much water he drank but didn't question it too much. Although we may have brought it up at a vet visit, we were however reassured enough not to worry. His faeces were also quite loose, unformed stool, but not exactly diarrhoea, and were extremely smelly. With the type of litter tray we used, it was obvious that he passed a lot of wee as well. Sadly, we did not realise these were symptoms of worsening health until early August 2012.

On 5/08/2012 we took him to the vet as he was urinating blood. Tests were completed by the vet, and medications prescribed. Royal Canin Feline Sensitive Sachets were also recommended to us, so we started feeding our cat with those. On Friday 31/08/2012 our cat was now urinating uncontrollably all over the house (he was incontinent), was drinking water constantly, and was clearly extremely unwell. We immediately took him to our local vet again, where urine and blood tests were completed, indicating that his blood glucose levels were dangerously high. He was diagnosed with diabetes mellitus. Surprisingly enough, we were told by the vet that our cat's illness was completely unrelated to his diet. We were told the only effective treatment was insulin injections, at an estimated cost of $350.00 initial treatment, ongoing $82 per bottle, which could last about 10 weeks, depending on dose, in addition to needle costs for each injection. The vet told us that without treatment our cat will become keto acidotic (ie, severe life-threatening condition requiring immediate treatment). We advised the vet that we would think about it over the weekend and return on Monday.

Fortunately for us and our cat, on Sunday we miraculously read an article in the Sunday Telegraph, 2/09/2012, pages 36-37 by Jane Hansen, titled 'Growth Industry' highlighting the fact that pets are big business, and discussing the high costs involved with pet ownership, particularly when they become seriously ill. The article quoted Dr Richard Malik, a Sydney University lecturer who ran a vet practice in Double Bay at the time of article printing. The article stated that Dr Malik blames many of the diseases he treats in cats and dogs, on their diet, and he is quoted as saying 'The great enemy of cats is dried cat food, it has way too much carbohydrate and now we see cats with diabetes and periodontal disease, a whole range of conditions due to being too fat.'

Wow, light-bulb moment for us—of course excess

grains in our cat's dry food could be linked to his high glucose levels causing diabetes. It made perfect sense. The article went on to mention vet Dr Tom Lonsdale, his clinic in Windsor, and his book 'Raw Meaty Bones.' Convinced we were onto something here, on Monday 3/09/2012 we took our cat to see Dr Lonsdale at his clinic, only 15 minutes' drive from where we lived. Tom suggested we try tablets first, rather than insulin, and prescribed a new diet—yes, raw meaty bones! We went home armed with medication, raw meat, and lots of information. Following Dr Tom's instructions, from Tuesday 4/09/2012, to Sunday 9/09/2012 we documented our cat's water intake—it had already halved in less than 7 days! We continued with the medication and the new diet, mainly raw frozen quail, rabbit and chicken. We never started insulin injection treatment as prescribed by our previous vet.

In the last 6 years since being on a raw meaty bone diet, our cat has become completely symptom-free from his diabetes, his eye discharge completely cleared up, his fur coat is much healthier, shiny and attractive, his faeces are well-formed and not nearly as smelly, and at nearly 11 years old he is still as playful as a kitten. He is no longer on any medication whatsoever and is at an ideal weight.

It has become clear to us that the Australian pet food industry is 'educating' or indoctrinating veterinary students on the apparent benefits of commercially produced dry pet foods, providing benefits to vet clinics who promote their products, and ignoring the field research of genuine vets who have seen time and time again the detrimental effects of feeding cats and dogs on a diet high in grains, and the real value of going back to the traditional diet of felines and canines in the wild—raw meat and bones. This is especially important for cats, as felines are known to be 'obligate carnivores'. Clearly the pet food industry is far more concerned with profits than the health of our pets, and needs a complete overhaul, or at the very least, requires an independent body to regulate pet food standards.

Thank you for the opportunity to provide this submission.

Yours sincerely,
Concerned Pet Owner[5]

George the Maine Coon got lucky because his owner happened to read a newspaper article about Titan the boxer dog who, also quite by chance, got lucky too.

Titan the boxer dog

Pet vet bills give paws for thought
The deep freezer out the back of Dr Tom Lonsdale's Veterinary Clinic in Windsor is a scary sight. Inside are sheep and goats' heads, rabbits, rats, guts, livers, lambs' hearts, you name it. For $2 a kilo, pet owners and patients stock up on the raw diet he believes nature intended our pets to have. Back in the '90s, Dr Lonsdale noticed many of his patients had stinking breath and rotten teeth.

He blamed the commercial diet of pets and wrote the book 'Raw Meaty Bones', which details the health benefits of returning dogs and cats to a carnivore diet.

'Dogs and cats are designed to chew, and they have been turned into little (junk food) addicts ... by eating stuff that is not for them' he says.

> Hayley Williams took her boxer to Dr Lonsdale. Up to the age of four Titan was fed a diet of standard canned and dried commercial dog food and got to a fat 32kg, became lethargic, had bad breath, flatulence and doggy dandruff. Titan boarded with Lonsdale for five weeks.
>
> 'He's lost six kilos, his coat is shiny and glossy, he has lost the dandruff and has so much more energy, and no doggy breath,' Williams says.[6]

Barbara O'Neill's elderly fluffy white dogs also, finally, overcame years of bad luck. Barbara read the newspaper article about Titan and made an appointment to see us. Given the age and failing health of her dogs, Barbara elected to have blood tests performed prior to multiple dental extractions and change of diet. Compare the pathologist's dry, detached interpretation of the blood test results with Barbara's close and nuanced assessment.

Connor (12 years) Maltese–Pomeranian cross

Pathologist's report: 'The results fail to reveal a specific aetiology.' Vet-speak for results are clinically insignificant. Barbara O'Neill's report:

> **Preoperative**
>
> Connor presented to Dr Lonsdale with severe gum disease and failing health. He had milky blue shadows across his eyes and was obviously having problems with his sight. His hair had become dry and coarse. Connor is a dog that imitates cats in his grooming habits and loved being spotlessly clean.
>
> I could not lift Connor without him yelping in pain and his hind legs were very stiff. He was becoming detached

from his surroundings and would stand for long periods staring into space.

Connor resisted chewing and was always lethargic. He had halitosis and little interest in food. He slept restlessly and urinated constantly throughout the night.

Postoperative

When I collected Connor on the day of the operation, he was running around following the vet nurse around the cages. That night he slept for 12 hours.

Upon waking he was given a raw chicken frame which he hungrily attacked. He then looked for more chicken frames, which of course he received.

Within a week the milky blue shadows in Connor's eyes had receded and they are barely there a month later. He is now alert and puppy-like in his playfulness and awareness of his environment. He does not yelp as much when lifted (I think he thinks he is going to hurt).

Connor now runs like a puppy and has a fresh clean smell in his mouth at all times. His coat is silky and beautiful; he prances around with his head held high. He is so happy.

My dog does not miss his teeth. I have noticed that the strength of his jaws has compensated for the missing teeth and he has no problems with bones.

I am however distressed that Connor had been to several vets to have his teeth fixed, with the result being a cosmetic polish and shine. I knew he was not well as a result of his teeth.

Connor no longer eats commercial dog food with the exception of Beneful meat and vegies once or twice a week;

> this is dependent on when I get home in the evening. Otherwise, it is raw meaty bones and nothing else.

Rosie (11½ years) Maltese

Pathologist's typically complex, convoluted and inconclusive report:

> Leucogram may reflect stress or inflammation. Increased red cell mass, albumin and sodium likely reflect dehydration at sampling. Non-specific liver enzyme elevations. Further interpretation is dependent upon the clinical appearance (underlying endocrine disease a consideration?) and thoracic imaging given the reported cough.

Vet-speak for the tea-leaves are being uncooperative. 'We're unsure what to make of the numbers. We're obliged to recommend more and more detailed testing and investigations.' Barbara O'Neill's report:

> **Preoperative**
>
> Rosie presented to Dr Lonsdale with severe gum disease and failing health. She had halitosis, was aggressive and irritable. Her hair had become very dry and coarse, and her skin was constantly itchy.
>
> Rosie had developed a meaty lump on her sternum which moved to the left and right across her chest regularly. She had developed chronic nocturnal breathing difficulties. During those episodes I had to assist her breathing by raising her chin and upper body.
>
> Rosie was diagnosed by a local vet with Congestive Heart Failure and was on permanent medication when I took her to Dr Lonsdale.

Postoperative

When I collected Rosie on the day of the operation, she was running around with Connor following the vet nurse. That night she slept for 12 hours.

Upon waking she was given a raw chicken frame which she hungrily attacked. She then looked for more chicken frames, which of course she received and which she proceeded to bury industriously. Previously she couldn't care and showed little interest in food.

Within a week the aggressive behaviour lessened and although she has now become aggressive in guarding her bones, her casual aggression to the other dogs in the family has markedly decreased.

Rosie runs like a puppy now; her coat is silky and beautiful, and she has a clean fresh smell in her mouth at all times. Her eyes are so bright, and she actually shows joy in her face. Rosie is loving life again and now enjoys playing games.

Rosie does not miss her teeth—nor do the other dogs and visitors! I have noticed that the strength of her jaws has compensated for the missing teeth, and she has no problem with bones.

Rosie has not had medication for her heart since the day of the operation. The lump on her chest is completely gone. I am however distressed that Rosie had been to several vets to have her teeth fixed—the result being a cosmetic polish and shine. In addition, with being diagnosed with Congestive Heart Failure.

Rosie no longer eats commercial dog food except for Beneful meat and vegies once or twice a week; this is dependent on when I get home in the evening. Otherwise, it is raw meaty bones and nothing else.

I am a strong supporter of Doctor Tom Lonsdale's theory and practice. I was reluctant to go through with the procedure, especially with Rosie being diagnosed with Congestive Heart Failure.

I did not think my dogs would be alive by the year ending 2013. I can now look forward to many more years of their unconditional love.

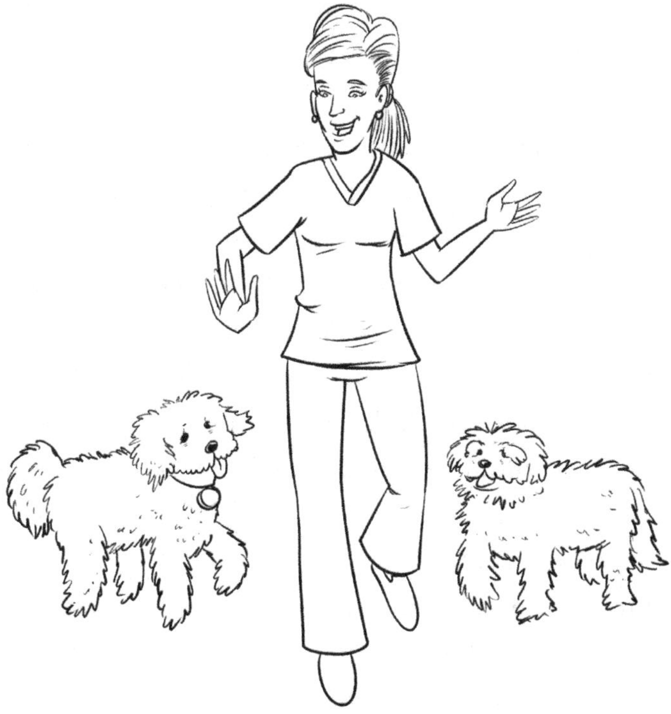

Rosie and Connor after extensive dental extractions.

Chances are, as you read this, that you are in a far-flung place remote from Bligh Park, New South Wales. Don't worry, be happy. Providing your dog or cat does not need any dental treatment, then visiting our practice may not be necessary. See what Tamara Rousso wrote from Oregon, USA.

Mac the cat and Zara the Labrador

I have been feeding RMB for about 2 years now. It began with my cat, Mac. At the tender age 4 years old he was diagnosed with cystitis. I had noticed for quite some time that he seemed to be somewhat uncomfortable. He would ask to go outside, and then back inside/outside over and over like he just couldn't get comfortable anywhere. He also didn't always use his cat box, but I chalked that up to living in a multi-cat house. Finally, one day Mac jumped up a decorative basket, and peed a nickel size pink drop of urine in front of me.

The vet diagnosed cystitis and sent him home on antibiotics (even though no culture for infection), and steroids. He was better for 2–3 weeks and then back in. This time she sent us home with Hill's Prescription Diet along with the medications. When I read the list of ingredients my heart sank as I could see this would not bode well for long life. Sure enough 3–4 weeks later we were back at the vet with the same problem even though I had fed the prescription diet. The vet really had nothing else to offer me other than more steroids and more antibiotics, so I started doing some research on-line and found someone who had experienced success with ridding their cat of cystitis by feeding a raw diet. We threw away the Hills, and I am happy to say it has been two years since Mac had any problems. He no longer has any inappropriate urinary issues, and he no longer asks to go outside, inside on and on. He is a happy, active, hunting, loving cat.

Once I saw how well the cats were doing, I felt guilty for not feeding the dogs a raw diet. I bought your book

Work Wonders and haven't looked back.

My dogs at that time ranged in age from 8 years old to 2 years old. The most amazing difference was seen with my 8-year-old Lab, Zara. She had really started to slow down and was having some difficulty rising from her bed. After about 2 weeks I heard Zara growling in another room. This was very odd. I couldn't ever remember Zara growling before. I went to see what was going on, and she was just standing there with a bone at her feet. Hmmmm. I went around the corner and the growling started again. No other dogs around—clearly not food aggression going on, which would have been odd in itself as she had never, ever exhibited food aggression. Back around the corner, and this time when she growled, I hurtled myself around the corner in time to see her throwing her bone in the air, growling at it and catching it! How cute!

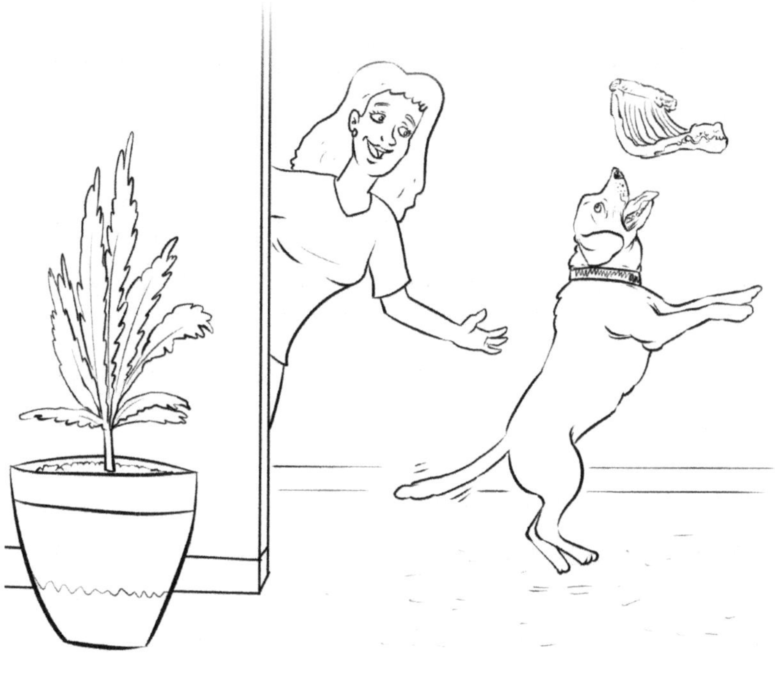

Not only had she started playing again, but her energy came back in spades. No longer did she appear as an old dog. She was rising from her bed with ease. In fact, a few months after we had switched her, I had to threaten her with putting her back on kibble! One day I walked from the back of the house to see what she was barking at outside to find she had bounded onto my dining room table where she had a view out the big window! Now at age 10 she is still active and happy. I often travel with my dogs and find since switching them to a raw diet I quite often have people ask to pet them. I attribute this to their shiny coats, clean teeth, and no stinky doggy smell. This didn't happen when they were fed kibble, and a high quality (read expensive) kibble at that!

Voiceless pets everywhere

The keen observations and astute interpretations by pet owners provide a glimpse of the constant suffering of pets forced to subsist on junk food. The comments above relate to end-stage diseases where organ systems are failing and where dramatic changes get noticed, even by 'dumb' humans. What about the chronic malaise and likely mental anguish affecting pets? Humans are not sufficiently in touch with their pets' feelings. And of course, pets have not yet learnt to speak. Clearly, it's incumbent on us to speak for them. In order to do so, we need to think long and hard about what it means to subsist on junk food.

Pets are exquisitely sensitive to their surroundings. Their senses of smell, sight and hearing far outstrip our puny abilities. Chances are they are exquisitely self-aware but cannot communicate to us their psychological and physical hurt. We need to think what it means to crave physical chewing, crave missing nutrients while simultaneously lost in a fog of chronic head and body ache.

Have you ever suffered a severe hangover or been chronically unwell? I suspect that's how pets feel when every part of their body is swimming in toxic metabolites from the junk food and the constant bombardment of toxins from diseased gums. Dogs and cats have a specialised organ immediately behind the upper incisor teeth known as the organ of Jacobson, or vomeronasal organ. It's my guess, this organ helps them sense changes in their saliva and thus the health of their mouth and their vulnerability or otherwise in the struggle for survival.[7]

I don't need to guess about the amazing precision with which dogs take liver treats from my outstretched hand. They cannot see the broken liver fragments, but they can sense where they are, simultaneously ingesting them while taking immense care not to bite my hand. They never make a mistake; they know in an instant if my fingers are between their teeth.

The junk pet food advertisements tell us dogs and cats are glowing with health and *joie de vivre*. The reality, for almost every pet from the moment it cuts its deciduous teeth to the moment it passes this world, is a craving for what's missing and a stoic acceptance of what must be endured.

Lessons in plain sight

Veterinary clinicians

By now, I'm sure you've seen the obvious. Vets, all vets, must change their approach to the treatment of dogs, cats and ferrets. They must stop doing harm. They must stop advising the feeding of highly processed pap to domestic carnivores. Simultaneously they must gain an awareness and clinical acumen regarding dentistry and obesity. If and when they make these essential adjustments, they'll be on the road to making amends for past failings. And for adult carnivores under their care, vets will be combining therapy and prevention in one. Raw meaty bones are easily the strongest, safest, most gentle, most effective therapeutic and preventative medicine for all domestic carnivores.

That being so, all puppies and kittens must be weaned off mother's milk onto the preventative medicine ordained by nature: whole carcasses or raw meaty bones, the subject of the next chapter.

Researchers, administrators, regulators

The testimonials from pet owners provide revelations galore about bountiful uplift in health and vitality not just on a few random occasions, but constantly, dependably over many years in my veterinary practice. Feeding a diet as close as possible to nature is the gift that keeps on giving. We need to stop and contemplate the magnitude of that realisation—if we have that realisation.

Eventually researchers, administrators and regulators woke up to the reality that Ignaz Semmelweis was right when he showed that by washing their hands doctors could save the lives of new mothers in the obstetric ward. Eventually the medical establishment accepted Lister's findings that by sterilising instruments, surgical outcomes could be dramatically improved. However, as important as those realisations are, childbirth and surgical interventions don't affect every person or every pet.

The results reported in the testimonials are applicable to *all* pets and by extension have implications for *all* humans *all* the time. The medical and research establishment should be inspired to ask questions, lots of questions, about why pets rebound in health and vitality as a result of a diet change. What are the patho-physiological mechanisms? What are the easy questions to ask leading to rapid discoveries? What are the aspects of deeper significance requiring more funding and more time to elicit nature's secrets?

Perhaps the question, above all, is 'Why aren't there already major research efforts being applied?' The answer to that question, unfortunately, is simple and disturbing. The dead hand of the pet food industry, enabled by the veterinary profession and fake animal welfare charities, conspires to (a) deny the bountiful research potential and (b) ensure that no researcher ever contemplates conducting research that would impugn the reputation and threaten the power of the junk pet food titans.

Educational and licensing authorities

You rightly point out that there are no 'educational and licensing authorities' when it comes to pet keeping. Anyone can buy a pet, receive one as gift or find it on the side of the road. No need for any formal or informal education and of course no need for a licence.

Clients, often by chance, arrive at our vet practice and are encouraged to unlearn their previous beliefs and take on a new way of caring for their pets—all in the space of a 15-minute consultation on an unrelated matter. You are reading this book, requiring many hours of study, and finding that there's an immense amount of information necessary to be a well-informed pet owner. And this book only deals with diet and health and has nothing to say about pet housing, governmental or municipal regulations or training.

How much better that folk should enrol in an educational course and receive a certificate, even a licence, at the end of the course ensuring that they know the basics sufficient to care for a sentient, carnivorous pet for its lifetime. Currently, that's a far-off prospect, but meanwhile maybe something to consider.

5

PRESCRIPTION FOR HEALTH

Building a new paradigm about nutrition, health and disease is a bit like building a new house. First clear the rubbish, level the ground and lay firm foundations. We want our house to stand the test of time without cracks opening up revealing poor construction on shaky ground. It's the same with our new way of seeing our pets and their nutritional and health needs. Make sure to avoid rubbishy old ways of thinking on unsound foundations.

Get going, get started

Now, with an open mind, let nature be your teacher. No matter the size, shape and outer packaging—whether a diminutive chihuahua, elongated sausage dog, or pink, permed poodle—your dog is a modified wolf. The same principles apply to your cat, a modified desert predator from North Africa. And if you own a ferret, it's a modified polecat from the forests and riverbanks of Europe. The job of carnivores—the reason for their existence, reason for living, etched in their DNA—is to track, hunt, kill and consume their prey, mostly herbivores and omnivores.

Carnivores living and breeding in the wild depend on the ideal *quality* of food in the right *quantity* at a suitable *frequency*. For domestic pets the same principles apply.

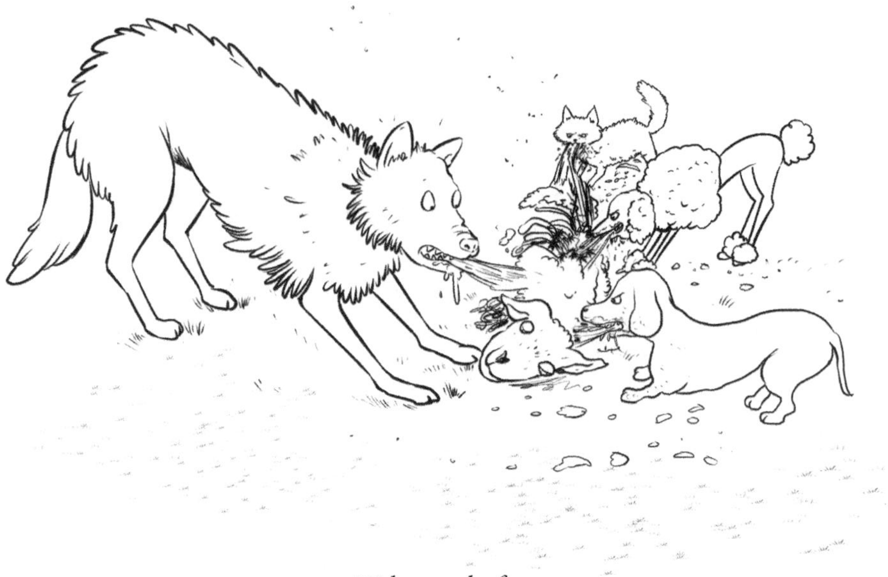

Wolves at the feast

Quality

Low-fat game animals and fish and birds provide the best source of food for pet carnivores. If using meat from farm animals (cattle, sheep and pigs) avoid excessive fat, or bones that are too large to be eaten—unless covered in lots of meat. Eating the meat but leaving the bone is standard carnivore behaviour.

Dogs are more likely to break their teeth when gnawing meatless large knuckle bones and bones sawn lengthwise than when chomping on meat and bone together.

Raw food for cats should always be fresh. Dogs can consume 'ripe' food and will sometimes bury valuable raw meaty bones for later consumption.

Quantity

Establishing the quantity to feed pets is more an art than a science. Parents, when feeding a human family, manage this task without the aid of food consumption charts. You can achieve the same good results for your pet by paying attention to activity levels, appetite and body condition.

High activity and large appetite indicate a need for increased food, and vice versa.

Body condition depends on several factors. The overall body shape—is it athletic or rotund?—and the lustre of the hair coat provide clues. Use your fingertips to assess the elasticity of the skin. Does it have an elastic feel and move readily over the muscles? Do the muscles feel well toned? And how much coverage of the ribs do you detect? This is the best place to check whether your pet is too thin or too fat. By comparing your own rib cage with that of your pet you can obtain a good idea of body condition—both your own and that of your pet.

An approximate food consumption guide based on raw meaty bones, for the average pet cat or dog, is 15 to 20 per cent of body weight in one week or 2 to 3 per cent per day. On that basis a 25 kilo (55 pound) dog requires up to five kilos (11 pounds) of carcasses or raw meaty bones weekly. Cats weighing five kilos (11 pounds) require about one kilo (2.2 pounds) of chicken necks, fish, rabbit or similar each week. Table scraps can be fed as an extra component of the diet (see below). Please note that these figures are only a guide and relate to adult pets in a domestic environment.

Pregnant or lactating females and growing puppies and kittens may need much more food than adult animals of similar body weight.

Wherever possible, feed the meat and bone ration in one large piece requiring much ripping, tearing and gnawing. This makes for contented pets with clean teeth. (See below for advice on dealing with possible mess.)

Frequency

Wild carnivores feed at irregular intervals. In a domestic setting regularity works best and accordingly I suggest that you feed adult dogs and cats once daily. If you live in a hot climate, I recommend that you feed pets in the evening to avoid attracting flies. If, however, your pets pester you, then consider making feeding times a random event.

I suggest that on one or two days each week your dog may be fasted—just like animals in the wild.

On occasions you may run out of natural food. Don't be tempted to buy artificial junk, fast your pet and stock up with natural food the next day.

Puppies, cats, ferrets and sick or underweight dogs should not be fasted (unless on veterinary advice).

Natural foods suitable for pet carnivores

Whole carcasses

- Rats, mice, rabbits, fish, chickens, quail, hens.

Raw meaty bones

- Chicken and turkey carcasses, after most of the meat has been removed for human consumption, are suitable for dogs and cats
- Poultry by-products include heads, feet, necks and wings
- Whole fish and fish heads
- Goat, sheep, calf, deer and kangaroo carcasses can be sawn into large pieces of meat and bone
- Other by-products include pigs' trotters, pigs' heads, sheep heads, brisket, tail bones, rib bones.

Offal

- Liver, lungs, windpipe, heart, tripe.

Table scraps

Wild carnivores eat small amounts of omnivore food, part-digested in liquid form, when they eat the intestines of their prey. Our table scraps and some fruit and vegetable peelings are omnivore food which has not been ingested. Providing scraps do not form too great a proportion of the diet, they appear to do no harm and may do some good. I advise an upper limit of one-third scraps for dogs and rather less for cats. Liquidising scraps, both cooked and raw, in the kitchen mixer may help to increase their digestibility.

Things to avoid

- Excessive meat off the bone—not balanced.
- Excessive vegetables—not balanced.
- Mineral and vitamin additives—create imbalance and are rarely necessary.
- Processed food—leads to dental and other diseases.
- Excessive starchy food—associated with bloat.
- Significant amounts of onions, garlic and chocolate—toxic to pets.
- Grapes, raisins, sultanas, currants—toxic to pets.
- Fruit stones (pits) and corn cobs—get stuck.
- Milk—associated with diarrhoea. Animals drink it whether thirsty or not and consequently get fat. Milk sludge sticks to teeth and gums.

Take care

- Old dogs and cats addicted to a processed diet may experience initial difficulty when changed onto a natural diet.
- Pets with misshapen jaws and dental disease may experience difficulties with a natural diet.

- Create variety. Any nutrients fed to excess can be harmful.
- Liver is an excellent foodstuff but should not be fed more than once a week.
- Other offal, e.g. ox stomach, should not exceed 50 per cent of the diet.
- Whole fish are an excellent source of food for carnivores but avoid feeding one species of fish constantly. Some species, e.g., carp, contain an enzyme which destroys thiamine (vitamin B1).
- There are no prizes for the fattest dog on the block, nor for the fastest. Feed pets for a lifetime of health. Prevention is better than cure.

Miscellaneous tips

- Feeding dogs, cats and ferrets the appropriate carnivore diet represents the single most important contribution to their welfare.
- Establish early contact with a dependable supplier of foodstuffs for pet carnivores.
- Buy food in bulk in order to avoid shortages.
- Package the daily rations separately for ease of feeding.
- Refrigerated storage space, preferably a freezer, is essential.
- Raw meaty bones can be fed frozen just like ice cream. Some pets eat the frozen article; others wait for it to thaw.
- Small carcasses, for example rats, mice and small birds, can be fed frozen and complete with entrails. Larger carcasses should have the entrails removed before freezing.
- Feeding bowls are unnecessary—the food will be dragged across the floor—so feed pets outside by preference, in a crate, or on an easily cleaned floor, for instance laundry or shower cubicle.
- Ferrets are small carnivores which can be fed in the same way as cats.

Puppies and kittens

From about three weeks of age puppies and kittens start to take an interest in what their mother is eating. By six weeks of age, they can eat chicken carcasses, rabbits and fish.

During the brief interval between three and six weeks of age it is advisable to provide minced chicken, chicken carcasses or similar for young animals (as well as access to larger pieces that encourage ripping and tearing). This is akin to the part-digested food regurgitated by wild carnivore mothers. Large litters need more supplementary feeding than small litters. (Minced meat can be fed, but only for a short time, until the young animals can eat meat and bone together—usually at about six weeks of age.)

Between four and six months of age puppies and kittens cut their permanent teeth and grow rapidly. At this time, they need a plentiful supply of carcasses or raw meaty bones of suitable size.

Puppies and kittens tend not to overeat natural food. Food can be made continuously available.

Problem solving

Junk pet food merchants and their vet proxies shout and holler about all the supposed problems with feeding a more natural diet. Their two main fixations are the feared bacteria they allege contaminate every mouthful and the perilous risks posed by bones. As with all things in life, risks need to be acknowledged and dealt with. Look both ways before stepping off the kerb. Buckle your seatbelt before take-off. Even when exercising all due precautions, risks remain, but risks we are willing to accept in exchange for the expected benefits to be gained.

Bacteria

The bacteria found in a jungle fowl perched high in a primordial forest would provide little threat to either us or our carnivore companions. Unfortunately, jungle fowl are becoming rare, and forests are on the wane these days. Food for the majority of humans and their pets comes from factory farms where the birds and animals are packed in close confinement ankle deep in their own excrement 24 hours a day. The meat in the butcher's shop and in your refrigerator is likely contaminated with bacteria including *Salmonella*, *Campylobacter*, *E. coli* and *Listeria* from the factory farm.

If the risks were inordinately high, abattoir workers, butchers and chefs would be in great and persistent danger. But it's just simply not the case. In our homes we manage such risks by washing our hands and kitchen surfaces and cooking meat and thus killing any microbes.

Since our pets need to eat their meaty bones raw, they come into closer contact with pathogenic bacteria and other parasites, some of which will pass through the pet and come out in the faeces. Avoiding loving licks from your pet and picking up the dog droppings are obvious ways to limit your exposure to germs. For cats, be sure to keep the litter tray clean and ideally wear gloves when disposing of used litter and washing the tray. This is particularly the case for women of child-bearing age when changing the cat litter. A protozoal parasite, *Toxoplasma gondii*, can be caught from cat and kitten faeces.

Fortunately for our pets, their digestive systems generally cope with a heavy bacterial load. Dogs, in particular, have evolved as scavengers that eat carrion and the faeces of other animals. In fact, faeces comes steaming and teaming alive with trillions of bacteria—microscopic live prey. For dogs fed indigestible, lifeless carbohydrate junk, the second time through complete with microbes and microbial enzymes tends to be the most nutritious—and apparently tastes better too! It's a useful fact that dogs tend not to be interested in eating faecal residue, either their own or that of other dogs, when fed raw meaty bones.

Occasionally when transitioning a pet from junk food to raw meaty bones a period of diarrhoea ensues. Usually this is a self-limiting problem that will disappear sooner if the pet is fasted for 24 to 48 hours. Mild, transient diarrhoea is not to be feared. Chronic diarrhoea as suffered by so many pets is a major problem, oftentimes simply and conveniently resolved by providing the medicinal benefits of raw meaty bones.

For kittens and puppies, the best time to introduce them to natural foods is while they are still in the nest. From three weeks of age, as their teeth cut through the gums, they can lick at natural food. By six weeks of age, when their deciduous teeth are fully erupted, they can rip and tear with gusto.

Two very important aspects contribute to their wellbeing. First, that they receive the diet evolved to provide optimum growth and development. Second, as newborns they gain protective antibodies against the bacteria and viruses common in the mother's environment. Colostrum, the first milk, is especially rich in antibodies and provides puppies and kittens with high levels of 'passive immunity'.

If mother dog or mother cat has been fed factory-farmed meat her milk will contain antibodies to the germs in her diet. 'Passive' antibody protection assists the newborns until they are exposed to pathogens in their environment. As the passive protection wanes the young animals gradually make their own active immunity to food-borne germs.

Bone risks

Bones, even raw meaty bones, as fed in a domestic environment may pose risks to pets. I acknowledge that. In a wild, natural environment bones pose little risk.[1] What's the difference?

In the wild, bones are never cooked. They always come raw, clothed in meat, tendon, hide, fur, feathers and fins. Bone is never presented shorn of meat in hard, small unchewable and indigestible pieces that can be bolted down and get stuck halfway. In nature the wolf pack departs the scene in search of the next prey deer leaving the long bones, spine and head behind.

The secret to gaining the benefits of feeding bones but limiting risks is to:

- make sure meaty bones are covered in plenty of meat and are of suitable size for the pet
- never feed cooked bones
- never chop bones into small pieces—choking hazard
- never feed large so-called 'recreational' bones—break teeth
- never cut long bones lengthwise—teeth-breaking hazard made worse.

Chicken wing and leg bones, even raw, can splinter and create a penetration hazard. Too much bone, especially splintering bone, can overwhelm the gastric acid supply with the result that sharp shards of bone pass down the intestine creating discomfort along the way and maybe even stabbing pain on the way out through the anus.

A preponderance of bone can also result in overly firm faeces or constipation. The solution, as ever, is to get as close as possible to the natural blueprint. Feed carcasses or raw meaty bones in large, large pieces. Better still feed carcasses wrapped in fur, feathers and fins. Alternatively, you can cheat a bit and feed some boiled pumpkin along with the raw meaty bones. The pumpkin is indigestible, absorbs water and thus bulks out the stool.

Your pet's behaviour will likely change for the better when fed raw meaty bones as opposed to the junk food offerings. Cantankerous cats become placid and content. Dogs tend to show their true nature—generally more compliant and easier to train. Occasionally, though, a previously placid dog may become more confident and thus more aggressive.

We know, of course, that dogs (and cats too) tend to be protective of their raw meaty bones with the risk that they may attack humans and other animals that approach too closely. I recommend that you teach your dog that the hand that gives the bone also is the hand that takes it away. Make sure that your dog sits patiently before you serve the daily ration and thus reinforce the message as to who is boss. Nevertheless, always take care to avoid conflict between feeding pets and people, especially toddlers and the elderly.

Another bone-related problem arises from the caching behaviour of wild carnivores. Dry indigestible kibble can lie exposed for days but domestic dogs fed juicy bones may seek to hide the leftovers. The soft earth of a flower bed is a favourite location in which to bury the precious bone with a view to disinterring the fermented, soil-encrusted morsel some days later—good for your dog, but not so good for the flower bed.

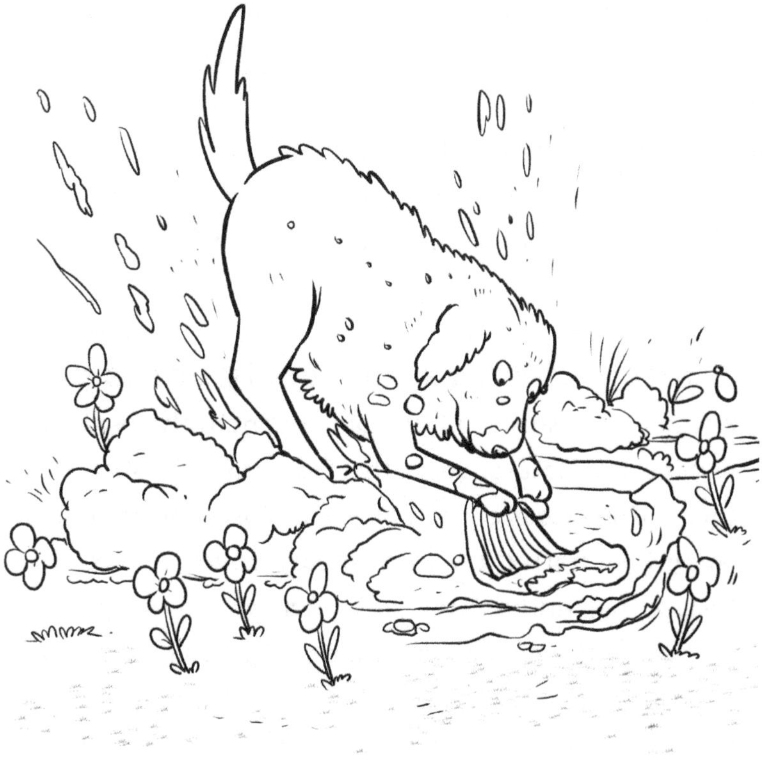

Refusing to eat

At the other end of the spectrum there are cats, ferrets and some small dogs that refuse to eat raw meaty bones. It's not their fault. They deserve our sympathy. Carnivores become imprinted by the foods they're offered to eat at an early age. If that 'food' comes out of a can or bag, then the pet may become addicted to it.

Owners are not to blame either. They feed what the advertisements, the vets and the culture tell them. And once their pet is addicted it can be very difficult to change established patterns of behaviour. Members of a household tend to accommodate an addict's needs—whether those needs are for alcohol, cigarettes or, in the case of the pets, Mars, Nestlé or Colgate manufactured junk. And to compound our problems, the junk food addiction seldom occurs in isolation.

Clearly, then, we cannot take the easy option. We must address the addiction issues at the earliest. It's a big deal. Cats, ferrets and small dogs are often uncooperative. Owners struggle to manage the psychological and physical challenges.

Our 'Switching cats' clinic handout—reproduced below—should help if your cat is addicted to junk food. With minor adjustment the same strategies work for small dogs and ferrets.

Starting cats on a raw meaty bones diet

Kittens and some adult cats instinctively recognise wholesome natural food the first time it's offered to them. Unfortunately, the great majority of adult cats when first started on a raw meaty bones diet tend to be less than enthusiastic and need some coaxing.

Making the change can be a tricky business and we need to get a good grasp of the task at hand. Do you rattle the packet before pouring the fishy pellets into a

bowl? What do you say to Kitty as she comes running? Maybe your feline seldom stirs except to nibble on the kibble sitting in the bowl 24 hours per day? Maybe the furry feline entwined round your legs signals the need for you to open the refrigerator and, with a tap on the tin, serve up the pungent canned food.

Feeding rituals differ, but timing, taste, texture, sight, sound and smell all play a part. Kitty is quite likely addicted to these powerful stimuli and you, as the carer, have likely grown accustomed to the ways that worked best for you. You have literally fed the addiction.

Now imagine the future with your lithe feline crouched low as she tucks into chicken necks, quail and whole raw fish. That's the successful end point. (See photos and videos at www.rawmeatybones.com.) If your cat is young and healthy you can start making the change. However, if your cat is overweight, suffers from dental or other medical problems, then you will likely first need to consult your vet before you embark on the diet changes. (Fat cats should not be starved, as it can lead to liver failure.)

Useful change techniques

Work with your cat, not with her addiction. Stopping 24-hour access to food is the essential first step. Instead, start a once-a-day routine at, say, 6 pm. Kitty's biological clock will soon synchronise, and her anatomy, physiology and behaviour will all line up, on time, in the kitchen. (Remember Pavlov's dogs with the 'conditioned reflex'? They salivated to order at the sound of a bell.)

Once the new routine is established, the switch to natural food can get under way.

There are several 'tricks' either singly or in combination that should help.

Hungry cats are always more willing to sniff, lick and ultimately eat new foods. So, reduce the amount of commercial canned or dry food offered. (Do not fast or starve your cat for more than 24 hours.)

Settle on one meat, for instance chicken, that you wish your cat to become accustomed to.

Taste and texture of raw meat are the two things you need your cat to accept. (Gnawing on bones comes later.) So, chop a few strips of chicken meat and cover with commercial food in a bowl.

Over successive days feed less commercial food and more raw meat.

When raw meat is accepted, try increasing the size of the pieces until chicken necks and wings replace the chopped chicken.

Other tricks involve slightly searing the meat in a pan or under the grill. You can try mixing canned fish juices with the meat or dusting it with powdered kibble.

Slitting the skin and making deep cuts into the meat of chicken wings or drumsticks and stuffing canned food inside may tempt your finicky feline. You can try tying a chicken wing on a string and playing a game of pounce and catch.

If you own several cats they can compete with and learn from each other.

Perseverance pays and ten days is usually sufficient time to switch the diet of a difficult cat. It's best to let

your cat become an accomplished chicken eater before introducing quail, rabbit, fish, day-old chicks or similar food items to the diet.

A further round of patience and trickery may then be needed.

Obesity

Pets fed on raw meaty bones tend not to overeat and are thus less likely to become obese. Increased body mass and large deposits of fatty tissue are almost always the result of feeding carbohydrate-laden junk foods. Complex carbohydrates from grains and potatoes are converted to glucose in the liver. And since dogs, cats and ferrets have no need for an external source of glucose, they need to deal with the surfeit. Excess glucose is converted into fat and deposited in tissues around the body.

Humans can develop sugar and carbohydrate cravings[2] and coupled with lack of exercise this contributes to obesity. From my observations the reason dogs and cats scoff more and more junk food is not a function of what's in it, but more a function of what is *not* in it. Animals are exquisitely sensitive to their dietary needs; for example, African wildlife congregate at the salt licks.[3]

In a 2020 paper, 'The unmapped chemical complexity of our diet', researchers estimate that there are more than 26,000 biochemicals in human foods that when consumed in adequate amounts and combinations contribute to good health.[4] At the biochemical level, we know that junk pet foods don't even slightly resemble the biochemical constituents of a natural diet. Denied essential biochemicals, perhaps thousands of biochemicals, I believe pets eat more and more junk hoping that somewhere at the bottom of the bowl they'll find what they need and crave.

A striking illustration comes to mind. A fat cocker spaniel presented at the clinic with a cooked chicken bone stuck in its mouth. The owner complained that the dog was a compulsive scavenger constantly raiding the kitchen bin. After removing the offending bone, I returned the patient to the owner with the advice to eliminate junk food and to institute a weight reduction diet—feed raw meaty bones on alternate days. That's to say one meal every 48 hours.

At the follow-up consultation I feared the owner might report that her fasting dog had become ravenous and even more driven to raid the kitchen bin. However, on the contrary, I was delighted to learn that as well as losing weight, the dog had transformed into a contented creature completely uninterested in the kitchen bin.

Of course, it's cruel and unfair to feed carnivorous pets on harmful junk in the full knowledge that they will become fat and subject to a litany of diseases. But reminiscent of the way the junk pet food industry and vet accomplices wrapped their tentacles around the periodontal disease problem, they are doing the same with pet obesity. The Mars Corporation, the world's biggest junk pet food maker, has enlisted Liverpool University veterinary school in its monumental trickery.

> **The Royal Canin Weight Management Clinic**
> Established in 2005, the clinic is the first specialist weight loss clinic for pets anywhere in the world. We are the world-leading experts in the field and, therefore, can provide a more comprehensive service than would normally be available through your usual veterinary practice. We aim to provide an outstanding service to clients and referring veterinary practices alike. The service includes:

- **A thorough consultation and clinical evaluation.** The initial consultation usually lasts 60 to 90 minutes, and covers all aspects of your pet's lifestyle and previous medical history.
- **Blood tests and urine analysis.** These tests check the health status of your pet, and assess whether there may be related problems (e.g. hypothyroidism: an under-active thyroid gland).
- **Blood pressure measurement.** All pets have their blood pressure checked at the time of the consultation.
- **DEXA scan.** Not available at standard veterinary practices, a DEXA scanner accurately measures the amount of adipose (fatty) tissue present in the patient and therefore calculates exactly how overweight they are. This is more precise than the standard estimates of obesity.
- **Regular follow-up contact.** Because a veterinary nurse runs the clinic full-time, we are able to maintain regular contact to ensure that the weight loss programme is a success. This includes telephone contact and regular 'weigh-in' sessions, all of which are free-of-charge.
- **Reports to your normal veterinary practice.** We keep your usual veterinary surgeon and nurse informed: writing reports after the initial and final visits.
- **Subsidised service.** All the consultations and tests directly related to the weight problem are free-of charge. In addition, you also get the first bag specifically formulated weight-loss food free![5]

At the website they go on to say:

> **How does the Weight Management Clinic benefit?**
> By agreeing to register with the clinic and participate in the work that we do, information relating to your pet and their health will be used to examine current obesity trends. The data we collect will be analysed alongside information from many other pets with similar problems. This helps us to spot key aspects in terms of common causes, problems and reasons for positive and negative outcomes. We can also assess the success of current management strategies to determine what works best and improve on methods which are less successful. This information is vital in establishing a 'best practice' in weight management.

Yes, the Weight Management Clinic 'data we collect' is vital to the calculations of Mars and their accomplices—billions of dollars are at stake.

The same venal self-interest informs the actions of Colgate-Palmolive, makers of Hill's junk food. In 2021, *Pet Gazette* reported:

> **Hill's Pet Nutrition launches new campaign to tackle pet obesity**
> The campaign will feature two short films highlighting the change in pets' quality of life as their weight increases, and how a healthy meal plan can support animals 'to live their very best life'.
>
> Hill's Pet Nutrition have launched a new national campaign to tackle the rise in obesity, placing a 'greater emphasis on helping pet parents take control of their animal's nutrition and address the poor feeding habits

amongst many owners, heightened by the pandemic'.

The company's new weight management campaign, 'Feed the Love, Lose the Weight' has been developed to 'raise awareness on the negative effects of too many treats, whilst educating pet owners on the full spectrum of aspects that make up their pet's health and nutrition'.

According to Hill's, obesity has been identified by vet professionals as one of the top five welfare issues amongst UK pets.[6]

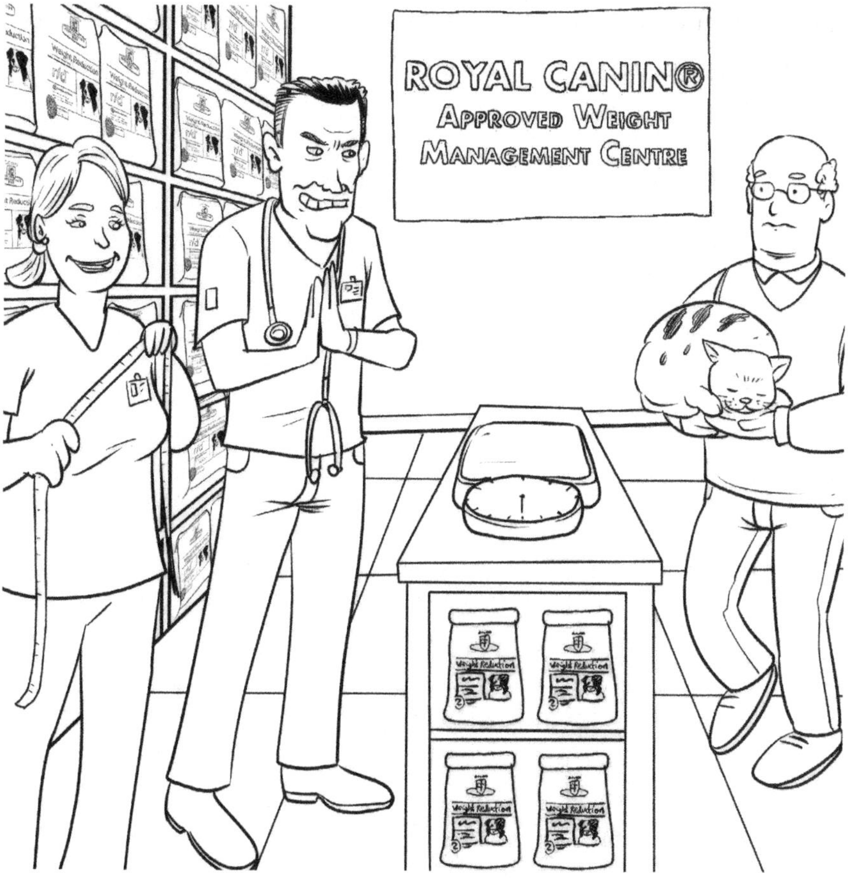

Vets, never known to pass up an opportunity to profiteer, sell 'weight reduction diets' and run 'weight reduction clinics'. Never, or almost never, do they mention that simply stopping the carbohydrate junk (that they themselves sell) would be the best first plan of attack. Never have I encountered a vet who recommends alternate-day feeding a diet of raw meaty bones. That's the way weight simply melts off rotund pets and that's the way pets gain a new vitality.

In our clinic we provided a weight reduction chart (see opposite page) to all owners of portly canines. Please make full use; share with friends and neighbours, it's wonderfully effective.

The same approach works for cats and ferrets. However, for cats and ferrets, it's important to change the diet to raw meaty bones *before* embarking on weight reduction. Fasting cats, especially overweight cats, for more than 24 hours can lead to liver problems—best avoided.

Weight watchers plan for ____________________

Many dogs are chubby and overweight tending towards obesity.

It need not be so and we're here to help.

Lack of exercise is a factor and genes play a part. But for the most part it's too much food or the wrong food (or both) that are the main determinants of pet obesity. Dogs, domesticated wolves, are designed to gorge and then fast – on a raw natural diet.

First, remove all junk food from the diet and introduce a healthy diet of whole carcasses or raw meaty bones.

Next, restrict the calorie intake. Feed one sizeable meal on alternate days only. Avoid titbits. Don't weaken. Your dog will soon settle into the new routine.

1. Starting weight: ____________________ Date: ____________________
2. Suggested target weight: ____________________
3. Weigh weekly
4. Keep a record

    Date

    Date

    Date

    Date

    Date

Visit vet Date: ____________________

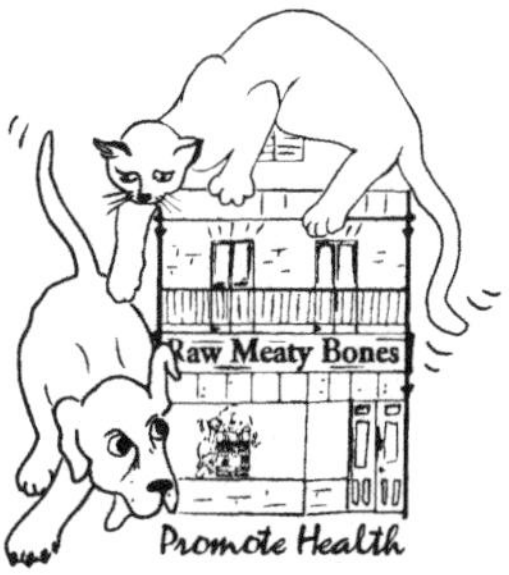
Raw Meaty Bones
Promote Health

Stop press

News just in. Money talks. The junk pet food industry, always ready to stage publicity stunts, seize the initiative and drive the agenda, spoke with British Members of Parliament.

> The Pet Food Manufacturers' Association (PFMA) recently held an event at the House of Commons to raise awareness of pet obesity ...
>
> Michael Bellingham, PFMA Chief Executive, advised: 'We held this important event to raise awareness of pet obesity, which is a life-limiting condition. Research has highlighted that dogs kept in lean body condition can live up to two years longer—surely that is the most persuasive fact of all time.'[7]

Michael Bellingham shared selective truths. Did he mention that, as with humans, a steady diet of carbohydrate-rich addictive junk food leads to morbid obesity? Probably not. Let's hope members of the UK parliament were paying attention.

PART III

CONFRONTING REALITY

6

VETERINARY SCHOOLS

If only half of what you say is true, then this is a very big issue.

Professor Stuart Reid 2014

If you have the sad misfortune to visit Sydney University Veterinary Teaching Hospital you will enter from Parramatta Road. The name in giant letters stretches across the upper façade. Picture windows give you a first look at the shelves laden with junk pet food in the junk pet food showroom—for that is what it is.

By the time you've waited in the showroom for your turn to see the vet, before you enter through one of the five consulting room doors with the Hill's logo, you will have been fully immersed in junk pet food propaganda. There will be no avoiding the Hill's (Colgate-Palmolive) and Royal Canin (Mars Inc.) slogans. And that's exactly how the monster companies like it. It's all part of the Faustian pact where the university accepts company oil and grease in return for 24-hour advertising and lifelong indoctrination of the students under their care.

You have skimmed this book and know better. But for thousands of vulnerable, trusting, Sydney pet owners their fate is sealed. They are lured into the trap. White-coated specialist vets minister to the fresh-faced students. They all seem so self-assured. Brand name junk

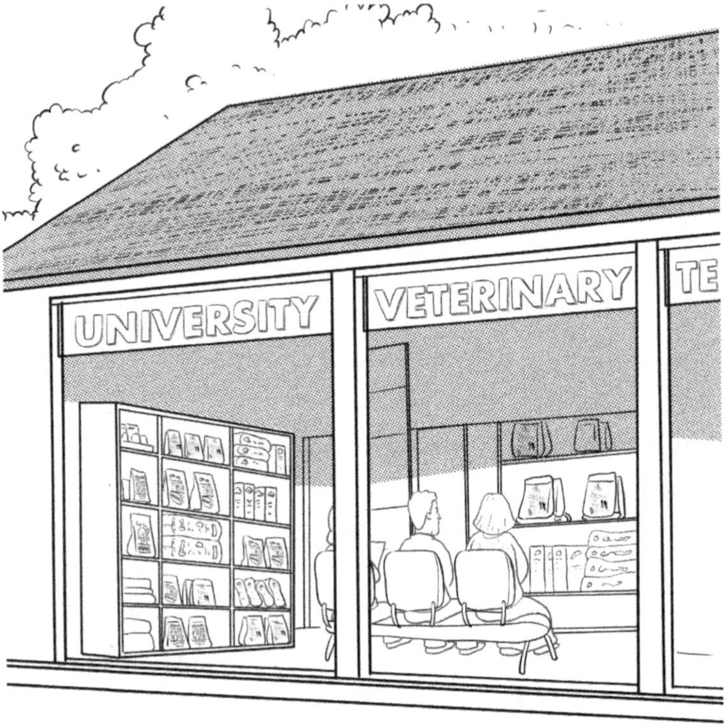

University Veterinary Teaching Hospital Sydney

products are spoken of approvingly. At reception, when paying the bill, there's an opportunity to buy those same shiny packaged products. Indeed, there's an opportunity to return time and time again to collect weekly supplies of the junk products *recommended* and *sold* by University Veterinary Teaching Hospital Sydney.

Cloaked in an aura of integrity and invincibility, the veterinary school is founded on fallacy, living a lie. Anyone drawn into its orbit becomes contaminated and damaged. We pity the poor pets at the bottom of the pile and then next the pet owners, who are all grist to the junk pet food mill.

Vet students are the chosen ones, or so they think. Overflowing with confidence, they have topped their class at high school and are now on the road to superiority, status and widespread acclaim. Selected for attitude and credentials, they are ripe for indoctrination within the university brainwashing machine. Unquestioning, rote learning is their *modus operandi*. Necessarily so, because memorising the mountains of facts—and junk pet food factoids—leaves no time for contemplation and intelligent debate.

The academic vets are both victims and victimisers in the disgusting mix. Of course, they have ascended the greasy pole of academic 'excellence'—no mean feat in itself. But to retain their power, prestige and profit they are compelled to toe the party line. To maintain a low profile and in all public utterances, subscribe to groupthink and group-speak. They enthuse about 'latest research' and 'evidence-based medicine' while ignoring the fact that only 'research' approved by the junk food sponsors is performed. Consequently, they ignore that the 'evidence-based medicine' mantra is but a

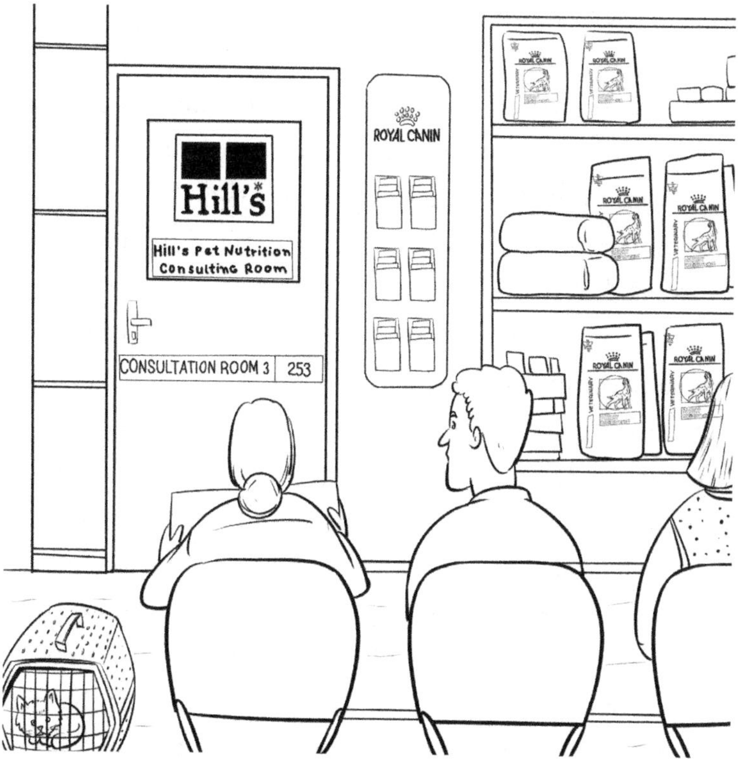

One of the five consulting room doors with the Hill's logo

smokescreen whereby the only 'evidence' available serves to protect and promote the products and influence of the pet food companies.

As victimisers of their captive audience, vet school academics deserve our scorn. They inflict untold harm on the students who then become vets and thence inflict lifelong harm on pets and their owners. Unfortunately for almost all concerned, the price of academic freedom is too great. Academic vets who dare to think differently do not last long. They dare not bite the hand that feeds them. The university controls the staff, and the junk pet food companies control the university.

'Surely not' do I hear you say? Yes, they do, just like parasites disarm their host's defences and commandeer the control systems.

For example, let me tell you about *Toxoplasma gondii*, a parasite that lives in the brains of rats and for part of its lifecycle lives in the intestines of cats.[1] As we know, cats are, generally speaking, a rat's worst enemy. However, rats infected with *Toxoplasma* develop a perverse predilection for cat urine. Unwary cat-urine-sniffing rats become easier prey for predator cats. And this is the moral of the story: by rewiring rats' brains and making them suicidal, the parasite secures its future in the intestines of cats.

University vet schools that sacrifice their students in the service of junk pet food companies can be likened to parasite-controlled rats.

Over decades, and in some cases over centuries, universities grow and develop. Bricks and mortar, administrative staff, academic staff, reputations and community standing are all built over time. In the case of veterinary schools, the very high cost of teaching students the basics of anatomy, physiology, pathology and biochemistry is largely met by taxpayers. That's all fine and the way it should be.

Where things go awry is with the clinical parts of the curriculum. Due to the ubiquitous nature of junk food, the vet schools slip into the easy assumption that all pet dogs, cats and ferrets are fed on junk. No matter that the mouth rot, the diarrhoea, vomiting and diabetes are all a direct result of the junk diets, the medical teaching skates over the 'root cause'. Worse than that, vet teachers appear ever mindful of the groupthink, ever mindful that junk food companies pay for academic chairs, research in their or their colleagues' department and junk products appear at the point of sale in the university clinic.

So the parasites, the pet food makers, by the application of very little financial oil and grease (profits extracted from unwitting pet owners) infiltrate and control university decision-making systems. Consequently, the companies turn universities into brainwashing machines, not just in Sydney but, on the available evidence, in every vet school on the planet. The output of those vet brainwashing machines are the legions of vets whose brains have been rewired in the service of Mars, Nestlé and Colgate-Palmolive.

Other factors contributed to the slow strangulation of the vet profession. Compare a frog sitting in a saucepan of cold water that only slowly, when it's too late, discovers the saucepan is on a hot stove. Vets, for the most part, previously ministered to the needs of sick horses and then farm animals. Pets were largely an afterthought that received little veterinary attention. However, a confluence of three things slowly occurred in the first half of the last century that wrought huge changes.

- The bottom fell out of the horse vet business, and factory farms put paid to the James Herriot style of vet practice.
- After World War II, large multinational corporations developed their manufacturing prowess. Purina developed the industrial extrusion of kibble in 1956.
- The fashion for keeping pets as status symbols in middle-class homes became a solid feature of modern life, driven by relentless junk pet food advertisements on the new medium of television.

For the vets, as the large animal door closed, the small animal door opened. Bear in mind this transition took place back in the 1950s and 60s. When I was at the University of London vet school from 1967 to 1972, our main subjects of study were horses and farm animals. When we turned our attention to the burgeoning trade ministering to the needs of sick pets, those pets were already fed on the commercial canned and dry junk offerings.

Almost overnight there were pets galore, all of them sick and getting sicker as a result of their junk food diets. Whether too busy or too preoccupied, vets concentrated on treatment without giving much if any thought to the origins of the widespread ill health. There was money to be made! And, what's more, you didn't need to get covered in cow shit!

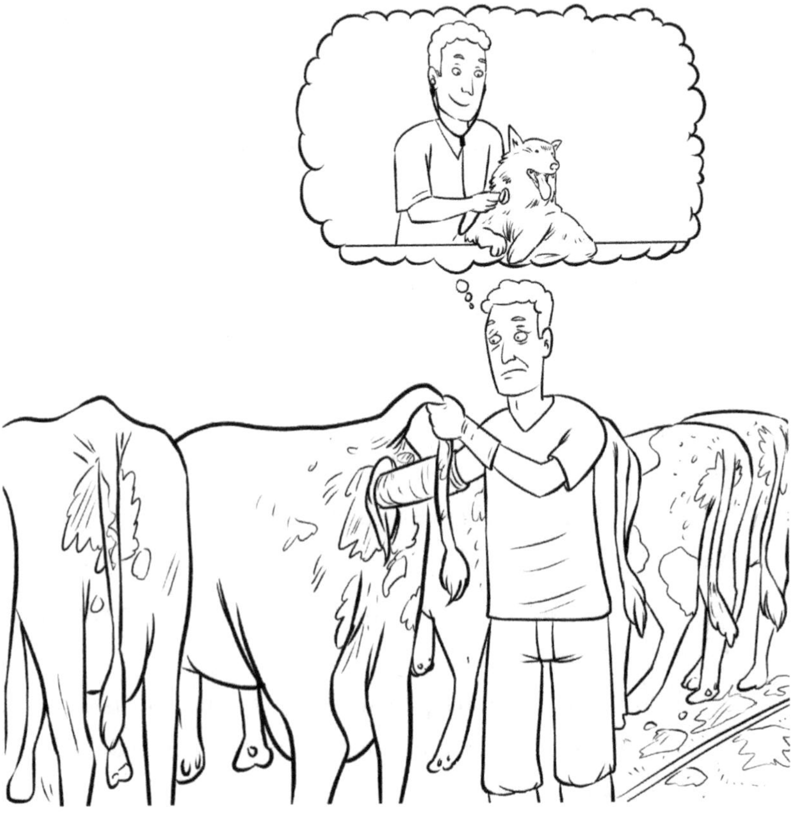

From an immediately practical and unthinking perspective, feeding pets became simply a matter of opening a can or bag of kibble. Vets, like everyone else, became accustomed to the ease and convenience of supermarket shopping—also an early 20th century innovation—and filled their trolleys with the packaged offerings. There was cultural transformation and, since cultural conditioning is so powerful, vets fell into line and became immensely well practised at doing the *wrong* thing.

Whether it be arranged marriages, female circumcision or the mass junk food poisoning of pets in the modern world, resisting cultural conditioning is nigh on impossible for most people.[2] Only the brave, bold or foolhardy go against the grain. Vets, being conservative, conformist types, tend not to want to blaze a new path. With endless repetition, no thought required, they become expert at opening cans and packets. Even the thought of reaching into a freezer, seizing a chicken frame or whole fish and handing it to a dog or cat leaves them perplexed and alarmed.

They have *no theory* about how to feed pets a natural diet. Consequently, they have *no practical know-how*. And thus, they have *zero experience* of how to feed pets for health and wellbeing. For most vets, the idea of feeding pets appropriately on whole animal carcasses or raw meaty bones is a foreign land replete with scary monsters, pitfalls and dangers galore. Better, they think, to stay safe and follow their vet school teaching.

It's a depressing tale—that gets worse. The issues are ginormous.

Lessons of history

> **Those who fail to learn from history are condemned to repeat it.**

As a backdrop to the veterinary myopia all the way through to rank corruption, we should take a look at the lessons of history. In 1847 Hungarian physician Ignaz Semmelweis was the first man to recommend the washing of hands as a means to reducing the incidence of 'childbed fever', a serious often fatal condition of women following childbirth. For doctors who attended the maternity ward and also performed post-mortems in the morgue, the fatality rate of their patients was three times that of midwives who did not visit the morgue.[3]

The medical profession at that time refused to accept the connection between dirty hands and medical disasters. That Semmelweis's empirical observations were rejected can be regarded as a form of 'belief perseverance', the psychological tendency to cling to beliefs even after they are disproved. This is particularly likely to happen when accepting a new theory means admitting one's own guilt in contributing to illness or deaths.

Semmelweis, unbowed, accused his colleagues of irresponsible murder. For their part they said Semmelweis had suffered a nervous breakdown and committed him to an asylum. He was beaten by the guards and died of a gangrenous wound believed to be the result of the beating.[4]

French chemist and microbiologist Louis Pasteur's work laid the foundations for our understanding of how microbes are often responsible for disease.[5] Back in the 1800s this amounted to a huge leap in understanding, forming the foundation of the germ theory of disease and how to 'pasteurise' milk to prevent spoilage.

Building on Pasteur's work, the British surgeon Joseph Lister

(1827–1912) revolutionised surgical outcomes by introducing antiseptic techniques for disinfecting wounds and surgical instruments.[6] Still earlier, Edward Jenner (1749–1823) pioneered the use of vaccines[7] and is said to have 'saved more lives than the work of any other human'.

In more recent times Alexander Fleming (1881–1955), quite by chance, discovered penicillin, the first antibiotic that could be injected into patients.[8] The discovery was termed the 'single greatest victory ever achieved over disease'.

Nowadays sterile surgery, vaccinations and antibiotics are all standard elements within the veterinary curriculum. The moral of the tale: simple ideas that overturn previous beliefs or simple chance discoveries can have immense impact, establishing whole new fields of treatment, discovery and research.

Food as medicine

Scattered through the scientific literature are numerous discoveries of the nutritional and medicinal benefits of food for humans. 'Let food be thy medicine, and let medicine be thy food' is often attributed to Hippocrates, the founder of modern medicine over 2000 years ago. The ingredients of food—proteins, fats, carbohydrates, vitamins, minerals and trace elements—are these days well researched and understood. And the specific medicinal benefits of food *ingredients* are increasingly well researched. British sailors were famously protected from scurvy by including limes and apples in their diet—both a source of vitamin C. And fish oil contains essential fatty acids beneficial in many body functions.

Recognition of both the nutritional and medicinal benefits of a carnivore's food is a relatively recent finding—actively suppressed by the vet establishment—and thus there is very little recorded information in the veterinary scientific literature. Actually, we need little more than the definition of dogs as modified wolves, cats as modified desert predators from North Africa, and ferrets as modified polecats from the forests of Europe. With a suitable admixture of common sense, vets should grasp the centrality of diet in the health and wellbeing of domestic pets.

Unfortunately, because there is little or no information, and because common sense is not so common, the world's vet schools deem it reasonable, even mandatory, that they do not teach the subject. When confronted, vet schools feign ignorance or lie. However, there are four university vet schools—Sydney Australia, London UK, Pennsylvania USA and Massey New Zealand—that cannot feign ignorance of the history of medicine, whether ancient or modern, as a flimsy defence.

Sydney Centre for Veterinary Education

The Centre for Veterinary Education (CVE) at the University of Sydney is a department of the Veterinary Faculty established way back in 1965. Dr Tom Hungerford OBE, grandfather of the Australian veterinary profession, was the founding director.[9] In 2001, when Tom was 90 years old, I sent him a copy of *Raw Meaty Bones*. Imagine my pride when a handwritten message arrived with the words:

> Tell the people who won't review their views that: 'The foolish and the dead never change their opinions.' Maybe that is an overstatement—as the 'brain-dead' may also refuse to revise. Anyhow there are many who adopt the stance of: 'Don't confuse me with facts, my mind is made up.'

Dr Douglas Bryden AM succeeded Tom Hungerford as director of the CVE.[9] His response when receiving the book included:

> Every graduate and undergraduate veterinarian should read the book for it has the potential to challenge the things they believe to be true and gives them the wonderful opportunity to step back from themselves and to look more dispassionately and more deeply at the science they practise and to realise how important it is to listen carefully to others who may have a pearl of wisdom to share.

Dr Michele Cotton,[9] director of the CVE during the years 2003 to 2007, wrote a review telling veterinarians:

> Tom Lonsdale has now published his book 'Raw Meaty Bones' and consequently kept the fires of his passion for this subject burning as brightly as ever. This Don Quixote of Dog Food has kept his quest alive and now stands to enjoy the credit for having had the courage of his convictions.

Dr Richard Malik, consultant at the CVE, bestowed an enormous honour on me. In 2004, he nominated me for the College Prize of the Australian College of Veterinary Scientists (ACVS).[10] In part he wrote:

> A further benefit of Tom's work has been the focus he has directed on the infrastructure and marketing that goes part and parcel with the pet-food industry. Lonsdale provides well documented information that confirms that some of these multinational organisations work through

> 'front' organisations to collect data, lobby, or otherwise influence public opinion as a marketing ploy. Importantly, these organisations sometimes employ veterinarians as consultants. Ironically, useful information concerning the data collected by these organisations is frequently not made available for the public domain, where it might fruitfully contribute to clinical epidemiology. By drawing our attention to the existence of these practices, Lonsdale has made us more aware that for these companies, 'business is war,' and this too is a valuable lesson for the profession.
>
> As the primary custodians of the human animal bond, it is our duty to make objective decisions about the nutrition and health of the patients under our care. Dr Lonsdale has focussed our attention on how as veterinary students, subliminal messages concerning 'normal' feeding practices, the value of prescription diets and the danger of feeding fresh meat or meat by-products can be influenced by companies providing free food for university teaching hospitals and positions for faculty staff. Although there may be nothing wrong with this in itself, the information, clinical data, and hypotheses promulgated by Lonsdale provides very useful counterpoint to information provided by companies that cannot help having bias towards an ethos of commercial feeding.

Douglas Bryden, as former president of the ACVS and former director of the CVE, was well placed to second the nomination:[10]

> Through his work as a veterinary practitioner Dr Lonsdale has identified a problem, researched the aetiology and

> the pathogenesis, introduced therapeutic and preventive procedures, and addressed, head on, what he saw to be a moral issue for the profession. In short, he has changed a paradigm and guided his profession in a more thoughtful and proper course of action.

Clearly high-ranking University of Sydney veterinary academics and administrators were prepared to make a stand. But high-level acknowledgement was not enough. The ACVS declined to bestow the Prize. And under the new CVE director, the junk food companies returned to prominence. A procession of junk pet food advocates led the CVE courses, often accompanied by company advertising.

Failed representations

I take the view that the University of Sydney CVE, despite being told the truth about junk pet food, nevertheless continues to ignore the evidence in a way that results in its students being insufficiently exposed to alternative views—in short, brainwashed.

In 2007 the CVE newsletter carried a letter from two pet owners who described their experiences at the hands of the vet profession. It offered a chance to open discussion, or so I thought. I wrote a letter for publication by the CVE.[11]

> Two owners recount the sorry tale of how a discharge from their cat Sefi's ear led them through an obstacle course of first opinions, expert opinions, bacteriological tests, radiographic tests, test therapies and radical surgery.
>
> After spending several months, and doubtless hundreds of dollars, the owners say:

> **We were highly concerned and frustrated at the lack of progress we had made, and the costs outlaid which had provided no answers as to why she had the condition or what was causing it. As a last resort, our vet told us about Dr Richard Malik at the CVE.**

Dr Malik recommended that the owners discontinue feeding the prescription dry cat 'food' and provide a more natural diet which straightaway had the desired effect: 'After changing her diet, it didn't take long for us to see a rapid improvement in the condition of her ear and the happiness of our cat.'

In conclusion the owners state:

> **We have learnt that while our vet went through appropriate routine testing to find the cause of Sefi's ear problems, there isn't always an obvious diagnosis and factors such as diet and environment should be investigated in the first instance.**

After reviewing the plentiful evidence that University of Sydney vets and vets more generally should re-evaluate the role of junk pet food I concluded:

> It seems to me that we know, or at least should know, the biological, ethical and legal imperatives regarding the veterinary treatment of carnivores in our care. Sadly though, in respect to Sefi the cat and thousands like her, these things are more honoured in the breach than the observance. What's to be done and by whom? May I suggest that perhaps the Board of the CVE may have a role to play?

> As a way forward, and in the first instance, I suggest that the Board could review:
>
> a) The content of CVE courses and publications, as they relate to both wild and domestic carnivores, in light of biological imperatives.
>
> b) The objectivity, affiliations and possible conflict of interest of CVE course teachers.
>
> c) The diverse legal implications of the pet diet and disease issue as may apply to veterinary clinicians, researchers and educators.
>
> Publication of the review findings would honour the good work started by Sefi's owners and would help the veterinary profession to learn from history, keep faith with Sefi the cat and better secure our future.

The CVE director at first hesitated, then consulted former director Douglas Bryden, who recommended that the CVE should 'bite the bullet', as that would serve to 'put the CVE on the map'. Unfortunately, Dr Bryden's advice went unheeded; Australian vets were denied access to the information—until now 15 years later.

What now? Will Dr Bryden's prophecy come true? Will the University of Sydney CVE gain a place on the map?

University of Sydney Senate and vice-chancellor

Surely someone somewhere at the University of Sydney can be relied upon. Sorry, the answer appears to be 'No', and the higher you go the worse it gets.

Sitting atop the university is the Senate, which 'oversees all major decisions concerning the conduct of the University'. Sitting atop the

Senate are the chancellor (a largely ceremonial role) and the vice-chancellor (equivalent to a US university president) with about 20 fellows forming the decision-making committee. The fellows are supposed to be right-minded people drawn from the ranks of academia, commerce and media. In 2010 the chancellor was Her Excellency Professor Marie Bashir AC CVO. I wrote to her at the Senate office.

> Since the early 1990s senior staff in the Veterinary Faculty and the Centre for Veterinary Education (formerly the Post Graduate Foundation) have known about and understood the ramifications of the junk pet-food scandal. In my opinion the Veterinary Faculty and the Centre for Veterinary Education, by their policies and actions, [have] become ever more deeply mired in the scandal.
>
> The costs to pets, pet owners and the community run into the $billions. I hope that you can help investigate and resolve the issues and thus help pave the way towards a scientific, medical and nutritional renaissance.[12]

Included with the letter were several supporting articles and a copy of *Raw Meaty Bones*. I duplicated the package 24 times, enough for the chancellor, vice-chancellor, each named fellow and one spare for the Senate office.

The Senate office and the vice-chancellor's office are housed in the same rooms. My wife and I delivered a cardboard box containing individually addressed packages to be handed to the chancellor and Senate fellows at the next available meeting. 'We don't have funding for that,' said the lady in the office. As to whether the documents and books ever reached their intended recipients, we may never know.

For a time, I believed that someone in the administration had simply intercepted the packages—stolen, if you like—and chucked them in the dumpster. Nowadays I'm more inclined to the view that someone connected with the Senate was in on the ploy. It seems that they pretended not to know and thus felt no obligation to respond. Instead, the vice-chancellor asked Professor Rosanne Taylor, the dean of the Veterinary Faculty and the subject of my complaint, to reply. Her statement included the following:

> Students do not receive biased instruction from pet food companies as we tightly control the content and delivery of our curriculum, however we do have partnerships with a variety of industry supporters including pet food suppliers, in common with almost all internationally accredited veterinary schools.[13]

On that last point Professor Taylor is undoubtedly correct—every last one of them turning tricks, in bed with the junk food makers.

Australian Freedom of Information inquiries

Over the years I have lodged numerous Freedom of Information (FOI) inquiries in Australia and the UK. Mostly it is a game with the odds stacked against anyone in search of information from government departments and instrumentalities. The various national and state-based FOI acts speak piously about a 'presumption in favour' of disclosing government information. After all, the government are presumed to be acting for and on behalf of us, the governed. We pay the bills and should get to see what we pay for.

In practice FOI Officers generally disclose limited information. Simultaneously, they provide elaborate reasons why they obscure information about the dirty deals struck by governments against the interests of the people. I've tabulated at www.rawmeatybones.com

some of the FOI information gathered on the seven Australian vet schools.[14] At www.ukrmb.co.uk you can see the UK vet school data.[15] All vet schools tried to obscure their dealings.

Paradoxically, I feel a tiny tinge of sympathy for the FOI office at Murdoch University in Perth, Western Australia. They fulfilled most of their obligations and released hundreds of pages of documents and several glossy brochures revealing the university's involvement with Hill's (division of Colgate-Palmolive). Here's an example.

Multi-Project Funding Program Hill's Pet Nutrition Australia
Proposal for 2013–2015 Partnership
Introduction

While Murdoch University and Hill's Pet Nutrition have been collaborating for many years, in 2009 we partnered to provide a multi project funding agreement to benefit nutritional education and student experience at Murdoch. ...

Hill's will be automatically named the major sponsor at the Veterinary Professional Life Conference

- Hill's Pet Nutrition will be acknowledged verbally at each event
- Hill's Pet Nutrition's logo will be displayed on promotional materials distributed at the events
- Hill's Pet Nutrition's logo will be displayed on course materials distributed at the events
- A representative from Hill's Pet Nutrition will be invited to attend and participate in Hill's sponsored Veterinary Professional Life events
- Hill's Pet Nutrition will be provided an opportunity to

provide a 'promotional' Hill's branded product to students at supported Veterinary Professional Life events, for example Hill's t-shirts at 1stYear Orientation Day

- Pet Nutrition Education for Students Nutritional lectures for students by a Hill's representative can continue to be part of an ongoing partnership.[16]

The shiny document spruiking the proposed *quid pro quo* with Mars company Royal Canin states:

> **Proposal for Partnership Opportunities for Royal Canin From Murdoch University College of Veterinary Medicine**
> **Three Year Sponsorship Agreement**
>
> This proposal recommends that Murdoch and Royal Canin focus on functions that would be consistently linked with Royal Canin sponsorship, providing mutually agreed benefits throughout the duration of the contract. The areas as detailed in the proposal are:
>
> - Pet Nutrition Education for Students
> - Clinical Skills Centre
> - KeePad Interactive Learning
> - Associate Lecturer Professor in Clinical Instruction[17]

However, it was the signed 2013 Agreement with Hill's that created the most consternation.[18] Seemingly the Murdoch FOI office should not have released the document due to it being 'commercial in confidence'. They tried to snatch the document back, I'm guessing because they didn't want Royal Canin to know the Murdoch price for prostituting its students to Hill's. But too late, I posted the entire document at www.rawmeatybones.com under the heading:

> **Murdoch University sells itself cheap and pimps its students to Colgate-Palmolive. Price: $123.28 per day and truckloads of Hill's dangerous junk food.**

Royal Veterinary College, University of London

The banner headline proclaims:

> **Royal Veterinary College voted world's leading vet school**
>
> The RVC has been ranked as the world's number one veterinary school in the prestigious QS World University Rankings 2019.
>
> This is the first time the RVC has occupied the top spot in this particular league table, after being ranked one of the world's top three veterinary schools within it for the past four years. It was listed as number one out of 401 institutions offering veterinary sciences. ...
>
> Established in 1791 and based in London and Hertfordshire, the RVC is the oldest veterinary school in the English-speaking world. The RVC is also the only veterinary school in the world to be fully accredited by the Royal College of Veterinary Surgeons (RCVS), American Veterinary Medical Association (AVMA), European Association of Establishments for Veterinary Education (EAEVE), and Australian Veterinary Boards Council (AVBC)—which allows graduates to practice as veterinary surgeons, researchers and scientists across the world.[19]

They say it's the best. I say it's one of the worst. My reasoning is simple. For over 25 years the RVC has known about the devastating effects of junk pet food and refused to do anything about it. On the contrary, they employ junk pet food proxies and perform 'research' with and for the companies.

Since graduating from the RVC in 1972 I have kept distant contact. I am proud to say that tutors Oliver Graham-Jones and Arthur Hayward, towards the end of their lives and for several years, both endorsed the raw meaty bones campaign. Commencing in 1997, they nominated me in Royal College of Veterinary Surgeons (RCVS) elections. The RCVS is the governing body for all vets registered to practise in the UK. In 1998 my manifesto asked all members of the RCVS:

> Does it concern you that modern small animal veterinary science is founded on information derived from artificially fed animals?
>
> Is it of concern that the majority of artificially fed animals suffer from periodontal and other diet induced diseases including an 'AIDS like' condition? (See web site.)
>
> Does the absence of naturally fed controls, in veterinary practice and clinical research, suggest a drift towards pseudo-science?
>
> The human medical and dental professions extol the benefits of a healthy natural diet, but the veterinary profession is influenced at every level by the junk pet-food industry. Does this matter?
>
> Do you want the Council of the RCVS to rise above the parochial and give priority to the biggest issues and hardest tasks?[20]

In 2001 Oliver Graham-Jones kindly provided the foreword to *Raw Meaty Bones*, in which he stated:

> Tom Lonsdale has written this book with his hand on his academic heart. He is refreshingly straight forward in his condemnation of convenience foods for pet dogs and cats.

In 2005 I coordinated the UK Raw Meaty Bones Group FOI inquiries of all UK vet schools. In respect to the RVC, we were interested to know about the employment of Lynne Hill, the then president of the Royal College of Veterinary Surgeons and previously European sales manager for Hill's junk pet food. In part our inquiry asked for details of:

- All professional and character references in respect to Mrs Hill's application for employment at the Royal Veterinary College.
- Current terms of employment including job title and description.
- Subject matter taught and examination questions set from the past two academic years.
- All correspondence between Mrs Hill and any processed pet-food company or companies from 1998 to the present.
- Details of any grants or sponsorships administered by Mrs Hill.[21]

In reply the RVC wrote:

> We are unable to disclose any information relating to point 1 and 2 as this is classed as personal information and

> would breach the data protection principle of processing information fairly and lawfully.
>
> With regard to point 4 we believe this is a vexatious request as it does not appear to have any serious purpose or value and will therefore not disclose any information.
>
> We also believe that point 5 is exempt from the Freedom of Information Act as disclosure of the information would prejudice the effective conduct of public affairs.[21]

We fired back addressing Professor Quintin McKellar, principal of the RVC:

> You will be aware of the public disquiet at the veterinary profession's involvement with the processed pet-food industry and that Mrs L V Hill, prior to taking up a senior position at the RVC, was a senior executive for a pet-food company. Mrs Hill is currently President of the Royal College of Veterinary Surgeons, the body responsible, under the terms of the Veterinary Surgeons Act 1966, for regulating the veterinary profession in the United Kingdom.
>
> We believe that, in the public interest, it is incumbent upon the RVC to respond to our enquiries with full, honest and transparent disclosure.[21]

Nine years later, in 2014, I travelled to the UK to visit family. I also made appointments to meet with senior veterinary administrators. Top of the tree was Professor Stuart Reid BVMS PhD DVM DipECVPH FRSE MRCVS, dean of the Royal Veterinary College and simultaneously the then president of the Royal College of Veterinary Surgeons. Clearly, he is a man of immense ability, connections and power, and in person Professor Reid was most charming.

The big takeaway from our meeting was his comment: 'If only half of what you say is true, then this is a very big issue.'

I can't remember the full extent of our one-hour discussion. But no matter, Professor Reid, in his capacity as dean of the London vet school and president of the RCVS, was surely aware of my 2014 RCVS election manifesto.

> Veterinary incomes mainly derive from treating pets—pets addicted to junk pet-food.
>
> Denied their birthright of appropriate nutrients, teeth cleaning and mental stimulation—raw meaty bones diet fundamentals—the junk food addicts' suffering begins with the first glutinous slurp. Thereafter nasty ingredients, vile mouth rot and obesity predispose pets to a litany of end-stage diseases.
>
> Unfortunately, arrogant veterinary schools deny the obvious in their monster display of the Semmelweis reflex.
>
> Veterinary associations, snouts deep in the junk pet-food trough, host conferences in partnership with multinational pet-food makers.
>
> Veterinary journals provide advertising and support for the pet-food industry. Bogus 'research' papers never mentioning the main determinants of pet disease extol the alleged benefits of artificial pet food and specifically condemn natural diets.
>
> Brainwashed veterinary students graduate to become blinkered practitioners over-servicing a population of junk food poisoned pets but seldom if ever confronting the key determinants of pet disease and suffering.
>
> Alas the RCVS when 'Setting Veterinary Standards' fails to see, hear or speak about the junk pet-food fraud—

> hypocrisy writ large and sinister manifestation of the rotten callous venal scam.
>
> In previous years I've called for a full parliamentary inquiry. Now I believe that the RCVS Council should be dismissed, and an administrator appointed pending the outcome of that inquiry. I recommend that there be legal proceedings against prominent companies, veterinary institutions and individuals in respect to breach of contract, animal cruelty, theft and deception.[22]

Yes, I suggested that Professor Reid was president of a Rotten Callous Venal Scam (RCVS) that should be investigated and prosecuted. He smiled and we had an affable meeting. He knew the issues and has done nothing—except continue to oversee the same curriculum which, in my view, brainwashes hundreds of trainee vets at the Royal Veterinary College, University of London.

USA veterinary schools

We're used to American exceptionalism. Things are bigger, better, glitzier in the land of Uncle Sam. To a degree it's true of veterinary care and veterinary education. American diagnostic acumen and clinical excellence set the standards for the rest of us. However, that is only one side of the story. On the other side there is the disgraceful level of junk pet food infiltration of USA veterinary schools.

In 1997 the *Wall Street Journal* carried a headline:

> **Colgate Gives Doctors Treats for Plugging its Food Brands**
> Borrowing a page from pharmaceuticals companies, which routinely woo doctors to prescribe their drugs, Hill's has spent a generation cultivating its professional following.

> It spends hundreds of thousands of dollars a year funding university research and nutrition courses at every one of the 27 U.S. veterinary colleges. Once in practice, vets who sell Science Diet and other premium foods directly from their offices pocket profits of as much as 40%.[23]

Professor Emerita Sandra Scarr is now retired and breeds Labrador retrievers in Hawaii. In her working life she was an eminent child psychologist at leading USA universities. Her opinion counts. Regarding UK FOI discovery of the University of Edinburgh's dubious dealings[24] with Mars and Purina, Professor Scarr let rip:

> To say it is shocking is a vast understatement.
>
> How can anyone, let alone a veterinary practitioner, fail to be thoroughly disgusted by the sale of veterinary education to pet-food companies—for a pittance, I would add.
>
> ...
>
> Surely, surely, if veterinarians knew how they had been sold to pet-food companies, they would revolt. The veterinary colleges sell them, body and soul, through pet-food-paid & provided nutrition lecturers, through paid & provided resident-supervisors, through measly donations of free and half-price pet foods, through free subscriptions to pet food propaganda, through pet food companies' prior review of lectures, research, and publications. The whole stinking morass is beyond my comprehension.[24]

Subsequently, in 2009, Professor Scarr commenced FOI inquiries in the USA. She told me: 'The FOI laws are providing a goldmine of information about pet food companies' direct subversion of veterinary education. It's astonishing to see.'

Amid the murk and stench of junk pet food corruption, Professor Scarr happened across an unexpected patch of clean air. In a four-page memo Dr Dale Hancock cautioned his Washington State University College of Veterinary Medicine colleagues about involvement with Hill's.

> I have included a number of citations which constitute a basis for my opinion that a long-standing conflict of interest exists within the curriculum of our College.
>
> When the majority of our two core dog and cat nutrition courses are given over to a person employed by a pet food company, there is *prima facie* evidence of an ongoing conflict of interest. The conflict seems especially problematical when this perennial service is provided to the College *gratis*, rather than on a one-time, fee-for-service basis to fill a short-term personnel gap. Would we consider giving over our core vet pharmacology course, in such a lock-stock-and-barrel manner, to a drug company in the name of saving money or reducing the faculty workload? ... Somebody explain to me how that would be different from what we are doing with core nutrition in our curriculum.[25]

For a fuller account of Professor Scarr's findings of US vet school corruption see her blog posts in Appendix E.

School of Veterinary Medicine, University of Pennsylvania

What did they know and when did they know it?

For 33 years until his retirement in 2013, Colin Harvey held the title of Professor of Surgery and Dentistry in the School of

Veterinary Medicine, University of Pennsylvania. As one of only two full professors of veterinary periodontology in the world, Professor Harvey was a role model for vet dentists and vets the world over. More immediately, at the university he occupied a senior position with a department staffed by numerous vets and technicians.

Back in 1993 he led the five-day course in veterinary dentistry staged by the University of Sydney. (See Chapter 2 and Appendix D.) Over those few days he and I developed a rapport based on our shared fascination with periodontal disease and the systemic effects impacting virtually all other body organs and systems. Professor Harvey gave me valuable help and support with papers I was writing. I helped him with raw meaty bones theory and practice.

Since we had both 'seen the light' about the junk pet food devastation, I figured that we were honour bound to communicate the information to dependent vets, pet owners and pets everywhere. Colin took the view that, for him, working within the system was a better option. For me, that decision of his was more than I could bear. As much as I craved interaction with the only person I knew with a shared scientific passion, I nevertheless ceased contact—for 28 years.

In 2021, in the hope that with the passage of time Colin Harvey may have changed his stance, I sent an email. Over seven short days our email exchange tells the tale. You can read within and between the lines at Appendix G.

January 2022 review article

Quite by chance, in January 2022, I happened across Professor Harvey's latest review article 'The relationship between periodontal infection and systemic and distant organ disease in dogs' published in *Veterinary Clinics of North America: Small Animal Practice.*

About the journal they say:

> *Veterinary Clinics of North America: Small Animal Practice* offers you the most current information on the treatment of small animals such as cats and dogs, updates you on the latest advances, and provides a sound basis for choosing treatment options.

Key points listed at the head of the article state:

> - Periodontal infection is common in dogs.
> - Bacteremia is common in dogs with periodontal infection.
> - Distant organ pathology associated with periodontal infection is seen in the kidneys, heart, and liver.
> - Stress indicators (serum CRP, serum amyloid A, white blood cell count) increase as the severity of periodontal infection increases.
> - Preventing accumulation of dental plaque is an important contributor to good health.[26]

So far, so good. But then, over the course of what in my view are 14 dreary, misdirected, meandering pages, Colin Harvey acknowledges and then tiptoes around the junk pet food elephant in the room.

> One likely reason for the high prevalence [of periodontal disease] is that many pet dogs have little or no natural daily cleansing of the surfaces of their teeth; the home-cooked food or canned convenience foods that many owners feed their dogs may be excellent nutritionally but provide little effective chewing activity. The need to chew plays a critical role. Switching from a minced diet to one

> that contains the same ingredients but requires extensive masticatory activity, such as chewing whole bovine trachea and esophagus, causes measurable changes in gingival tissues within 24 hours.[26]

However, rather than recommend the prevention of life-threatening gum disease at source with 'the need to chew' requiring 'extensive masticatory activity', Professor Harvey switches emphasis. In conclusion he tells North American vets:

> Obtaining optimal oral health in our patients is a challenge, because they cannot brush or floss their own teeth. Although brushing remains the gold standard, fortunately effective oral hygiene methods can include more than brushing. The Veterinary Oral Health Council ([VOHC] www.VOHC.org) provides a list of products that have met the pre-set VOHC standards for retarding accumulation of plaque and calculus (tartar); in addition to brushes and dental wipes, these products include dental diets, treats, water additives, gels, and toothpastes. The key is daily use, which is much easier to accomplish if the owner can find a way to make daily oral hygiene a fun interaction with her or his dog. Making use of more than one modality improves the result.
>
> An oral care regime and twice-yearly veterinary dental health checks should be provided from an early age for breeds with high likelihood of developing periodontitis (see Fig. 1). While waiting for confirmation that the periodontal-systemic associations are indeed cause and effect, it would be prudent to practice prevention; this consists of the following 3 steps:

1. Periodic, at least annual, oral examination (including 'lifting the lip' every time a veterinarian see the patient for any reason) should be performed. Six-month intervals are recommended for dogs that early on are recognized as heavy plaque or calculus formers.
2. Effective daily oral hygiene, starting from completion of eruption of the permanent teeth, is recommended. The options should be described to the owner and use of VOHC-accepted products should be demonstrated.
3. The teeth should be treated professionally when indicated, again starting from an early age.

Disclosure
There is no conflict of interest resulting from publication of this article.[26]

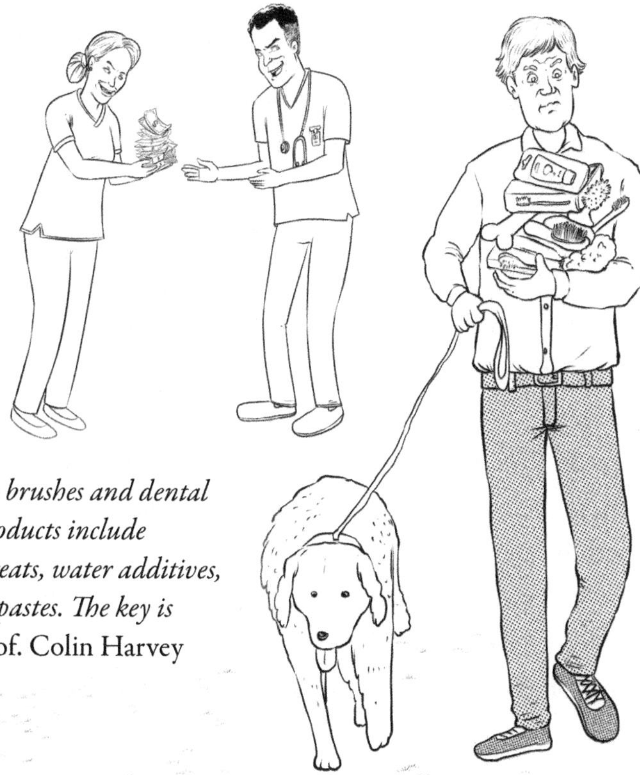

'In addition to brushes and dental wipes, these products include dental diets, treats, water additives, gels, and toothpastes. The key is daily use.' Prof. Colin Harvey

So that, dear reader, is the January 2022 'most current information' regarding prevention and treatment of the most prevalent disease affecting dogs, as published by the long-time director of the Veterinary Oral Health Council and renowned professor of dentistry at one of the world's foremost veterinary schools.

What percentage of puppy owners know about or sign up for 'making use of more than one modality' every day of their pet's life? What about other carnivores—cats, ferrets, zoo animals? What are their owners supposed to do? Is tooth brushing the 'gold standard' for those animals too? The mind boggles. These and a raft of other questions must wait for another day.

First-year University of Georgia veterinary student comments

> OK, we just started Nutrition on Monday and it's already absolutely unbearable. I guess I am just hopelessly naive, but I'm not sure I actually believed until I got there, that they could think it was worth anyone's time to devote a whole class to pouring dog or cat food out of a bag and into a bowl. And that a woman who spent seventeen years of post-high school education in veterinary nutrition studies could honestly think that commercial food is the only viable option to feed pets. She's not even making an attempt to teach us anything except how to evaluate dry foods, how to read dry food ingredient lists, how to do all these ridiculous calculations about Kcal, resting energy requirement, etc.
>
> We had two hours of it today, once at eight and once at four. I didn't go to the eight o-clock class, because every time I go, it literally ruins the rest of my day. But, two

friends, one raw-feeding and the other doing her research to start, spoke to the professor at the end of the class about some things she said that they questioned or didn't agree with. They tried to pose their questions politely, but apparently the conversation degenerated pretty quickly.

One of the things they asked about was her mantra, which she regularly asks the class to _chant_, 'pets need nutrients, not ingredients', meaning, of course, that it doesn't matter what's in the food as long as the companies guarantee certain nutritional content. My friends brought up some non-species-specific ingredients, like corn, soy, wheat, etc. and asked if she didn't see a problem with that. Her reply was that corn gets a bad rap, that it's a perfect healthy ingredient and that Native Americans survived on it well enough, so why not dogs? (I'm not joking) She also told them that high cooking temps/extrusion doesn't have any effect on the health of the food at all. When they mentioned raw and some good results they'd seen with it, she said that George Burns smoked and drank every day and lived to be 100, but that didn't mean those were healthy things to do.

She also said that raw is dangerous because of food borne pathogens, referencing an E coli 01:57 outbreak at a Jack In the Box as proof, even though that deals with _humans_ eating _cooked_ meat?!? She then told them that they're just being influenced by fad diets on the Internet with no science behind them, and that she shouldn't just believe everything they hear or read. When they tried to stand up for themselves, she fell back on the 'I'm one of only 50 certified veterinary nutritionists in the country' as if that ended the argument. They were both so furious they could hardly speak when I got there.

Then, for our second hour this afternoon, she taught us the nine steps she uses to evaluate a commercial food if a client wants her opinion. See what you think of these:

1. The bag, box, or can should contain the phrase 'complete and balanced'.
2. Products that contain this claim must also follow with one of two AAFCO statements, i.e. the product was tested through feeding trials or the calculation method.
3. The label should contain a toll-free phone # so you can ask the company questions if necessary.
4. The product should have a digestibility of at least 80% (you may have to call the company to get this figure).
5. If you are feeding a dry product, it should contain a preservative (all of which are completely safe according to her).
6. Reputation of the company.
7. Cost.
8. Animals require nutrients not ingredient (this one has about three paragraphs explaining why corn, soy and other ingredients are perfectly suitable for dogs).
9. How is the pet doing while consuming the product?

That's it. Nothing about what the ingredients are, ingredient sources. As long as it fits the above criteria, it's fine in her book. The really ridiculous thing is, she keeps contradicting herself. She told us about the experiment where they made a food out of leather boots, old tires, peanut hulls, whatever, that met the pet food companies' nutrient requirements, but then she stressed that she thought

> Purina is a really quality brand of food that has an unjustified poor reputation (she's basing this on the fact that they claim their digestibility is 84%, which is supposed to be good, I guess). She also talked about ingredient splitting and how bad it is, but then showed us several labels of acceptable (to her) pet foods that had five or six split fractions of one ingredient.
>
> I could go on with this forever, but I think this letter's long enough already :) I just need to blow off some steam; I think I'm going to have a sneer permanently affixed to my face after a couple months of that class.[27]

Massey University School of Veterinary Science, New Zealand

What did they know and when did they know it?

In 1993, in the days before email, a letter arrived from Professor Peter Stockdale, dean of Massey University School of Veterinary Science. He had noticed the vigorous raw meaty bones debate in the Australian Veterinary Association newsletter and was keen for his staff and students to hear more. Although not part of the formal curriculum, Massey had a tradition of inviting speakers on hot topics who gave evening lectures.

Apart from the thrill of being invited to deliver what, I believed, was the first formal university lecture on the most important topic to confront the veterinary profession, there was the added offer of half the flight costs and motel accommodation. I set to work researching and writing. I wanted my audience to be left in no doubt about pet foods.

Pet Foods' Insidious Consequences
(A modern veterinary snafu)

Summary

A recurring theme is that both content and form of the pro-pet food argument is flawed, making invalid conclusions the rule. The euphemistic use of the term 'pet food' is deplored and the cynical manipulation of the rules of logic, mass psychology, politics and economics is described. Insidious environmental consequences are listed. Veterinary science is seen to be corrupted due to an uncritical appraisal by those responsible for animal health care.

The state of health is dependent upon the correct balance of quantity, quality and frequency of chemical and physical requirements provided by food intake. Examples of failure are provided with the emphasis being placed on periodontal disease. Recent case surveys and research findings are presented on Foul Mouth AIDS, Feline Eosinophilic Disease Complex, Plasma Cell Pododermatitis and FLUTD.

The limitation of the clinical diagnostic pathways are shown to perpetuate the insidious process. A 'Cybernetic Hypothesis of Periodontal Disease' provides an evolutionary, ecological perspective casting the modern feeding practices in a grim light. Arising out of this dark and corrupted phase a renaissance is predicted providing beneficial insight into health and disease.

Introduction

Unrecognised, and therefore undefined, problems have the potential to be the most sinister. This paper is intended as

> an introduction to the insidious consequences of the processed pet food industry. It should dispel the propaganda myth proclaimed in the TV advertising and replace it with a strong revulsion.
>
> Given the assiduous way that the monster spreads its tentacles one could be forgiven for subscribing to a conspiracy theory. It is more likely that cultural conditioning and the coincidence of economic and environmental factors have facilitated the growth. Now in a dominant position, the industry enjoys super profits which are then directed to maintenance of its grip on the market.
>
> There does remain a whiff of conspiracy when one considers that the problem is in the main unrecognised and undefined by the veterinary profession. Veterinarians gain legitimacy and privileges as guardians of the public welfare in respect to animal health. The profession has failed badly in its duties. Recent experience has confirmed that rather than admit failure of function the profession would rather deny it has missed the obvious.
>
> The Australian Veterinary Association, for example, has adopted an aggressive stance. The Association was in receipt of direct and indirect sponsorship from two large multinational pet food companies. This occasioned bitter criticism of the implied conflict of interest. Rather than limit or stabilise their involvement the AVA has recently entered a sponsorship agreement with a third American multinational pet food corporation.[28]

The vet school staff and students were respectful, perhaps a tad wary. The presentation went to schedule. And following on, late into the night, my wife and I shared pizza and plentiful red wine with

Massey veterinary nutritionist Dr Grant Guilford. Apparently, according to Dr Guilford, in response to the raw meaty bones campaign, there had been a marked increase in periodontal disease research projects in universities and pet food laboratories around the world. It was news to me. I scoffed that instead of communicating the wondrous health benefits of raw meaty bones the vet establishment was secretly assisting the junk pet food makers in damage control.

At the end of the evening and our enjoyable 'meeting of the minds', we said our goodbyes. Dr Guilford took with him a bundle of some 50 lecture monographs ready printed for distribution to the students. It was, perhaps, a chance to reach a handful of students about pet foods' insidious consequences and the global veterinary snafu: **S**ituation **N**ormal **A**ll **F**ucked **U**p.

7

WHITE-COLLAR CRIMINAL COLLABORATION

Those who can make you believe absurdities can make you commit atrocities.

Voltaire

The white-collar criminal collaboration between the junk pet food industry and vet profession was here first, before any of us were born. The collaboration defines the pet-owning culture and all elements of the ecosystem—the regulatory bodies, vet associations, pet associations, welfare bodies, rescue groups, insurance companies and guide dog training organisations. All elements have evolved and adapted in the polluted environment that depends upon the mass poisoning of pets and the widespread consumer fraud.

Knowingly injuring the health of animals and deceiving consumers both carry severe criminal penalties. But few if any of the elements of the ecosystem are doing anything about limiting their involvement or seeking to expose and resolve the issues. On the contrary, there are significant and powerful elements, comfortable in their role and devoted to perpetuating the collaboration. Some are front organisations and some are the more passive elements that go along for the ride with a 'What's in it for me? I'm alright Jack' outlook. Let's take a look at a few.

Australian Veterinary Association

Veterinary associations are the equivalent of trade unions, established and committed to pursuing the interests of their members. That's laudable when everything is open, above board and honest. It's scandalous when an association acts as a front organisation engaged in a racket.

As I write this in 2021, I think about the reach and influence of the Australian Veterinary Association (AVA) and thus the reach and influence of its junk pet food industry bedmates. AVA members dominate each of the Australian state veterinary boards. They hold influential positions in government regulatory bodies. And in all instances known to me they abide by the Mafia code of *omertà* often defined as 'loyalty and solidarity (or silence) in the face of authority'.

Of course, the Mafia, an underground organisation, seeks to clandestinely corrupt regulators, police officers and judges. Vet associations perceive no need for secrecy. They operate in plain sight. They are the smug, loyal, controlling face of authority.

Another way of understanding the associations is as subcults within the wider vet cult. A cult is a social group that is defined by its unusual religious, spiritual or philosophical beliefs, or by its shared interest in a particular personality, object or goal.

Back in the early 1990s Breck Muir and I—rather naively it now seems—attempted to change the AVA. We stood for election to the AVA board by appealing to the members' better nature. My manifesto statement for each of the years 1995, 1996 and 1997 stated:

> Our most pressing problem of self-regulation is that thirty years ago, due to lack of vigilance, we allowed economic colonialists free entry to develop their pet-food culture. At the time we were scientifically and socially naive and, as a

> community, we were persuaded to favour foreign-owned, expensive items over the superior, cheap local produce. Given the difficulty of correcting culturally conditioned errors it must be a concern to all Australians that the AVA and various government departments are still in denial over this issue. When we stop the internal battles over this absurdity, we can redirect our resources for the good of the community. Everyone from either side of the debate will have a role in retrieving our credibility and setting about the task of re-education. ...
>
> For the future I envisage a renaissance for the profession as we show a lead in animal welfare, the human economy and the natural environment. New environmentally friendly industries should emerge for the feeding of the world's pets. Spin-off benefits would likely include solutions for our feral goat, rabbit and kangaroo problems. Our farming communities and our children should obtain a sounder economy and a better environment. Veterinarians working in primary industry, government, teaching and general practice should all gain a new importance.[1]

In 1998 Breck and I appealed to the membership in our election manifesto.

> Back in December 1991 we published articles pointing to the devastating effects of diet and periodontal disease on the health of domestic pets. The AVA and the Pet Food Manufacturers Association attempted to quell the discussion but soon the *AVA News* letters column became a place of spirited debate. The matter was placed before the 1993

AGM where members voted to set up a $7,000 'Diet and Disease Committee' to investigate some of the allegations. The February 1994 AVA News advised that veterinarians, 'need to be concerned about the relationship between diet and disease' and that, 'Periodontal disease is arguably the most common disease condition seen in small animal practice and its effects on the gums and the teeth can significantly affect the health and well-being of affected animals. This is sufficient in itself to give reason for concern. Proof of additional systemic effects is not necessary to justify further action.' The December 1995 edition of the Journal of Small Animal Practice carried an article on additional diet induced systemic effects akin to an 'AIDS like' condition.

We in the Raw Meaty Bone lobby are proud of our record. As a result of our efforts in print and on TV and radio we have done much to overcome the propaganda of the artificial pet food industry and their veterinary advisors. At the same time, we have highlighted the medical and dental professions' promotion of healthy natural food and clean teeth. In turn the medical and dental professions have leant us support with their discovery that periodontal disease is a prime risk factor for heart disease, premature and still births and overall mortality.

It is worth putting on the record some of the activities of some of the AVA Board members. The President Roger Clarke has published several internet messages extolling the benefits of artificial pet food and was even seen in the pages of a pet food company magazine. Dr Jill Maddison, consultant to Friskies, appeared in a TV programme in which she promoted artificial pet food and denied the

> existence of a diet induced 'AIDS like' condition. She also appeared in a Medical Benefits Fund article along with Board member Jonica Newby in which it was alleged that pet ownership is worth huge savings to the Australian health bill. This claim was central to the Newby book but as two objective research projects have since shown the savings are not 1.5 billion but in fact zero. Mr Stuart Littlemore QC was most unhappy with the Newby incognito performance on the ABC. He said that she should not have been on the ABC at all. Ian Denney the director of the Western Plains Zoo presides over the feeding of liquid pet food to cheetahs, an endangered species, as part of a sponsorship arrangement with a pet food company. Garth McGilvray AVA spokesman on the Channel 9 Money Programme said, 'The AVA would consider the best diet consists of 80% dry food and 20% perhaps of raw bones.' ...
>
> When elected to the AVA Board we shall straight away initiate steps to discontinue the arrangements with the pet food company sponsors. In 1992 legal advice was published indicating that vets and by extension the AVA could be held legally responsible for promoting dietary substances which give rise to periodontal and other diseases. At an early stage we would take steps to minimise that risk to the Association.[2]

At each election around 10 per cent of AVA voters, in a secret ballot, supported our calls for reform. None came forward; none stood up to be counted. And of course, 90 per cent of voters were either indifferent or opposed us.

At the head of my manifesto in 2003, the last year in which I stood for AVA elections, I tried ridicule.

Kamikaze pilots fly for the honour.
Mercenary soldiers risk death for the dollar.
But perish the thought,
professional suicide for nought,
with no saving grace, only dogma.[3]

Simultaneously I tried to involve the New South Wales Board of Veterinary Surgeons, the state government regulator. I sent the board a letter.

Excuses and falsehoods

Members of the NSW Board of Veterinary Surgeons are likely aware of the allegations of scientific and consumer fraud perpetrated upon an unsuspecting Australian public by an alliance of pet food companies and veterinarians.

The implications are numerous and serious.

Any right-thinking person knows that the slow poisoning of the nation's pets by junk food manufacturers, aided by veterinarians, is against the interests of pets, pet owners and the wider community.

Unless the allegations can be proven false, they deserve the widest airing leading to timely resolution.

The correspondence below reveals a series of excuses and falsehoods serving to postpone and perhaps suppress news of the scandal.

The Australian Veterinary Association (AVA) has financial ties to pet food companies. For ten years the AVA has sought to stifle news of the scandal. ...

Given the magnitude of the alleged fraud it would appear incumbent on government authorities to take the necessary steps to protect the public.

> Despite the complicity and efforts of some, the allegations are now a matter of public record.
>
> Will the NSW Veterinary Surgeons Board investigate and report on the alleged widespread fraud?[4]

Protecting the public, investigating and reporting on alleged fraud were clearly not at the top of the AVA or NSW Veterinary Board agendas. The AVA Executive moved to cancel my membership and no amount of lawyer's effort could reverse their decision.

Paul Lynch, lawyer and member of NSW Parliament, rose to speak in parliament on 13 May 2004. In conclusion he stated:

> Tom Lonsdale was expelled from the AVA on the basis of an anonymous complaint in relation to which further particulars were not provided at a hearing at which he could not have legal representation. The whistleblower was punished.[5]

For more on this issue, see Chapter 10, 'Politicians and regulators: let dog food companies lie'.

Self-regulatory disasters

> **Power tends to corrupt and absolute power corrupts absolutely.**
>
> **Lord Acton**

At core, enabling and facilitating the white-collar criminal collaboration is the universal self-regulatory status of the vet profession. I say 'universal' for as far as I know, in all states and territories of Australia and in all countries of the world, vets enjoy self-regulatory status. A long time ago, politicians trusted vets. Simultaneously they took the view that since veterinary proficiency only arose from several years of university study, therefore only vets could fully understand veterinary matters. Accordingly, government regulation is delegated to veterinary boards that keep a register of vets licensed to practise in their geographical area, set and maintain standards of vet performance and conduct disciplinary actions against those who are deemed to have fallen below 'current accepted standards'.

Although vet boards are *given* the power to regulate, you could say they *captured* that power. They behave as if it were a God-given right, never open to question. That would be OK, even efficient and admirable, if the boards behaved with integrity, honesty and truthfulness. But alas, the boards themselves on many levels tend to be subject to 'regulatory capture' by the prevailing junk pet food culture.

Why do you, a pet owner, need to know about this stuff? Simply because this is the number one issue that cements the entire corrupt junk pet food culture in place. Wikipedia defines 'regulatory capture' as 'a corruption of authority that occurs when a political entity, policymaker, or regulatory agency is co-opted to serve the commercial, ideological, or political interests of a minor constituency, such as a particular geographic area, industry, profession, or ideological group'.[6]

So, in the veterinary sphere, the fox is well and truly in the henhouse and Dracula controls the blood bank. You and your pet are vulnerable. Vet regulators across the world don't protect you. They protect the *status quo*, the fake animal welfare alliance between the pet food industry and the vets.

NSW Board of Veterinary Surgeons

Although the Veterinary Practitioners Board of New South Wales, as it is now called, is an arm of the state government, it is predominantly made up of AVA nominees approved by the Minister of

Agriculture. In all the years since 1991 that the vet board has been told about the junk pet food fraud, they have done nothing to resolve the issues. They have, however, harassed me on behalf of the AVA and junk pet food industry vets through four separate disciplinary actions.

Threatened with deregistration, a year in prison, a fine of $2000 or both, I came to see legal defence strategies as my top priority. Documents on file weighed a combined 12 kilograms (26 pounds) and represent years of hard work and countless hours spent in lawyers' offices—not to mention the costs, personal and financial. The first complaint arrived in May 1994.

> Dear Mr Lonsdale,
>
> The Board has received a complaint concerning statements allegedly made by you in the media.
>
> While the Board does not wish to enter into the scientific controversy surrounding the matter, the Board is concerned that the statements, if made as presented in the media could place you in breach of Clause 10.1 under the Code of Professional Conduct. This Clause states that – 'Veterinary Surgeons have an obligation to their colleagues, individually and collectively, and to the public, to conduct themselves at all times in an acceptable manner.'
>
> Such claims as –
>
> 'A Sydney veterinarian, Dr Tom Lonsdale, said 75 percent of the income vets earned from treating dogs and cats was derived form ailments caused by inadequate diet'
>
> 'dog and cat food should be banned because it causes shocking tooth and gum disease in 85% of pets'.
>
> May imply that the veterinary profession as a whole is

> negligent in not advising against the use of proprietary foods or performing adequate dental and other health checks.
>
> It is the Board's opinion that before such claims or statements can be publicly made, there should exist sound scientific evidence supporting them. Otherwise, such claims could be detrimental to the veterinary profession and misleading to the public.

My lawyer responded:

> We act for Tom Lonsdale to whom you wrote on 9 May 1994.
>
> We advise as follows:
>
> 1. Your letter does not require a response and therefore raises a question as to why it was written. Perhaps you would be good enough to enlighten us.
>
> 2. It is cowardly and unprofessional of the complainant not to release a copy of his letter and thus prevent a professional colleague from defending both his actions and reputation.
>
> 3. It would be most improper of the Board to take action which might, and very probably would, adversely affect our client's professional standing and thus his livelihood and at the same time refuse even to provide a copy of the complainant's letter so as to give at least some semblance of foundation for the Board's stance.
>
> Any action taken by the Board prejudicial to our client in the present circumstances would constitute a complete denial of natural justice and would be treated accordingly.
>
> It is or should be a basic tenet of the approach of every

> professional regulatory body in Australia in these circumstances that no action will be taken based on anonymous complaints and that every member of a profession has a fundamental right to be able adequately to defend charges levied against him especially if those charges are wilfully, mischievously, falsely or stupidly based.
>
> Accordingly, you are requested within seven (7) days to provide a precise statement of the Board's stance on this matter together with a photocopy of the complete letter of complaint.

The Board refused even this straightforward request. My lawyer, angry by now, wrote again.

> The Board's response ... is considered unsatisfactory ...
>
> The Board's continued protection of the anonymity of the complainant must be challenged ...
>
> This is the more critical in the context of one professional making derogatory remarks or allegations about another ...
>
> It would be doubly unfortunate if members of the veterinary or any other profession were given the implied assurance from its professional body that as long as they request allegations of impropriety or unprofessional behaviour be kept confidential, they are at liberty to make such allegations ...
>
> Allowing the anonymous and undisclosed allegations to lie in the Board's files like a time bomb to ensure to Dr. Lonsdale's detriment in the future is likewise unfortunate and inequitable. ...
>
> You will appreciate that it is essential that members of

> the veterinary profession should hold your Board in high esteem. The corollary of this is, of course, that the Board at all times should act in such a way as to deserve that esteem.
>
> We trust that our client will not have to resort to the processes of the Freedom of Information Act in order to enjoy natural justice. ...

And so it came to pass, three years later, our resort to the Freedom of Information Act provided the details of the complaint from Dr Barbara Fougere BSc BVMS (Hons) Grad Dip Bus Mgt. Her letter began:

> PO Box 474
> ROZELLE
> 2039 NSW
>
> Dr Dick James
> Veterinary Surgeons Board
> Locked Bag 21
> Orange NSW 2800
>
> Dear Dick,
>
> I would like to register a complaint against Dr Tom Lonsdale of Riverstone Veterinary Hospital. I am concerned about Dr Lonsdale's recent media attack on processed pet foods. ...
>
> His statements in the media directly undermine the professionalism and credibility of practitioners who recommend processed foods to pet owners. ...
>
> Dr Lonsdale's proposition that periodontal disease leads to the ultimate death of pets implies veterinarians

> are not routinely checking dental health. He is therefore making public the assumption that veterinarians are not performing routine dental checks. ...
>
> I believe a suitable resolution of this complaint would be the prevention of further publicity of Dr Lonsdale unless authorised by the veterinary surgeons board. ...
>
> Good quality petfoods have undergone AAFCO protocols for suitability as a solus diet. They provide a complete and balanced ration. ... [7]

Barbara Fougere wrote from her home address and was on first-name terms with the chairman of the vet board. For her, there was no need to mention that she was a Mars company 'consultant'. Mars use front people to fight their battles. Straight away I understood why the vet board and Dr Fougere tried to keep her identity secret.

Harassing me, a whistleblower, and giving comfort to the junk pet food makers and their vet protective cordon has been the government vet board *modus operandi* right up to the time of writing. You could say that in New South Wales, the mass torture of pets and the incompetence and overservicing by the vet profession have been part and parcel of the NSW Board of Veterinary Surgeons' maladministration.

By way of illustration, let's take a look at the vet board's failure to oversee the activities of the Small Animal Specialist Hospital.

Small Animal Specialist Hospital (SASH)

These days specialist vet hospitals provide a place of referral where general practitioner vets can send their difficult, hard-to-diagnose, hard-to-treat cases. Staffed by highly trained specialists in vet medicine and surgery and supported by sophisticated MRI and CT scan technology and vast nursing staffs, their services don't come cheap. The hospitals are part of a luxury trade for the few that can afford them and for those with pet insurance (i.e. for veterinary health care). In the US the Mars Corporation owns 53 specialist hospitals across 18 states employing more than 3,000 people, including over 600 veterinarians.[8]

Whether Mars own SASH or whether they merely own SASH *allegiance*, I cannot be sure. I do know that in 2018 the owners of Dozer, a Jack Russell terrier puppy, were advised to feed him 'a high-quality commercial diet such as Hill's or Royal Canin. Dozer should not be fed raw food for the rest of his life.' SASH make promotional videos in conjunction with Mars company Royal Canin, who they describe as their 'nutrition partner'.[9] And, rather conveniently for SASH and Royal Canin, the NSW Minister of Agriculture appointed a SASH vet to the NSW Board of Veterinary Surgeons.[10]

Ordinarily pet owners, having been to see the SASH folks, don't then go looking for first-opinion practitioners like me. Owners feel that they've been to the top of the tree and that vets on the lower branches don't have much to offer. Even if owners are not happy with the outcome of a specialist's recommended treatment, no-one likes to throw good money after bad.

Dawn Vale was the exception. Her opening remarks when presenting Jiminy, her 10-month-old kitten, were: 'I hope you can help, you are the fifth vet I've consulted, and no-one seems to know what to do. I took Jiminy to three local vet practices and then, when Jiminy was just six months of age, I was referred to SASH who charged me almost $6000.' Dawn went on to say: 'SASH told me that the probable best hope was to remove all of Jiminy's teeth—I don't want to do that!'

Jiminy's breath stank. His gums were a fire engine red. I told Dawn I thought she had booked a consultation with me just in time, but only just. Thankfully, we were able to remove some minor teeth and most importantly persuade Jiminy to overcome his junk food addiction and convert to a raw meaty bones diet. We made a video, posted on YouTube, showing Jiminy back to health, ripping into a rabbit head with a soundtrack of parrots chattering in the trees above.

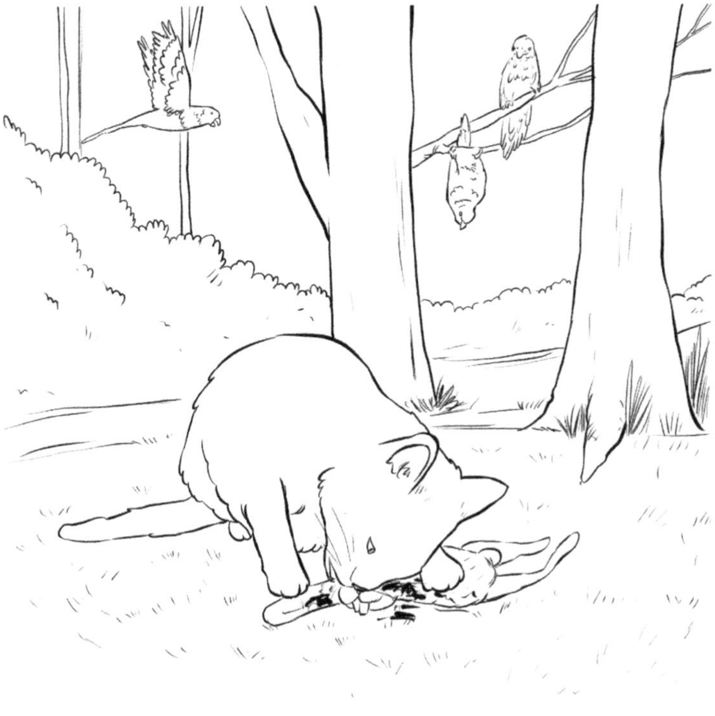

The YouTube caption reads:

> **Feline gingivostomatitis: Nature's best medicine—raw meaty bones—to the rescue**
> Take home messages
>
> 1. Jiminy eventually got lucky. Luck frequently plays a part.
> 2. Vet incompetence and over servicing is the norm.

3. Vet dentistry incompetence is the norm.
4. Junk processed pet food/vet conspiracy should be investigated.
5. Junk raw pet food/vet/holistic/barfer/prey model self-styled experts (with zero vet dental know-how) should be exposed.
6. Raw meaty bones are key to the carnivore code—ripping, tearing, consuming raw meaty bones validates the carnivore compact.
7. Jiminy's case provides strong supporting evidence for the Cybernetic Hypothesis.[11]

Three years later, events took an interesting turn. Tim Hopkins, SASH 'veterinary relationship manager', made an appointment to see us. SASH was promoting their latest oncology services and Dr Hopkins was keen to receive feedback from first-opinion practitioners.

Tim Hopkins waited in the reception area, reading the displayed material, seeing the photos and watching streaming videos—his jaw beginning to drop and his eyes beginning to pop. Nevertheless, he maintained his composure and after watching the Jiminy video and chatting with head nurse Sandra and me, he agreed that potentially SASH could learn much from our experiences. We even discussed how SASH could potentially lead the vet world by reversing course from their junk food endorsements. Waving goodbye, Tim Hopkins said that he would consult with the SASH team and return soon.

At Appendix F you can see how the SASH team were not so keen on any repeat interaction. Apparently, SASH do not recognise fundamental biological definitions and the evidence of their own eyes. We can assume all patients visiting SASH have teeth and eat food. Assessment of oral health and diet, in line with biological determinants, should be integral to every consultation—especially in a high-priced specialist hospital. However, SASH say:

> As a specialist referral centre, we believe it is our duty to outsource these questions [about diet and dentistry] in the absence of specific nutrition or dentistry qualified staff members.

My lawyer and I worked on a response:

> This is an important public issue for all vets: feeding pets the wrong foods injures their health and in my view amounts to cruelty to animals (a criminal offence).
>
> Further, failing to alert pet owners to the consequences of harmful diets and then proceeding to provide elaborate and costly treatments, should be viewed as over-servicing, and should be viewed as representing a further level of fraud.

Royal College of Veterinary Surgeons (RCVS)

By now you know the odds are stacked against you. You know that the junk pet food issues transcend mere hypocrisy and reach the standard of a monumental fraud protected and perpetuated by legions of vet collaborators.

In the United Kingdom, vet self-regulation began with a Royal Charter in 1844 and continues to this day. The 2015 update states:

> The objects of the College shall be to set, uphold and advance veterinary standards, and to promote, encourage and advance the study and practice of the art and science

> of veterinary surgery and medicine, in the interests of the health and welfare of animals and in the wider public interest.[12]

If their statement were remotely true, then the mass poisoning of UK pets and fraudulent overservicing of pet ailments would be hot-button topics. But they're not and never will be as long as the junk pet food proxies run the show.

Way back in 1995, Henry Carter, former president of the RCVS, wrote:

> For 45 years I have observed Pedigree Petfoods [Mars Inc.] (and its predecessor, Chappie Ltd) seeking to influence veterinary students and practitioners.
>
> For over 25 years I have observed Pedigree Petfoods and other pet food manufacturers exerting what some may consider undue influence on the British Small Animal Veterinary Association (BSAVA).[13]

And since the council of the RCVS is mostly made up of BSAVA and British Veterinary Association vets, Henry Carter could have said Mars and Co. have undue influence—nay complete control—over the RCVS.

Certainly, Mars would have been feeling confident of avoiding scrutiny while Professor Neil Gorman, the head of their Waltham research establishment, was president of the RCVS. Similarly, Colgate would have been delighted when Lynne Hill, their European sales manager, was president and sitting on the RCVS Council for many years.

In 2004 vet Roger Meacock and I had a rather futile meeting with the then president of the RCVS, Professor Richard Halliwell

MA VetMB PhD MRCVS. I sent Professor Halliwell a contemporaneous record of our discussion:

> I suggested that the artificial pet-food industry, in alliance with the veterinary profession, is responsible for the mass poisoning of domestic pets.
>
> As the UK regulator of the profession, I implored the Royal College to act, and thereby save itself from public contempt. I indicated that my colleagues and I, when we discovered that we had previously misadvised our clients regarding the suitability of processed foods, quickly set the record straight, apologised and moved to remedy past wrongs.
>
> I suggested that around 9% of veterinarians agree with my analysis judging by the votes I have received at Royal College elections in each of the past eight years.
>
> You vehemently denied that the votes carried any validity—and spoke as if this was the collective view of the College Council. You asserted that a hamster, if it should stand for election to the Council of the Royal College, would receive as many votes....

The mass poisoning of domestic pets by their health care providers cannot be condoned.

As self-appointed guardians of the public interest, where pet health is concerned, the leaders of the veterinary profession have obligations:

- To research and advise on the extent of the damage caused by artificial diets—they have not.
- When presented with the evidence, to clarify and act upon that evidence—they have not.

- When presented with the evidence, at an early stage to alert the veterinary profession and wider community—they have not, but instead have taken steps to suppress the evidence.

These failings of the veterinary leadership serve to inflict great cruelty upon the animals under our care, cost £billions in unnecessary food and veterinary costs and stand in the way of major human health care advances.[14]

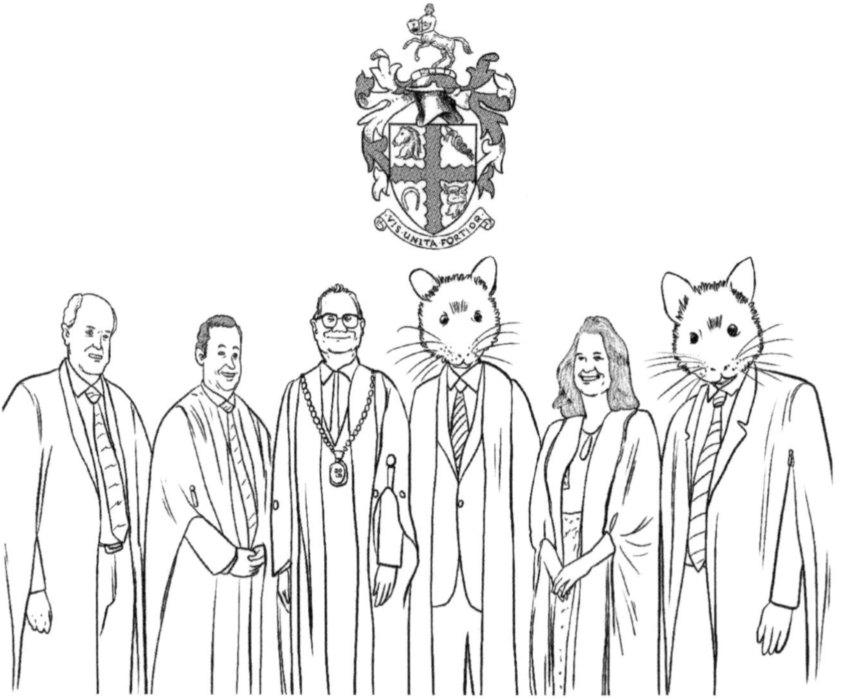

Councillors of the Royal College of Veterinary Surgeons

From 1997 to 2020—a total of 24 consecutive years—I contested elections for a place on the council of the RCVS. Most years I received between 8 and 10 per cent of the vote. Never did I expect to get elected, but at least it was a chance to air the largest, most consequential issues facing the veterinary profession. (The veterinary press refuses to air the issues; election manifestos are harder to suppress.) I shared tales with my elderly mother about the RCVS's refusal to even discuss the issues. 'What about the animals?' she'd say, shaking her head.

Veterinary Oral Health Council (VOHC)

Today the June 2021 *Dental Solutions* catalogue dropped into my inbox. With August designated as Pet Dental Month, Australian vets are encouraged to stock up with artificial products facilitating the belief that vets should and do care about pet dental health.

> We know how important it is having regular conversations with clients around Dental Homecare and preventative solutions, to assist with this we have a comprehensive article on Toothbrushing Tips—training pets & owners on toothbrushing on page 2, as well as a great article on page 16 detailing Chewing Temperament and Dental Health to help you discuss which Dental Dog Toys are right for your clients.[15]

In the catalogue chock-full of junk chemicals and plastic toys Dr Rebecca Nilsen BSc BVMS (Hons) MANZCVS (Small Animal Dentistry and Oral Surgery), president of the Australian Veterinary Dental Society, holds forth on the pet toothbrushing scam:

> Overall, an increase in the awareness of dental disease will lead to an increase in requests for more professional dental treatments which can significantly increase profits and build greater relationships with clients. Although owner

> compliance will always be a confounding factor, the recommendation for tooth brushing should continue to remain the gold standard.

About the Veterinary Oral Health Council (VOHC) she says:

> Homecare products can be classified into mechanical, chemical, dietary and dental sealants. The Veterinary Oral Health Council (VOHC) was established in 1997 and consists of independent board-certified veterinary dentists who award the VOHC seal of approval to those products that were shown in controlled studies to reduce the development of plaque and calculus.

However, from my perspective, the VOHC (www.vohc.org) is a protection racket whereby manufacturers of junk products, *if they pay the VOHC*, gain a 'seal of approval'. Consumers gain false assurances that the products (gimmicks) work. And the entire VOHC enterprise serves to distract from and suppress the truth about the devastating effects of junk pet food.

The evidence is clear; nature got it right, raw meaty bones are the key to the carnivore code. It's the essential ripping, tearing and gnawing at raw meaty bones that keep teeth clean. The VOHC got it wrong. Promoting ineffectual vegetable chews, plastic toys and tooth brushing for dogs and cats is commercially inspired confidence trickery, but they continue with the trickery. Here's a recent advertisement aimed at vets.[16]

Introducing NEW VeggieDent® FR3SH Dental Chews for dogs

NEW VeggieDent® FR3SH Dental Chews offer a healthy solution to bad breath in a great tasting dental treat that dogs love. Featuring innovative FR3SH Technology, VeggieDent® FR3SH Dental Chews target the causes of bad breath in 3 ways:

- CLEANSE—Addressing oral causes of bad breath
- COOL—Freshens breath with cooling action
- DIGESTIVE—Promoting balanced and healthy gut flora to help address the digestive causes of bad breath

VETERINARY ORAL HEALTH COUNCIL
VOHC Accepted®
HELPS CONTROL TARTAR
HELPS CONTROL PLAQUE ®

New VeggieDent® FR3SH has been awarded the VOHC® Seal of Acceptance to help control plaque and tartar following review of data from trials conducted according to strict protocol guidelines.

Available in 4 different sizes.

Exclusive Vet launch deal buy 3 of each size and get 1 of each size free (buy 12 get 4 free) that includes a free counter display unit and support material*

Fake animal welfare and rescue groups

Given the success of the junk pet food industry and vet collaborators at encouraging a largely urbanised community to keep dogs (modified wolves), cats (modified desert predators) and ferrets (modified polecats), it comes as no surprise that problems beset the community. Lacking proper appreciation of the biological and management needs of carnivores leads to a vast oversupply of pets and discarded pets.

In simple terms, the community is encouraged to keep pets as if they were furry toys with daily maintenance needs being conveniently met by the brightly packaged formulas on the supermarket shelf. In the event of need, there's the pet hospital at the end of the street. However, if things become too inconvenient, expensive and troublesome there's always the council pound, the fake animal welfare bodies and rescue groups ready to mop up the discards.

Plot the flow of funds through this system of abuse and you'll find that it's the junk food makers and their vet allies who make the money. In all instances it's the community that pays—pays to buy the pets, pays for the junk food, pays for the fake vet services, pays for the local pound and pays for the fake welfare and rescue groups. The animals, of course, have no say in this as they sit in solitary confinement obliged to eat industrial pap and finally paying with their lives.

Welfare groups, if they were honest, would campaign against the cruelty and suffering. But never in my experience has that happened. Instead, they develop elaborate, expensive systems dependent on donations, legacies and bequests.[17] Yes, even after death the community pays for the highly paid operatives within the oversupply and discarded pet system. Adding further insult to injury, the welfare groups set up cross-promotional deals with the junk pet food makers. In Australia, the Royal Society for the Prevention of Cruelty to Animals (RSPCA) sought out funding from Colgate-

Palmolive and sell and promote Colgate (Hill's) junk products through their clinics.

Rescue groups depend for their operation on donations of money and countless hours of volunteers' time and effort. Most receive donations of junk pet food and in turn recommend industrial concoctions. And of lasting and greater benefit for the junk food makers, every extra pet rehomed by a rescue group is an extra mouth worth thousands of dollars to the junk food makers. During the COVID-19 pandemic *Pet Gazette* reported:

> **Royal Canin warns of rescue centre struggles post-lockdown**
> To help support these centres, Royal Canin has supplied over £200,000 of food to over 250 rescues and food banks across the UK and Ireland during the last year.[18]

Pet Gazette subsequently reported:

> **Mars Petcare launches £1.3m TV campaign**
> Mars Petcare has announced that it will launch a £1.3m TV campaign from Pedigree, as part of its global ambition of 'ending pet homelessness by 2030'.
>
> The advertisement will feature the tagline 'Feel the good. Adopt'. Mars said the advert aims to highlight the 'good' that can come from pet adoption, showcasing the 'unconditional love and happiness that adopted pets can bring to families'.
>
> In addition, the group will also work in partnership with the Association of Dogs and Cats Homes (ADCH) and its members, to provide a 'comprehensive programme of support to shelters across the UK.'[19]

Clearly turning off the tap, stopping the flow of unwanted pets by stopping the promotion of sentient creatures as if they were animated toys, stopping the false junk pet food advertising would be the best preventative strategy. Unfortunately, on the evidence, the fake welfare groups and most rescue groups would rather work with Mars, redirect the flow of discarded pets and keep themselves in the game—money for all and kudos all around.

Assorted niche marketers

The bubble economy of the junk pet food industry and vets spawns plenty of niches into which enterprising people fit snuggly. I'm thinking of the dog groomers, hydro-bath makers, pet sitters, doggy day care and boarding establishments, pet magazines, animal transport companies and the list goes on.

Vet pharmaceutical companies thrive in their lucrative niche supplying vets with an ever-expanding range of medicaments. Pet cremation services swing into action at the end of pets' lives. One group of opportunists, the pet insurance companies, rely on the increasing numbers of ailing pets and mounting vet bills. More sick pets and hefty vet bills means more and higher insurance premiums.

You might think that at least some animal welfare lawyers would focus on cruelty and corruption induced by junk pet food. There may be lawyers whose practice depends on prosecuting the mass animal poisoners, but I've yet to meet them.

Broadly speaking, the niche marketers' activities are not unethical or illegal. They are, however, dependent on the junk pet food bubble economy, the white-collar collaboration and failure of the veterinary self-regulatory system. No-one with a pet business wants to see their niche disappear. Unfortunately, despite the inherent cruelty of the system, I don't know of any people who campaign for change.

Outside experts

Given the magnitude of the junk pet food scam and the numerous niche marketers supportive of the system, it is nigh on impossible to find honest, objective professionals who will make public comment. From time to time I've tried to reach out to outside experts whose field of study overlaps with my concerns. Outside experts are not part of the junk pet food cult and could perhaps offer insight and advice while simultaneously obtaining data of benefit to their discipline. I've communicated how the junk pet food debacle provides a rich seam of information with immense potential to be mined by biologists, zoologists, ecologists, environmentalists, periodontists and human nutrition experts.

By way of example, dogs' mouths, relative to the size of their bodies, are about eight times the size of ours. Dogs live on average 15 years compared with our average 75 years. Consequently, the effects of oral disease and dependent diseases are more dramatic and occur in a compressed time frame. Simply stopping feeding junk foods often provides remarkable health improvements observable *in real time*. Old dogs and cats become miraculously like puppies and kittens again, verging on the biblical 'picking up their beds and frolicking'. Research professionals could take note and discover why.

Occasionally an outside expert has replied to my introductory email. But that's not usually the case. A wall of silence, a failure to respond has been the norm. Members of other professions don't want to stray onto veterinary turf outside their field of expertise. They don't want to tangle with vets and junk pet food makers. For the experts, the perceived benefits would be minimal and the potential reputational and other damage not worth the risk.

8

FALLACIES IN THE ALTERNATIVE

Nature abhors a vacuum

BARFers, prey-modellers and holistics

If the alliance between junk pet food companies and vets represents a bizarre global cult, then that cult provides numerous niches for subcults. The new wave of alternative diet proponents assert the benefits of 'golden grains', 'organic', 'range-fed', 'natural', 'fresh' and 'preservative-free' pet food. Some of the touted concoctions are freeze-dried, even sealed in a can. But most recipes call for raw ingredients. RAW (Righteous And Wrong?) feeder groups assert their authority in websites and Facebook pages. Opportunist marketers operate alongside, emphasising the word 'raw' as self-evident justification for their pulverised packaged concoctions bearing the image of a wild wolf.

'How do they get away with the subterfuge?' you may reasonably ask. Apart from the evident lack of regulation, there is one important aspect that the niche marketers rely on. Their products appear to improve the health of the pets, often greatly. However, the health improvements only partially derive from the raw ingredients. The main improvements derive from owners *stopping the feeding* of heat-treated, industrial junk from the can and packet.

It's the same if you stop bashing your head against a wall. Taking a deep breath or taking an aspirin or other pill may appear to help. But the main contributor to your improved health is that you *stopped* bashing your head.

Born Again Raw Feeders (BARFers)

These days thousands of unsuspecting pet owners fall prey to the BARF mythology. The acronym is said to stand for Biologically Appropriate Raw Food, or Bones And Raw Food. Most people are unaware that the acronym 'BARF' was first coined by followers of vet and raw feeding guru Ian Billinghurst in the early 1990s. At that time followers were filled with quasi-religious zeal. They had discovered the benefits of *stopping* the feeding of industrial junk and were busy in their kitchens and garages grinding and mincing fruit, vegetables, meat and supplements according to the recipes of the new messiah. With self-deprecating humour, they referred to themselves as Born Again Raw Feeders, contracted to BARF, which in American parlance is slang for vomit, puke or spew.

Ian Billinghurst, in his 1986 writings, did not promote his diet in its current form. Relying on the 1982 book *Dr Pitcairn's Complete Guide to Natural Health for Dogs & Cats*, and the 1970 book *The Complete Herbal Handbook for the Dog and Cat,* he advised dog owners:

> **Midday: A Carbohydrate Meal**
>
> Rolled oats soaked in hot water until like porridge. Alternatively Weet Bix or muesli or vegetables. Add to this such things as dates, sultanas, prunes, raisins, grated apple or carrot. Add honey.

> **Evenings: A Protein Meal**
> Raw meat e.g. mutton (excellent for dogs with skin conditions), beef, chicken, rabbit, kangaroo. Feed in large chunks to exercise the jaws and alert the digestive system. Sprinkle wheat germ, brewers yeast and bran over the meat.[1]

Two years later the Billinghurst musings included:

> **Fruit and Vegetables as Dog Food**
> Fruit and vegetables are an essential part of every dog's diet. An essential part, not an optional part. Meat is optional, fruit and vegetables are not. ...
>
> If a dog has never eaten vegetables before, it is amazing how a little hunger, e.g., several days without food, will stimulate an appetite for anything, including vegetables.
>
> Start off with the vegetables lightly steamed, and over a period of time, reduce the steaming period, presenting them eventually in the raw state. When raw, they should be cut very finely, grating being an excellent method. Prepare them freshly just before they are fed.[2]

In a complex world filled with competing theories, concepts and snippets of information, both good and bad, it should not surprise us that Billinghurst conveys some important truths. In his book *Give Your Dog a Bone* he comments:

> In addition to exercising and healthily stressing a dog's muscles and bone, all that ripping and tearing at big lumps of meat—on or off the bone, helps with a dog's digestion.
> ...

> The bone eating dog contrasts strongly to a dog fed it's [sic] food in a minced up, soft and soggy dollop. One or two gulps and it's gone. No work is required. The poor creature does not even have to go to the bother of standing up to eat. There is very little time for messages to be sent to alert the digestive system which remains unprepared. This mass of mush, slides past the tartar covered teeth which have not had to chew food for years, arriving as a leaden, lifeless lump in an unprepared stomach. Poor digestion, indigestion, and quite commonly diarrhoea result.[3]

Unfortunately, a few pages later Billinghurst returns to his vegetable theme in a chapter title.

> **Green Leafy Vegetables—an Essential Part of a Healthy dog's Diet**
>
> Because dogs are omnivores, vegetables, particularly green leafy vegetables should form a substantial part of their diet. They are not essential, however. Dogs can live and survive without such fare. There is only one problem. They will never be totally healthy. Their lives will be short, disease-ridden, and painful. In other words, vegetables are essential for dog's health. It is impossible for a dog to be totally healthy unless it spends a lifetime eating vegetables as a major part of it's [*sic*] diet.[4]

It's small wonder that the BARFers were rendered cross-eyed and confused. Science tells us that dogs, modified wolves, are carnivores. But according to Billinghurst they are 'omnivores'! In the headline he says vegetables are 'essential'. Then in the second sentence 'They are not essential' and in the second last sentence Billinghurst again asserts 'vegetables are essential'!

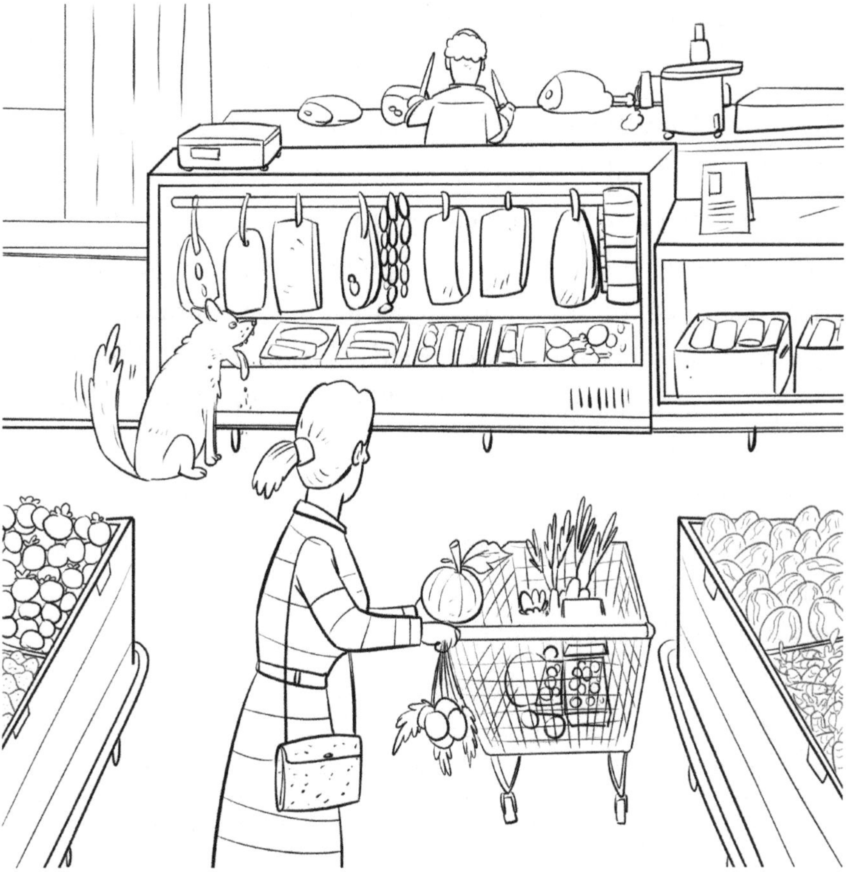

No matter the vegetable word salad jumble, BARFers were on the march. They had stopped feeding industrial cooked junk—with the magnificent resultant health benefits. A little bit of confusion as to whether dogs are carnivores and whether salad vegetables are *essential* did not deter them. Their dogs and cats were already showing health improvements. Billinghurst basked in the warm glow of sainthood, his halo burnished bright, as he planned his commercial future.

Raw Meaty Bones Lobby Group

I never knew the motivation for Ian Billinghurst's request to join the Raw Meaty Bones Lobby Group of concerned veterinarians. He told me he had seen my earlier writings and agreed wholeheartedly that raw meaty bones were key to the health and wellbeing of domestic dogs and cats. The lobby group, comprised of vets Breck Muir, Alan Bennet and me, were engaged in the political and scientific struggle against the junk pet food collaborators. The three of us, acting in concert, gained some credibility, and perhaps our united front provided a measure of defence against our opponents. We welcomed Ian Billinghurst as further reinforcement of our position.

Our media releases were intended to gain maximum impact. In September 1996 we drew attention to failings in the Australian Broadcasting Commission (ABC).

> We would draw your attention to the employment of a Dr Jonica Newby as a part time reporter on the ABC Science Show. Dr Newby's other occupation is as consultant to the Pet Care Information and Advisory Service (PIAS). PIAS is owned by the giant multi-national confectionery and pet food Mars Corporation. Dr Newby is also a Director of the Australian Veterinary Association which is sponsored by and promotes the interests of divisions of the Mars Corporation.
>
> PIAS devotes considerable resources to school visits throughout Australia. It is unlikely that primary school children would know of the connection between PIAS and its parent company. When a PIAS employee appeared in an infotainment segment (which we believe served to promote the interests of the Mars Corporation) on ABC

> Radio 2BL on 5 February 1993 there was no mention of the parent company. Coverage on the ABC and in schools carries connotations of official approval and is of correspondingly greater value to the advertiser.[5]

On 5 March 1997 we continued shining a light on the Mars Corporation front Petcare Information and Advisory Service.

> **Pet food front**
>
> There is a 'wolf in sheep's clothing' roaming through Australian primary schools.
>
> Masquerading as an educational organisation the 'Petcare Information and Advisory Service' (PIAS) was exposed by Stuart Littlemore (ABC Media Watch 3/3/97) as: 'nothing more than a front for the multi-national pet food manufacturer Mars, through its Australian subsidiary Uncle Bens.'
>
> Media Watch demonstrated how a PIAS vet targeted the listeners of the ABC Radio National Science Show with a 'crudely subtle pitch'. Littlemore said, 'Jonica Newby didn't tell us to buy Pal in so many words, but to keep pets. Well, we have to buy food for them don't we!'
>
> If the Science Show audience, made up of scientists and administrators, can be duped what hope is there for our primary school children?
>
> PIAS visits schools with its 'flip charts' carefully programming our children to become docile consumers of Uncle Bens products.
>
> A particularly disturbing development is the use of a programme called 'PetPEP'.
>
> Purported to be an educational programme this is a

joint Australian Veterinary Association, PIAS venture. There is a classroom module for each of years K to 6 complete with activity suggestions and PIAS/Selectapet promotional material.

Many issues are raised by this woeful state of affairs. Apart from the obvious indoctrination issues there is the matter of artificial pet foods damaging the health of our pets, the national economy and the natural environment.

These matters have been repeatedly drawn to the attention of the relevant authorities, but they refuse to act. Why?[6]

Unfortunately, no sooner had Billinghurst joined the lobby group and given us increased strength than he resigned by letter.

Dear Tom,

I am writing to you because it is the only way I can collect, organise and present my thoughts with clarity and coherence. I have been giving a lot of thought to why I feel uneasy being involved in the politics of the 'natural food/raw meaty bones question'. I want you to understand my role is totally different to yours. I am not a political animal. I am not a stirrer. It is not in my nature to attack people or institutions or commercial organisations. ...

If I am to be of use, I need to be seen as outside the political arena. Someone who has the respect of the profession, whilst retaining strong views and unequivocal beliefs—supported of course by good evidence. My aim is to make a positive difference in this debate, and continue to make a living.

As a consequence, I cannot continue as a signatory to the political activities of the Raw Meaty Bones Lobby. ... [7]

For a time, Breck, Alan and I continued distributing our media releases. Our opponents—Mars, Nestlé, Colgate and the Australian Veterinary Association—were doubtless pleased to see that the lobby, always small, was now depleted and on the wane.

Billinghurst's stocks, however, continued in the ascendant. Numerous internet chat groups sprang up extolling the alleged benefits of Billinghurst's diet—pre-eminent among them the BARF chat group with many thousands of members, mostly resident in the USA.

Subscribers to the group posted their questions, for instance about green leafy vegetables, bottled supplements and where to buy meat grinders. A select group, BARF moderators, dispensed their wisdom to the 'Newbie BARFers' from 1997 until March 2002.

BARF trouble brewing

A couple of chat group postings in November 2001 heralded the storm ahead. A post under the heading 'Dr B's new web site' alerted list members to the establishment of BARF World, Billinghurst's new North American commercial venture selling frozen BARF products and bottled supplements. Another wrote: 'I have noticed that a lot of people on this site don't feed their dogs veggies or feed very little of them. I am confused ...' As consternation grew among the list participants, behind the scenes the chat group administrators were reading the newly published book *Raw Meaty Bones: Promote Health*. They surely took note that, among other things, the book undermined their BARF mythology. They invited me to appear as guest author on the discussion list.

Over those three days in December 2001, we enjoyed a lively and respectful internet discourse regarding raw meaty bones essentials. My lingering recollection, however, was the sound of a collective 'jaw-drop'. From the questions and comments received, it was clear the BARFers were suddenly not so sure of their rigid beliefs.

In February 2002 a list member wrote:

> Now, he [Billinghurst] has his own brand of 'complete and balanced' food 'and supplements' ... He's done the raw feeding movement a 'huge' disservice by turning his back on it and going over to the 'prepared pet food' side, one remove from the dogfood companies that have wrecked the health of so many dogs. You don't honestly believe that most people will see a difference, do you? They'll simply think of the B—— diet as one more of the more expensive and presumably quality pet foods on the market.

Another wrote:

> I don't begrudge anyone, including Billinghurst, the ability to make a living. ... BUT when you start trademarking words like BARF and BARF World, I think a line has been stepped over. He is trademarking a name for the diet that someone else thought up. He is also trademarking a name that is another word for vomit. This is not 'his' diet, it is nature's diet. In my opinion the very worst thing that could happen to the raw diet movement and the battles we have with pet food companies and veterinarians is for one of the main spokespeople to sell out.

Clearly the BARFer throng were annoyed and plotting revenge. We didn't have long to discover their solution: close down their BARF chat list and regroup elsewhere. They migrated *en masse*. Their new place of residence: the Rawfeeding List. Their new holy mantra: 'Prey model'.

BARF spew across the globe

Ian Billinghurst, despite being rejected and discarded by his previously adoring fans, pushed on with ever-expanding zeal. Whether under his banner or as imitators, numerous companies jumped on the get-rich-quick bandwagon.

In Australia, his trademark-protected 'minced up, soft and soggy dollop' came in a box labelled 'Doctor B's BARF' and bearing three technicolour pictures of Doctor B. Accordingly, the technicolour 'Beef recipe' seems especially apt.

> Beef, finely ground chicken bone, beef liver, whole egg, yoghurt, cabbage or bok choy, celery, spinach or silver beet, carrot, ground flax seed meal, dried alfalfa leaf powder, beef heart, unbleached beef tripe, whole apples, dried kelp powder, garlic, oranges, salmon frames.

Interested to know more, I bought a pack and waited for the reddish-purple contents to thaw. I scooped some into my hand and felt the gritty, greasy slime ooze between my fingers—reminiscent of boysenberry ice cream spilled in a child's sandpit.

The Hong Kong BARF website asks the rhetorical question:

> **Why choose Dr. B's Genuine Aussie R.A.W. B.A.R.F. patties?**
> Switching to the BARF diet can be a daunting experience. That is why Dr. Billinghurst developed a safe and easy BARF diet which is as convenient as feeding dry dog food.
> ...
> The product has been a sold-out success in Australia, the UK, the USA, Japan, Singapore and Taiwan.[8]

In the UK, Nick Thompson, vet and BARF company marketing man promoted the company wares. Back in March 2003 he had this to say:

> Today I flicked through the ukbarfclub discussion forum; the discussion site affiliated with AMP and saw that there was some discussion on the non-meat (fruit and veg) component of dog diets—quality and quantity. I just thought I'd give you my penny's worth.
>
> Firstly, I have to state that dogs are not carnivores. Tom Lonsdale, in his book *Raw Meaty Bones*, gives guidance for cats and dogs as if they were had similar eating habits. I'm sorry Tom, cats are not just small dogs, they have a completely different nutritional need, dental pattern, gastrointestinal set up and behaviour, reflecting their differences. Cats are carnivores, yes. Dogs are omnivores; carnivorous omnivores, perhaps, but omnivores all the same.
>
> Omnivores eat meat (including everything else in a carcase—perhaps we should call them carcasivores?) and non-meat. Even in the frozen wastes of Siberia or Northern Canada they will eat mainly herbivore carcases—carcases full of vegetation. Even if, in these extreme circumstances, wolves can survive, they do not thrive as the diet is minimal in quantity and quality. We can feed our dogs a lot of good quality fruit and veg to optimise the diet. I think we should.
>
> Man has survived on a sub optimal diet for his/her entire evolution until about 100 years ago. This does not mean we should continue eating roots and the odd rabbit. One of the major contributors to human health, alongside the sterling work of Mr. Crapper and all the other san-

itation engineers through the ages, is diet (not doctors, vaccines and antibiotics as some will tell you). Improved diet means improved health. Always. Incontrovertibly—always. If we are doing it for us, why not for our dogs? Eating well is easy to do and makes so much sense.

Dog's digestion is more like man than a cat's, so this is why I suggest a 30-50% inclusion of meat in the diet I recommend. Raw meaty bones are on top of this, so at a push the meat proportion could reach 60% for the very fit and very young (if high protein suits them). Fruit, vegetables, seeds, nuts and herbs all contain components that are not found in carcases. Offering a good variety of all of these things takes our wolf model from scraping an existence on the nutritional edge to thriving in nutritional plenty.

Blending the fruit is a good idea. The same goes for root and leaf veg. Plenty of variety is a good thing. Most meals should have a green tinge if you can. Colour is a good way to ensure variety—if you're giving a good variety of colour, then you can be pretty sure you're getting all the food groups. Grinding the nuts and seeds mimics the action of herbivore teeth allowing greater digestion of these things. Herbs are not just for flavour—they contain minerals and vitamins and contribute to a rounding of the diet.

If you find preparing fruit and veg a bit of a pain, then please note that those nice people at AMP have thought of this and done all the dirty work for you. Nature's Menu Frozen Range offers a choice of diets where raw meat and veg have been mixed and frozen for you. They are ideal for those too busy to do the whole BARF diet or for those who can but find holidays and trips difficult.

> So, I hope this helps to clarify my position on the how much non-meat should I feed my dog question. Please feel free to write to Jon and I via the Anglian Meat Product website.
>
> Nick Thompson BSc. (Hons), BVM&S, VetMFHom, MRCVS[9]

In more recent times Dr Thompson presides over the Raw Feeding Veterinary Society. Their website proclaims:

> The gold standard diet is as close to the evolutionary diet of dogs and cats as is practically possible, is made from fresh frozen raw meaty bones, meats, organ meats, fruits and vegetables, minimally processed by mincing and freezing. The diet contains no added synthetic supplements, additives or preservatives.[10]

They say approvingly that:

> The number of raw pet food manufacturers has increased from five in 2013 to ninety in 2018.

and:

> The majority of raw pet food companies in the UK are using high quality raw meaty bones, and organ meats, sourced from the human food chain, of known provenance. There are currently nine raw pet food companies listed on the PFMA [Pet Food Manufacturers Association] website. These companies are following the *Guidelines for the Manufacture of Raw Pet Food in the UK*. As raw pet food

> has become more popular with dog and cat owners, so too has demand for hard evidence as to its nutritional adequacy and safety. Veterinary professionals, in particular, seek reassurance. Naturally, they do not wish to recommend anything that could have adverse health implications.

As you are now a reader well versed in the biological imperative for pet dogs and cats to rip and tear at raw meaty bones, I wonder about your opinion on the current state of play—Mars, Nestlé and Colgate in control with *manufacturers* of raw pet food multiplying and joining the Pet Food Manufacturers Association club.

Prey-modellers

The original BARFer leadership tore off their BARF labels and affixed another: 'Prey Model'. What, you may well ask, is a prey model?

In ecological science 'prey model' describes the dynamics of ecological systems in which two species interact, one a predator and the other its prey—for instance fox and rabbit, cat and mouse.[11] That, however, is not what the prey-modellers use as their standard. Instead, they have manufactured a completely new definition in which the imaginary 'prey' of cats and dogs can be reduced to a 'model' recipe of 80 per cent meat, 10 per cent offal and 10 per cent bone.

Righteously, they berate anyone who dares to disagree with them. Of course, whether a rabbit, a mouse, a fish, a bird or an elephant, no prey animal is comprised of this 80–10–10 formula. Equally absurd is their denouncement of feeding raw meaty bones because, they say, that leads to too much bone!

For a time, I tried to persuade them of the raw meaty bones essentials. I tried to explain the need for ripping and tearing and how chicken carcasses, after most of the meat has been removed for human consumption, come from six-week-old birds. Bone is non-toxic and full of nutrients in the Haversian system, the network of tubes within the bone. And in any case, young birds' bones are soft and comprise much cartilage—which for carnivores is readily digestible protein. Staying pragmatic, securing the balance of affordability, availability and health benefits are the critical issues when deciding how best to feed a domestic dog or cat.

But I was silenced, banned from their discussion list and accorded pariah status. When pet owners ask which books are best for helping with diet matters, the prey model high priests declare: 'There are no good books, all you need do is follow our prey model advice'.

Holistics

An incessant din rises up from the hordes of 'holistics' and other niche marketers. They swarm over the battlefield, trampling raw meaty bones principles.

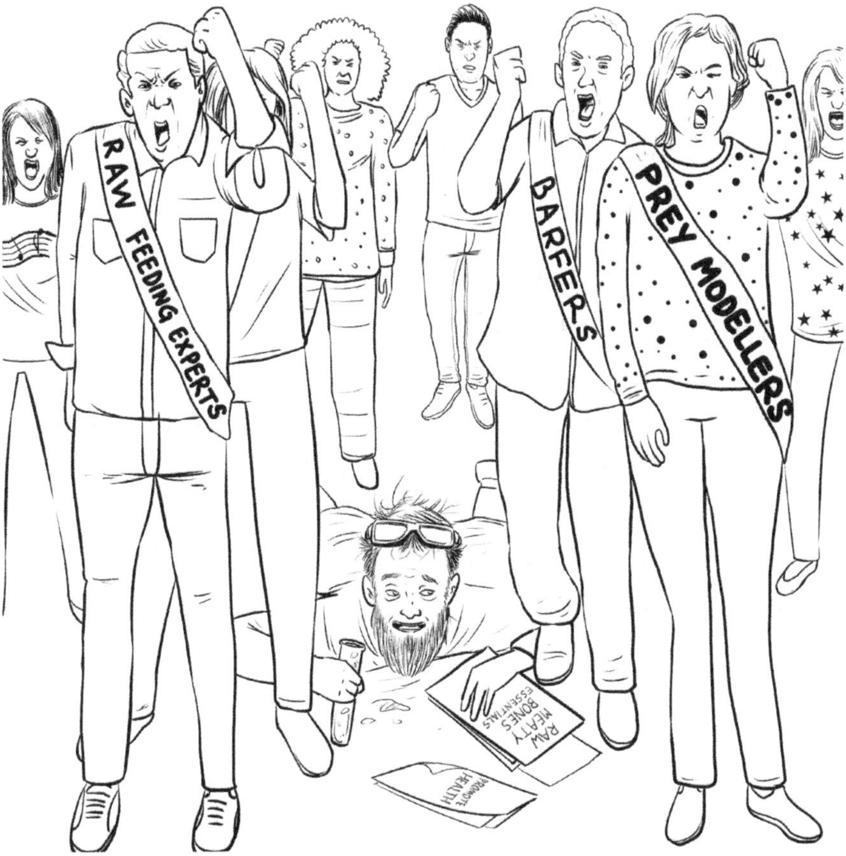

They claim to have discovered the truth, become enlightened as to the inadequacies of junk foods and conventional vet practice. But instead of combining forces to defeat the junk pet food manufacturers and their vet enablers, they pontificate on the minutiae of Bach flower remedies and the virtues of shark cartilage extract. It's another instance of 'more a part of the problem than part of the solution'. The Mars Corporation, Nestlé and Colgate must be delighted.

Dr Marty Goldstein tells visitors to his website:

> I've been a frequent guest on many national television shows, like The Oprah Winfrey Show, The Martha Stewart Show, and Good Morning America. I'm also the author of The Nature of Animal Healing—one [of] the most widely read books on pet health.[12]

Of his freeze-dried products he says:

> **Dr. Marty Your Pet's Best Friend**
> For over four decades, Dr. Marty has been a leading voice in veterinary medicine. Many experts—and thousands of satisfied clients—consider him to be America's foremost integrative veterinarian. Dr. Marty knows what your dog needs to stay their healthiest. That's why our premium pet food is always grain free, with multiple protein sources and essential vitamins and minerals to keep your best friend healthy and happy.

Have a look at what USA company Volhard Nutrition says on its website.

> AM Porridge is part one of a two-part dehydrated foundation mix (AM/PM) which eliminates prep work and allows maximum control over ingredient freshness and vegetable choice. NDF AM/PM gives you the flexibility to meet any special dietary needs your dog may have. The uniqueness of this recipe separates certain digestible nutrients so that a dog having issues digesting different ingredients at the same time are completely eliminated.

Why Feed Protein and Veggies Separately?
Regardless if you are feeding a Raw Diet or a Kibble based diet, you should be feeding raw fruits and vegetables separately from the protein in your dog's diet. Protein is digested at a much slower rate and when fed together, the fruits and vegetables will 'push' the protein through the GI tract much quicker than the nutrition can be absorbed. Feeding fruits and vegetables separately in the day allows them to have a chance to be well on their way out of the body before you introduce the protein for the day.[13]

Sundry false prophets

By now you've seen enough false prophets. I'll spare you the pain of listing more who are intent on separating you from your hard-earned cash.

However, beware; the wellbeing of your pet depends on you. Beware the many with the indifference to animal suffering who sell packaged pap supported by claims that are too good to be true. Beware the writers of books who suppress biological imperatives and push fantastical recipes.

Nature got it right, is honest and unimpeachable. Nature sets the rules. The con artists who break the rules should be prosecuted for animal cruelty and consumer fraud. Good luck.

9

THE MEDIA: GOOD, BAD AND UGLY

Much pet-feeding and pet-keeping information comes by word of mouth, frequently handed down from generation to generation. However, it is the media that supplies the bulk of the information informing our daily lives. In past times printed newspapers, magazines and books were primary sources. These days it is mostly the electronic media that cycles and recycles information—television, radio, film, social media, blogs, online news, magazines and ebooks. Since most information about feeding pets is variously misleading, false and harmful, the media in all its guises bears heavy responsibility.

The media, we can assume, knows its audience, and knows what the audience wants and will pay for—with advertising revenue sometimes running into the millions of dollars. Watch the pet food ads, the lifestyle programs and vet reality shows. The media holds up a mirror to the wider public who either see themselves reflected or wish to see themselves reflected. It's a winning formula that plays on an endless loop. Dogs, cats and ferrets are the unwitting props, the status symbols and fashion statements whose ancestry and biology seldom get a mention.

Besides informing, educating and entertaining, the media is supposed to fulfil another very important role as investigators and gatekeepers of the public interest. Sometimes referred to as the Fourth

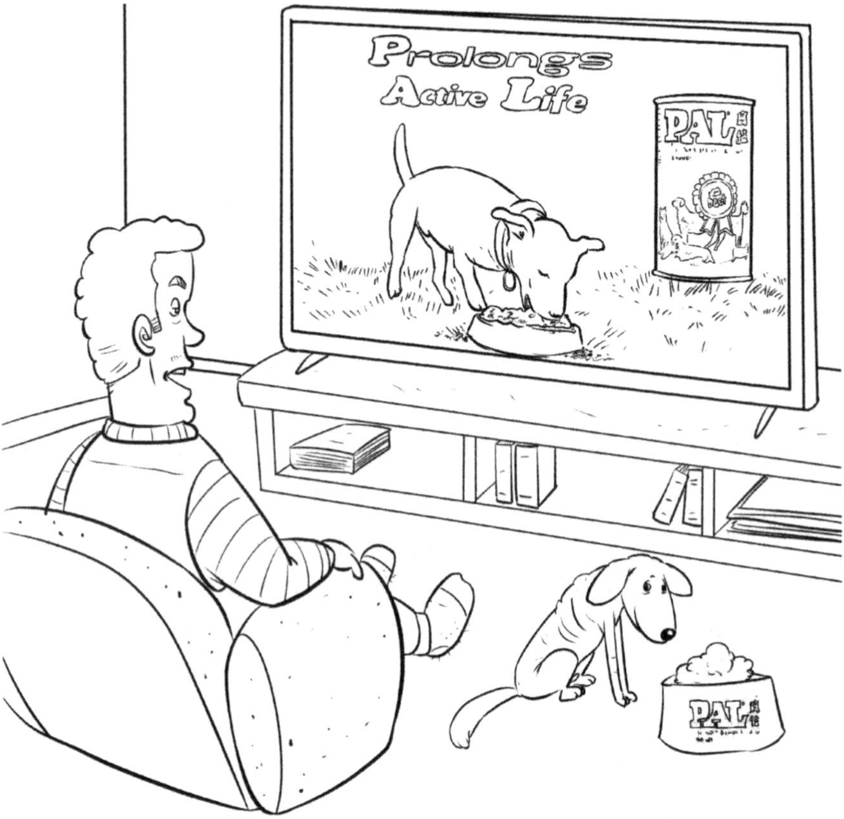

Estate of the realm, media organisations as watchdogs are supposed to interrogate the holders of power; they are supposed to frame debate and in general protect the welfare of the wider community. Plainly, then, in respect to the junk pet food criminal collaboration the media fails dismally.

Brainwashing the community has been going on, courtesy of the media, ever since Jack Spratt manufactured his Wheat Fibrine Dog Cakes in the 1860s. Since when, of course, media moguls have got rich and so have the junk pet food makers—principally the Mars family,[1] Nestlé and Colgate-Palmolive. With their fortunes so closely intertwined, it is no surprise that the media moguls and would-be media moguls are reluctant to rock the boat. And if a media outlet were sufficiently ethical to run a campaign on the junk pet food issue, it would not only jeopardise its junk pet food advertising revenue but also all the other lucrative ads across numerous categories and product lines belonging to Mars, Nestlé and Colgate.

Already we see that the media is next to useless in the fight against the mass pet poisoners. And alas, as we shall see in the next chapter, politicians are no better. Social, scientific, humanitarian gridlock is the order of the day. Hans Christian Andersen provided a beautiful illustration of this in his parable *The Emperor's New Clothes*.[2] All the onlookers could see that the emperor, parading before them, was stark naked. The emperor had been duped into believing he was wearing robes of the finest woven thread. The onlookers, for their own reasons, could not bring themselves to admit the evidence of their own eyes. Finally, a small boy in the crowd broke the spell. He exclaimed that the emperor wore no clothes. In protecting our pets we need to be that 'small boy'. We cannot rely on the media; we must sound the alarm and publicise the naked truth ourselves.

The good

The Veterinarian

Here and there some good information has made it into the media, but it has been mostly short-lived.

In 1993, a new Australian vet magazine, *The Veterinarian*, was launched. The first edition carried a prominent headline: 'Diet debate opens more than just a can of worms'. See how the central issues were the same in 1993 as now:

> For the past six months, Dr Lonsdale has been writing about the toxic effects of periodontal disease in pets. A job which he has taken up full-time.

> Dr Lonsdale said his passion for the issue was so intense because he believed it was the 'greatest consumer fraud in the western world'.
>
> 'And vets are up to their necks in it,' he said. ...
>
> 'Despite the debate, thousands of vets are not only advising pet owners to feed their animals processed food, they are also profiting from its sale. They then further profit in the treatment that ensues.' ...
>
> 'It is not me who determines the suitability of food for animals, it's nature. I'm just drawing attention to a reality that everyone else is choosing to ignore.' ...
>
> He said his fight against the 'evils' of processed pet food would continue to the grave, or until the pet food manufacturers folded—whichever came first.'[3]

The same edition carried the statement:

> Pet food manufacturers and many veterinarians rejected Dr Lonsdale's claims on the basis they were unsubstantiated and ran counter [to] the proven knowledge of leaders in the fields of pet nutrition and dentistry.

In interview sessions for the inaugural edition, *Veterinarian* journalists were friendly and communicative. But, as if a switch had been flicked, straight after publication they became cold and remote. Clearly those with 'proven knowledge' in the fields of pet nutrition and dentistry were back in control.

ABC Television

Also, in the dim and distant 1990s there was a flickering on *The Investigators*, a consumer affairs program broadcast on ABC television.[4] The ABC is government-owned and does not run pet food advertisements. Over a period of three months the *Investigators* journalists did a fine job. They got to the crux of the issues.

A shopper in a supermarket junk pet food aisle was asked 'Do you ever feed your cats bones?' He replied matter-of-factly 'No, never'. Another shopper with a beaming smile giggled 'Our vet suggested we brush our cat's teeth'. The president of the Australian Veterinary Dental Society provided viewers with a mixed message:

> Most dogs now are on more convenience food, and we have to accept that. But the best thing to do would be to go and give your dog probably an oxtail with the hide still on it once a week, but that's just socially not acceptable.

The big cats at Taronga Zoo were less constrained. Video of them ripping and tearing at raw meaty bones sent a clear message—further endorsed by the zoo vet:

> We haven't seen any signs of periodontal disease in any of our big cats or canids and some of these big cats can be up to over twenty years of age.

And they filmed me pulling the teeth from a badly diseased Maltese terrier. The accompanying journalist's voiceover delivered with heartfelt emphasis:

> Sydney vet Tom Lonsdale believes it's through that very change of diet that today's pet lovers are condemning their carnivorous companions to a life of ill-health and misery.

At the time we were elated with the prime-time television exposure. We received word that the Australian Veterinary Association president had seen the segment on Qantas in-flight entertainment. Could we expect some shift in attitude? Alas, no. There was no follow-up; no desire on the part of the ABC to explore further. Subject closed.

Sydney Morning Herald

Elizabeth Farrelly writes with flair. Her July 2013 column in the *Sydney Morning Herald* carried unmistakable truths about her two cats.

> Cats are carnivores, and carnivores hunt. Even Jack and Diesel hunt. Twigs. Leaves. Cockroaches (crunchy!). Bogongs. Baby rats. Inadvertent mynahs (rare) and, despite long-term lizard-aversion therapy, the occasional drop-tail skink.
>
> Frankly? Half a can of jellified ex-meat spooned out with the evening news doesn't cut it in the thrill department.
>
> There's also this. That can of Purrfect Pussy is like putting your kids on a Maccas three times a day.
>
> Jack, age four or five, was diagnosed with feline urinary tract disease. He had trouble peeing and needed a scientifically formulated biscuit diet, $66 a bag. To feed him anything else, the vet said, risked hospitalisation and death.
>
> It got worse. A couple of years later, Diesel developed dreadful smelly breath. He grew listless and refused food. The vet diagnosed feline stomatitis. Said he needed antibiotics, possible dental surgery and regular tooth cleaning.
>
> I'm sorry, what? Me, twice a day with a cat toothbrush? There had to be a better way.
>
> Meanwhile Jack, on his exorbitant science-nosh, was

> permanently ravenous. He lost weight and, under the big fur, became bird light. He was anxious, and started escaping over the back fence at night, hunting. At least once a week I'd find a baby rat, or a tail, or just a blood-smear, on the bathroom floor.
>
> Before re-mortgaging the house, I did what you do. Googled, found a website called Raw Meaty Bones. The message was obvious and compelling. I decided to try it. For a month, I gave them each a daily, raw chicken wing. Period. Pretty soon both cats were bouncing. No trouble peeing. No bad-breath or sore inflamed gums. Their coats became thicker and glossier. Two happy cats.[5]

Did you notice the reference to 'exorbitant science-nosh'? It's my guess Elizabeth Farrelly was referring to Hill's Science Diet but chose not to antagonise Colgate-Palmolive by naming and shaming their nasty product.

The bad

I characterise the media performance as good, bad or ugly, not in respect to the performance of individual journalists but according to published outcomes. Pre-eminent New York journalist John Swinton well knew, in the 1880s, that bad outcomes were the norm. He advised his colleagues:

> There is no such thing, at this date of the world's history, in America, as an independent press. You know it and I know it.
>
> There is not one of you who dares to write your honest opinions, and if you did, you know beforehand that it

> would never appear in print. I am paid weekly for keeping my honest opinion out of the paper I am connected with. Others of you are paid similar salaries for similar things, and any of you who would be so foolish as to write honest opinions would be out on the streets looking for another job. If I allowed my honest opinions to appear in one issue of my paper, before twenty-four hours my occupation would be gone.
>
> The business of the journalists is to destroy the truth, to lie outright, to pervert, to vilify, to fawn at the feet of mammon, and to sell his country and his race for his daily bread. You know it and I know it, and what folly is this toasting an independent press?
>
> We are the tools and vassals of rich men behind the scenes. We are the jumping jacks, they pull the strings and we dance. Our talents, our possibilities and our lives are all the property of other men. We are intellectual prostitutes.[6]

In 2001 a brave Australian journalist attempted to announce the launch of *Raw Meaty Bones: Promote Health.* The journalist well understood the significance of the book and took the unusual step of allowing me to see an advance copy of the proposed article:

> Well-meaning cat and dog owners are causing long-lasting damage to their pets by feeding them commercial pet foods, according to a new book. Veterinarian Tom Lonsdale claims in a new book that all cats and dogs need bones as part of their diet to keep them healthy. But he says many vets promote and sell the processed foods despite the problems they cause, because of their close links with

the multi-billion-dollar pet food industry.

'If you own a dog or a cat which you feed with processed food from the supermarket or corner store, you will probably find this book deeply disturbing,' Dr Lonsdale said in the preface.

The launch of the book coincides with a campaign by the American pet food company, Ralston Purina, using Sydney University veterinary students to promote its products in supermarkets.

The company claimed last week it had hired the students to promote its 'optimal nutritional excellence' pet foods because Australian consumers were the most uneducated in the western world about pet nutrition.

But Dr Lonsdale argues in detail, using his own experience as a vet at South Windsor, the experience of other local vets and overseas research that dogs and cats need to chew on bones to prevent mouth disease. According to pet-food company Hill's, seven out of 10 adult pets have some degree of dental problems.

Without bones, their gums quickly become diseased, leading to tooth problems, bad breath and an array of systemic problems including a drop in white blood cells. As a result, they could develop serious immune deficiencies which Dr Lonsdale likened to the AIDS in people, although it is not caused by a virus.

'It's not a matter of whether artificial pet foods and food-induced periodontal disease give rise to ill health, it's more a matter of which disease, when and how,' he said.

Dr Lonsdale advocates giving cats and dogs raw chicken wings, chicken necks and ox tail to young kittens and puppies when they most need to chew. 'Older larger dogs need raw bones and cats need raw meat on the bone,' he says.

Dr Lonsdale said the book was intended to give pet owners the information to challenge their vets and overcome the most common problems for cats and dogs. He said pet owners often did not notice the problems until they were far advanced, especially in dogs which intuitively hide ailments. Although opening a can or a bag of dried food was convenient, he said most pet owners cared deeply for their animals and wanted the best for them.

'People have been led to believe that owning a cat or dog is a simple matter and feeding can be dealt with using commercial offerings,' he said. 'But if they start to see themselves as responsible zookeepers, looking after animals without bars, they will enjoy pet ownership much more and have fewer problems.'

Dr Lonsdale had to fight the veterinary profession to make his claims, which included that the Australian Veterinary Association had become too closely involved with commercial pet food companies. When he first raised his concerns in 1996, he was accused of professional misconduct and threatened with being struck off the veterinary register.

He was even threatened with jail if he revealed the nature of four complaints which were made about him to the NSW Veterinary Surgeons Investigating Committee (VSIC), all of which were later dropped. The investigatory committee claimed then that Dr Lonsdale was 'stating extremist views in a very public forum that he has not supported publicly by scientific data'.

NSW MLA Paul Lynch has raised Dr Lonsdale's treatment by the VSIC in Parliament several times as well as other concerns about the committee.

Another of Dr Lonsdale's targets is the Petcare Information and Advisory Service, which promotes dog and cat ownership. Although it does not declare this, Petcare is funded by Uncle Ben's, a subsidiary of Mars Group (which also makes Mars Bars), Australia's biggest pet food company. A Petcare spokeswoman declined to comment on Dr Lonsdale's views and said the service did not really advise people on nutrition. However, its website strongly advocates the use of commercial foods.

'The most reliable and convenient way to provide a balanced and palatable diet is to feed high quality prepared dog food, both canned and dry,' it says on its website. 'Puppies have different nutritional requirements to adult dogs and for this reason it is essential to feed your puppy with specially formulated puppy foods in canned and dry forms.'

AILMENTS WHICH PROCESSED PET FOODS CAN CAUSE IN DOGS:

Source: Dr Tom Lonsdale, author, 'Raw Meaty Bones'.

1. Bad breath. This is not natural in dogs and is a sign of 'mouth rot'.
2. Lack of a shiny glossy coat, itchy skin. Dog looks poor, unkempt, unhappy.
3. Prolonged sleeping, dull eyes, too thin or too fat.
4. Gastroenteritis, persistent diarrhoea. liver problems,
5. Arthritis, stiffness, poor circulation, collagen disease.

Upon submitting the article for proofreading and final editing, the journalist received a nasty shock. He was called into the boss's office and told, among other things, that the article would *not* be published.

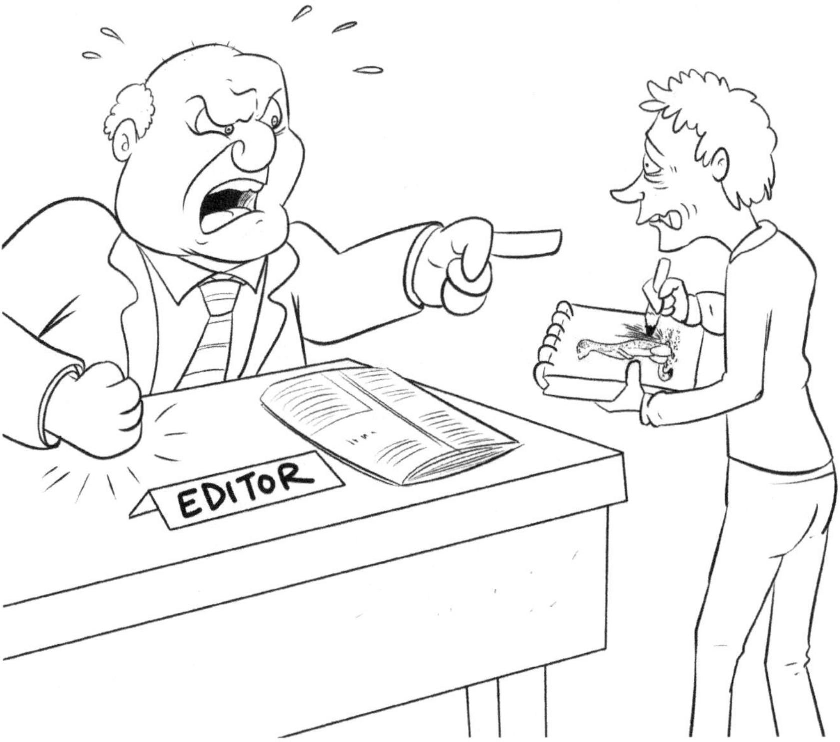

Now, 21 years later, that ruling has been finally overturned and the article is publicly available 'on the record'.

Of the threats levelled at the journalist and the reasons given, history does not relate. We do know, however, that a Mars Corporation promo for its forthcoming 'patent pending' junk appeared in the newspaper disguised as a news item. Note the false assumptions and weasel words laying the groundwork for the next Mars-generated con.

> **New Food Helps Pets Live Longer**
> An experimental pet food makes cats and dogs live longer by reducing the damage done to genetic material linked to the disease of ageing.
>
> Preliminary evidence was presented recently to a gathering of academics and vets in Vancouver, Canada.
>
> Patents are pending on the food, which mixes antioxidants, notably vitamins C and E which mop up damaging chemical intermediates, called radicals.

Simultaneously, in August 2001 the science writer for the *Weekend Australian*, a Murdoch newspaper, wrote an article complete with photographs publicising the launch of *Raw Meaty Bones*. However, you guess correctly, the article failed to appear. Subsequently the journalist, to whom I had provided reams of accurate, essential information, refused to discuss reasons for the about-face and thereafter refused to take my calls. Discussion closed.

Sunday Independent

A lengthy, thoroughly researched article by UK *Sunday Independent* journalist Jonathan Owen met a similar fate—twice.

Journalists mostly try to keep a detached separation from their sources. So, I was most pleasantly surprised when Jonathan Owen telephoned from London to tell me his article was due to be published that weekend. Surprise soon turned to disappointment. The article failed to appear in the paper. I wrote to Jonathan:

> Thanks for your call the other evening. I appreciated that extra effort at the end of lengthy and detailed investigations.
>
> You are likely as disappointed as we are about the

> absence of the article in Sunday's paper. Is this part of the process where features sometimes get delayed or is it part of editorial policy meaning it's been vetoed?

By return Jonathan wrote:

> The story was bumped off at the last minute due to something else coming in that was deemed more topical for that week and it was in no way vetoed. It is on the list for this Sunday and, given the number of articles about fat dogs in the UK recently, I am confident/hopeful that it will go through.

That Sunday and several more Sundays passed and still no sign of the article. Indeed, the London *Sunday (not-so) Independent* newspaper, having thoroughly researched the issues, cannot pretend ignorance. They knew the significance for their readership and wider community; they knew the monetary and editorial costs of researching the truth. They chose to throw away their costs and jeopardise their integrity. They vetoed the article. But why?

Throughout the research phase they could have but did not activate their self-censorship button—they could have simply closed their eyes and pretended that they never knew. My guess is that the *Sunday Independent* sought comment from Mars/Nestlé/Colgate or their proxies about the proposed article critical of junk pet food. It is the way media outlets protect themselves against being sued. They invite those criticised to present their side of the argument and to correct factual details before going to press.

Until whistleblowers tell us or until there are government inquiries, we are left with guesswork as to the pressures brought to bear by the mega-rich junk pet food makers. Do the companies threaten legal action? Do they threaten to remove advertising revenue? Do they promise to increase their advertising spend if the newspaper agrees to publish a series of photos and articles promoting dog ownership?

Over the years I've contacted lots of journals and newspapers in an attempt to interest them in the pet food fraud. Mostly I've been given the cold shoulder. Briefly there was a flickering of interest from *National Geographic*, but it soon flickered out.

Reader's Digest Magazine

David Hurst, a freelance journalist working for the *Reader's Digest*, contacted me, with an invitation to help him with 'a large in-depth article on pet food testing for *Reader's Digest Magazine* to appear in the UK and 50 further countries'. Almost too good to be true, I thought, while hoping to be proved wrong. Over succeeding months my confidence increased. David posed numerous questions. I provided comprehensive answers. He got the full unvarnished truth about the collaboration between junk pet food makers and vets. After he completed his article, fact-checker Angelika Romacker took over. She wrote:

> The British edition of *Reader's Digest Magazine* is planning to publish an article on pet food. I understand you were interviewed by our journalist David Hurst, and you are now quoted in this article. As we have a policy of checking articles for accuracy before publication, I'd be grateful if you could let me know that what we are planning to publish is accurate. Please find the text below. I have included a few questions in square brackets which I hope you might be able to answer.
>
> If you let me have your address, we will of course send

> you complimentary copies upon publication.
>
> As I'm working to a tight deadline, I'd be grateful if you could get back to me at your earliest convenience.

In total I counted 86 emails sent back and forth between David Hurst, Angelika Romacker and me. Clearly *Reader's Digest* invested heavily in the article. It was sure to have a big impact, I believed and hoped—up until Angelika sent the message:

> Well, the article has been postponed; I think there was another article that came in that was more urgent. I understand editors are planning to revisit the issue in the near future.

That was back in November 2007. The previous 'tight deadline' turned into a very long wait!

Over the long wait what has *Reader's Digest* been doing about the junk pet food fraud? With photos and articles, they have been continuing the relentless drip-feed of junk pet food propaganda. Just today I stopped at the newsagents to pick up a copy. As the saying goes, 'a picture is worth a thousand words' and hence the photo glorifying a small fluffy dog on the front cover. Inside there was an article by 'Our regular pet columnist, Dr Katrina Warren, ... an established and trusted animal expert'. Dr Warren advises in bold block capitals: 'INTRODUCE YOUR PET TO TEETH BRUSHING'. The accompanying photo depicts a cutesy toy dog with pink toothbrush and red ribbon in the topknot.[7]

Keeping vets in the frame, Dr Warren assures pet owners there's no need to worry: 'Professional dental checks by your vet may include an X-ray, thorough cleaning under anaesthesia and occasional tooth removal.' Good, that's settled, everything's OK then!

The ugly

Pet owners beware. The blogosphere, pet feeding books and magazines are overpopulated with vanity publishers intent on gaining (illicit) power, prestige and profit from their specious reasoning. Some of the worst offenders start out with a clear understanding of the dietary needs of pet carnivores, but then lose track and lose focus with meandering commentary piling confusing notions upon confusing notions.

One online magazine, I recall, commissioned me to write a definitive article on the dietary needs of pet cats and dogs for their first edition. In subsequent editions the published information became increasingly watered down, misleading and harmful. This is a function of the vanity press. It appears that once truth is told, it cannot be retold and still hold the interest of the readership. By deliberately suppressing known truths and replacing them with false and confusing factoids, the vanity press draws its readers into a sticky inescapable web with a life of its own.

A case can be made for including in this 'ugly' section all media outlets that suppress truth and simultaneously push junk pet food propaganda. However, I draw attention to the *Veterinarian*, the Australian Broadcasting Corporation and the *Sydney Morning Herald* as prime examples for the simple reason that years ago they knew and understood the gravity of the issues. At that time, they resisted threats or inducements from vets and junk food makers and published accurate, critical articles. Unfortunately, ever since, over many years, they have *chosen* to be more a part of the problem than of the solution.

The Veterinarian

The 1993 'Diet debate' article published in the *Veterinarian* set a high standard—never to be repeated. When, in 2001, *Raw Meaty Bones: Promote Health* was published I tried again to catch their attention. I sent a review copy with a covering letter. They said that the book did not arrive. I sent another copy and was assured it would be reviewed in the February or March 2002 issue.

In all, I did battle with the *Veterinarian* for 21 futile, energy-sapping months until finally giving up with one last gasp. I wrote to the editor.

> On 15 October 2001 the then editor of *The Veterinarian*, Annette Basile, wrote: 'Send the book in and we will review it'.
>
> That was twenty-one months ago. Since when I have provided three copies of *Raw Meaty Bones* and written innumerable emails. *The Veterinarian*, when prompted, has made excuses and false promises, but otherwise has done nothing.
>
> Over the same period several journals have reviewed the book and supported the recommendation: '*Raw Meaty Bones* is a book that all pet owners and veterinarians should read.' (www.rawmeatybones.com)
>
> Please advise what is the attitude of *The Veterinarian* and whether you have any intention of honouring your undertakings?[8]

No, no further answer was forthcoming. Subject closed.

The ABC

When seeking coverage of the junk pet food issue these 30 years past, I have become accustomed to the silent treatment, the journalists' failure to respond about current and important issues. Have you ever tried to contact the media about anything? Likely you'll find they don't reveal their email address. It's a one-way street. The media suck details from the community about matters large and small, but they themselves don't like to provide reasons for any of their decisions. That's the system—like it or lump it. If you want publicity for your campaign, it will be on their terms.

After the ABC *Investigators*' wonderfully well researched and presented exposé I asked if they would be doing a follow-up—for instance to show how pets thrive once moved from a junk diet to a raw meaty bones diet. 'No,' came the reply, 'no current intentions'.

Of course, there can be legitimate reasons why media outlets cannot or should not follow up on stories. They can argue that once they have covered a topic their viewers and readers may not want second helpings. Further, it is important that media companies do not appear to be running vendettas against targets, however large and deserving of exposure those targets are.

Passively failing to follow up on vital stories is one thing. Actively suppressing those stories for many years and deliberately, knowingly, pushing false or misleading narratives is another—especially if you happen to be the government-owned ABC. That, however, is what happened after I wrote to Robyn Williams, doyen of science journalism at the ABC.

I sent him recordings of two ABC Radio programs featuring the pet food scandal and the monograph of Pet Foods Insidious Consequencies: A modern veterinarian snafu (See Chap. 6, p 148).

Mr Williams replied on 5 November 1992.

ABC RADIO

Science Unit

Australian
Broadcasting
Corporation

ABC Ultimo Centre
Level 4
700 Harris Street
Ultimo 2007

GPO Box 9994
Sydney 2001
Australia

Tel (02) 394 1407
Fax (02) 394 1414

5th November, 1992

Mr Tom Lonsdale
Tom Lonsdale and Associates
Riverstone Veterinary Hospital
Garfield Rd
RIVERSTONE NSW 2765

Dear Tom,

Thank you for your cassette and letter on "Insidious Consequences" it looks fun but unfortunately I'm about to go overseas and don't have time to look at it yet so I'll try to deal with it when I get back.

Kind regards,

ROBYN WILLIAMS
(Science Unit)

RW:JAL

Unfortunately for Australian pets and their owners, Robyn Williams never followed through, and letters went unanswered. I wondered why and fretted, until one day the radio provided the answer. Young, comely, ambitious Mars company vet Jonica Newby, daughter of the Mars Corporation chief lawyer,[9] was the guest presenter on a Robyn Williams program *Ockham's Razor*. It was the first public sign of bigger and 'better' things to come for Williams and new girlfriend Newby.

Newby moved in with the then middle-aged Williams and together they presented a four-part radio series on 'Why we should keep pets'. Eminent lawyer Stuart Littlemore QC told ABC viewers:

> Oh! they didn't admit that was the subject, but it was. Written and narrated by a publicist for something called 'the Pet Care Information and Advisory Service', which it seems fair to say, is nothing more than a front for the multi-national pet-food manufacturer Mars, through its Australian subsidiary Uncle Bens.[10]

Next came books by Newby published by the ABC and then a permanent berth as presenter on the *Catalyst* ABC television science program.[11] The glamour couple were regulars at award ceremonies and other fashionable events.

Efforts by Breck Muir and me, futile as you would expect, centred on trying to get the ABC management to reconsider their infatuation with Jonica Newby. In 1999 we wrote:

> Mr Williams and the ABC have provided extensive opportunities for Dr Jonica Newby, a pet-food company publicist, to broadcast radio programmes, publish books and produce TV series favourable to the artificial pet-food industry. Mr Stuart Littlemore said that Jonica Newby 'shouldn't have been on the ABC at all'[10] and labelled the radio programmes 'arrant tosh, highly insulting to her audience's intelligence'.
>
> - We are concerned that Mr Williams and the ABC appear to have chosen not to investigate and report on matters of scientific, economic and environmental

> significance for the Australian community. Please provide reasons for these apparent decisions.
>
> - We are concerned at the decisions to provide wide opportunities for a pet-food company publicist to air 'arrant tosh' helpful to her wealthy employer. Please advise why ABC resources have been allocated in this way.
> - Please advise how ABC policy and conduct in these maters has been 'responsive to the need for fair and accurate coverage of matters of public interest'.

As recently as 2020, 23 years after first joining the ABC, Newby published another book and Williams promoted it on air. An indignant fellow ABC reporter raised questions about the duo: 'Now, surely the ABC can do better than this, a host plugging his partner's upcoming book on his own show without being up-front with his listeners?'[12] ABC management responded:

> Dr Jonica Newby is an award-winning television producer, writer, director and presenter with some 20 years' experience in science journalism. Her personal relationship with Mr Williams had no bearing on the decision to commission her as a freelance contributor to the 'Climate grief' series, which was approved by ABC editors.[13]

On the back of the latest Williams and Newby double act I tried again to get *Four Corners*, the ABC investigative television program, to take an interest in the multi-billion-dollar pet food fraud. Predictably they replied: 'Unfortunately, this would not be a topic which *Four Corners* could pursue at this stage.'

The Sydney Morning Herald

Back in 2013 the *Sydney Morning Herald* published Elizabeth Farrelly's article containing the words: 'Before re-mortgaging the house [to pay the vet bills], I did what you do. Googled, found a website called Raw Meaty Bones. The message was obvious and compelling'.

Elizabeth Farrelly told her readers that 'exorbitant science-nosh' had devastated the health of her two cats and that raw meaty bones restored their health. But by 2021 the paper contradicted its previous reporting.

What the experts want you to know about your pet's diet

We love our pets and want them to be as healthy as possible. But knowing what to feed them to achieve that outcome isn't always clear.

So, we asked Dr Lee Danks, a veterinarian with a particular interest in companion animal nutrition, and part of the technical services veterinarian team at pet food producer Black Hawk, to answer a few questions.

Should I be giving my pet raw foods?

My view is no, but I understand that many will take this approach because they have a passion for feeding their pet, having 100 per cent control over what goes into their bowls and because of a negative perception of the manufacturing process that creates kibble.

The decades of research from many, diverse experts that informs us what is 'good' and needed by our pets to survive, also keeps our pets safe, informing safety criteria such as the need to heat and cook food to eliminate potentially harmful bacteria.

Not only do well put-together, complete and balanced pet foods deliver what pets need without excess or deficiencies, but they also provide food safety advantages.

Many vet and medical authorities around the world have expressed concerns over raw foods and feeding.

What about meat? Should I be giving them plain mince, or tinned or sausage-type meats?

Before giving mince to my dog or cat, I'd need to know what nutrients are contained in it and how they interact with the other 30 to 40 nutrients that they need to survive, and that's just way too difficult a task.

A tinned, or 'dog roll' format food from a reliable manufacturer will iron out issues of nutritional imbalance. While we won't be cooking in our own kitchen as many pet owners like to do, we will have the confidence in knowing that our four-legged family members are getting the nutrients that they need.

Feed your pet: food for pets. It's pretty simple.

Can a pet be healthy if it eats only dry food?

Of course. Most of the pets across the globe are fed dry food, also known as biscuits or kibble. When it's made by a manufacturer with high quality standards, dry food in this format is well balanced with nutrients that will ensure they not only survive on a day-to-day basis, but will help them truly thrive.[14]

Small italic print indicated that '*This is sponsored content for Black Hawk*'. Not just product placement subterfuge, but a full-on advertorial—that I say is false and misleading to its core.

Who might notice or care? Not many, I would wager, including the owners and editors of the *Sydney Morning Herald*.

Books and blogs

In your wanderings through the internet, bookstores and libraries you will likely encounter many publications that properly should be catalogued in the 'ugly' category. Be on your guard. Book covers and webpage illustrations sprouting green leaves, with bowls full of minced junk, will tell you straight away that the contents within are fictions—mostly deliberate fictions designed to sell you junk raw products.

Back in 2006, in the *Raw Meaty Bones Newsletter*, I suggested a three-part test to help pet owners protect themselves and their pets.

> Unfortunately, these days, there's a multiplicity of quacks, opportunists, niche marketers and false prophets seeking to turn a buck and gain kudos peddling nonsensical gibberish and weird incantations that do little to help companion carnivores in their time of need. How can we spot the well-meaning and ill-informed and those with more cynical intent? How can we protect ourselves and our pets against slick presentations and marketing hype?
>
> Maybe it's not so difficult. Maybe by applying the Three-Part Test false prophets can be identified and thus resisted.

Here's the test:

Does the speaker/proponent/prophet affirm and invoke the need for:

1. Carnivores to have a regular full belly of whole prey or something akin to the same?
2. Carnivores to maintain a pearly white set of teeth and salmon pink gums?
3. Every effort to overturn the junk pet-food industry/veterinary alliance?

Check out the articles, the websites, the books and the sly rhetoric of a multiplicity of barfers, herbalists and pushers of supplements and quack cures? Do they pass one, two or three parts of the Three-Part Test? Or do they fail abysmally?[15]

10

POLITICIANS AND REGULATORS: LET DOG FOOD COMPANIES LIE

A lie can travel halfway around the world while the truth is putting on its shoes.

Attrib. Mark Twain

A monstrous set of lies defines the existence of pet dogs, cats and ferrets at this stage in human history. It's an incontrovertible fact that carnivores—whether wild, feral or domestic—depend on a diet of whole carcasses, or at least raw meaty bones. Unfortunately for pets, pet owners, the wider community and natural environment that fact has been turned on its head relentlessly over the past 160 years.

Politicians and regulators

Where once manufactured products were seen as barely acceptable partial substitutes for meat and bones, the emphasis gradually changed such that those products are now claimed to be *good, beneficial, safe*—indeed the essential way to feed pets. Simultaneously vets and junk pet food makers say raw natural foodstuffs are *bad, harmful and dangerous.*

Doubling down on this crazy inversion, in the US the Food and Drug Administration (FDA) and the Centers for Disease Control

(CDC) 'have recommended not feeding dogs and cats a raw meat diet, meaning meat that is not cooked to a proper temperature'.[1] At the highest levels of the US federal government, the FDA and CDC have been hoodwinked and brainwashed into becoming docile promoters and protectors of the junk pet food white-collar criminal collaboration. Effectively, then, politicians and top-level bureaucrats in the US and other developed countries make laws and administer laws favourable to the junk pet food industry. If perchance existing laws work against the interests of the criminal collaborators, those laws are simply not enforced. I'm thinking of animal welfare and cruelty laws and consumer protection laws.

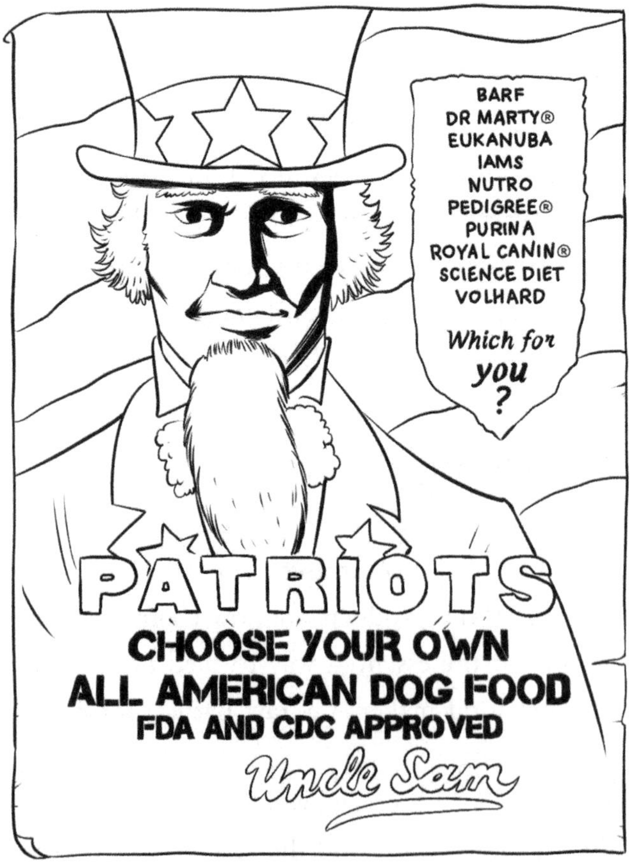

In Chapters 6 and 7 I placed the responsibility for the current lamentable state of affairs primarily at the feet of the veterinary profession. Vets take an oath to protect the patients under their care and are best placed to understand the science underpinning animal welfare. However, it's politicians who make laws and it's governments who administer laws and who have, over decades, deferred to vets.

With so many pillars in place supporting the junk pet food fraud it is damnably difficult to get politicians and governments to take another look. Although laws and conventions were established long ago by legislators who have since retired or died, the matter of sorting out the mess now falls to existing politicians and regulators. And that's a problem.

All those in current positions of power and influence ascended the ranks thanks to the system as it is, to the *status quo*. They operate within the bounds of accepted conventions, the current definition of 'normal'. They tend not to be wild-eyed revolutionaries keen on dismantling systems that protect powerful interests of, for instance, junk food makers, vets, welfare groups and media. Those in power recognise a population of complacent, contented consumers who subscribe to the fashion for keeping pets and feeding them according to the advertisements on television.

Most politicians belong to parties and must generally toe the party line. Anyone working in a bureaucracy knows groupthink and group-speak are an integral part of the job. Another important impediment to getting the junk pet food fraud examined relates to the competing work schedule of the politicians and regulators. 'Let sleeping dogs lie' is a political tradition popularised by Robert Walpole, the first prime minister of Britain in the 1700s. These days the *laissez faire* attitude comes with a sinister new twist. Politicians and prime ministers of all political persuasions: let dog food companies lie and lie and lie.

Generalisations apply to the political game where those in power, from either side of the political divide, want to stay in power and thus defend the *status quo*. Opposition parties, of course, wish to gain power and thus get into a position to defend the *status quo*. They don't want to burn their bridges in advance. They know who and what will be waiting for them once they gain power. When I met with a shadow minister of agriculture (the opposition spokesman) in an attempt to gain some assistance in the fight with the government, the vet profession, Mars Inc., Nestlé and Colgate-Palmolive, he told me point blank: 'I won't be doing that' and quickly showed me the door.

Political independents and those from the smaller parties sometimes express support, but seldom or never commit time and resources to the struggle. And sadly, this overall lack of commitment on the part of politicians, those we elect to defend us against the $multi-billion fraud, continues even when those politicians keep pets. *The Guardian* newspaper reported:

> Second only to babies, pets are a choice weapon for politicians who want to soften their image. Their canine best friend holds a special role: to project the image that the politician wants the public to have of them.[2]

When the Reverend Raphael Warnock campaigned for the US Senate, he didn't own a dog. His advisers found a solution. They borrowed a beagle and made a campaign video showcasing Warnock walking 'his' dog on a lead. The *New York Times* commented:

The dog had a lot of work to do.

He was co-starring in a political ad that had to showcase the candidate's good-natured warmth. But the ad also needed to deflect an onslaught of racialized attacks without engaging them directly, and to convey to white voters in Georgia that the Black pastor who led Ebenezer Baptist Church could represent them, too.[3]

Glimmers of hope

Back in 2004 a small group of UK pet owners helped in spreading the word. Through astute lobbying two magnificent early day motions (EDMs) were tabled. The UK Parliament website helpfully informs us:

> **What are early day motions?**
> Early day motions (EDMs) are motions submitted for debate in the House of Commons for which no day has been fixed.
>
> As there is no specific time allocated to EDMs very few are debated. However, many attract a great deal of public interest and media coverage.
>
> **What are EDMs used for?**
> EDMs are used to put on record the views of individual MPs or to draw attention to specific events or campaigns. Topics covered by EDMs vary widely.
>
> By attracting the signatures of other MPs, they can be used to demonstrate the level of parliamentary support for a particular cause or point of view.[4]

Early day motion 335 tabled on 7 December 2004 gained 55 signatures.

> **Processed Pet Foods and Vets**
> That this House deeply regrets the professional endorsement of processed food for domestic dogs, cats and ferrets by some members of the veterinary profession; is concerned at the level of incidence of malodorous gum disease and associated diseases of the kidneys, liver and other organs amongst the domestic pet population; recognises that their health and welfare is best served by foods, such as raw meaty bones, that reflect the full range of nutritional need; applauds and recommends the work of veterinary surgeon Tom Lonsdale and others in this field; recognises also that vets in the UK are trusted and independent advisers on the health of our pets; is therefore concerned by the nature of the relationship between some vets and producers of foods that cause illnesses in pets; and calls upon the Royal College of Veterinary Surgeons to make a definitive statement on the active endorsement and promotion of processed pet foods by vets.[5]

Early day motion 1003 tabled on 11 November 2005 gained 34 signatures.

> **Raw Meaty Bones Group**
> That this House notes the controversy surrounding the promotion and sale of processed pet foods by veterinary surgeons; acknowledges the evidence and analysis in the book *Raw Meaty Bones* by Tom Lonsdale; commends the UK Raw Meaty Bones Group's public awareness campaign; and calls for a wide ranging inquiry into that group's serious

> concerns relating to human and pet health, the economy and the environment and the adequacy of the current veterinary regulatory system to investigate these issues.[6]

Sterling stuff that should gladden the hearts of all those interested in ending the multi-billion-dollar fraud. Elected representatives must ultimately enforce existing laws and make new laws. The two EDMs show that, in the UK at least, there are MPs who understand the length and breadth of the issues.

Australia

How does Australia compare? Overall, and despite 30 years of intense lobbying, the Australian performance has been mostly dismal and disappointing—with two standout exceptions reproduced here.

When I was harassed and expelled from the Australian Veterinary Association for daring to criticise the vet profession, NSW State Labor Member of Parliament Paul Lynch rose to speak in parliament on 13 May 2004.

> **MR TOM LONSDALE AND THE AUSTRALIAN VETERINARY ASSOCIATION**
>
> **Mr LYNCH** (Liverpool) [5.39 p.m.]: Tonight, I inform the House of the plight of veterinarian Tom Lonsdale. Several of my constituents are interested in the case of Tom Lonsdale, which raises issues of relevance to my electorate, as it does for the electorates of all honourable members. Simply put, Tom Lonsdale complained to the Board of Veterinary Surgeons [BVS]—a State body. Somehow that complaint was made known to the Australian Veterinary

Association [AVA]. As a result, after some inadequate processes, he was expelled from the AVA. This is relevant to the House in two broad ways. The first is the behaviour of the BVS, a State body, and the second is the behaviour of the AVA which, while technically being a non-government body, is treated by the Government in a particular way—that is, it is regarded by the Government as representative of veterinarians generally—and representatives of the AVA are placed on various boards by the Government.

It is fair to say that Tom Lonsdale is a controversial figure within veterinarian circles. He has regularly run in elections for the AVA, getting about 10 per cent of the vote fairly consistently. No-one can argue that he has majority support among veterinarians but a consistent vote of 10 per cent suggests significant minority support. His most controversial position stems from asserting the need for dogs and cats to be fed more than canned and dry pet foods: they need to be fed bones. The lengthiest exposition of his argument is in his book, published in 2001 and appropriately entitled *Raw Meaty Bones*. The preface to the book contains the following comments:

> **If you own a dog or a cat which you feed with processed food from the supermarket or corner store, you will probably find this book deeply disturbing ...**
>
> **The book is about what happens to dogs and cats if their diet is inadequate. These days most pet owners give their animals processed pet food. It may seem a convenient way of feeding but such a diet on its own is likely**

> **over time to cause the pets considerable ill health and suffering. And the signs of the ill health may not be obvious to many owners.**
>
> **But ask yourself the question: Is it likely that a carnivore—a meat eater—whose species evolved on a diet of the whole carcasses of other animals, will benefit from bland processed food with never a bone in sight?**

Needless to say, such views have done little to endear him to the very large, seemingly multinational, companies that mass produce pet food. He has also done himself no favours with veterinarians who do not share his views. Vets and any of their associates who are funded by pet food companies would be likely to be pretty hostile towards him. When his book was published in 2001, Tom Lonsdale sought to have it reviewed in a journal called The Veterinarian. I have seen the email correspondence this generated. Despite promises or suggestions that the book would be reviewed, an interview with Tom Lonsdale published or a feature article printed, nothing eventuated. After two years of this frustration, Tom Lonsdale sent copies of what he regarded as this highly unsatisfactory email correspondence to a number of bodies, including the Board of Veterinary Surgeons of New South Wales. He received an email from Maria Linkenbagh, registrar of the board, asking why he had sent it to her. He replied in an email dated 18 July 2003, which he also sent to almost all members of both Houses of the New South Wales Parliament, part of which stated:

> **Members of the NSW Board of Veterinary Surgeons are likely aware of the allegations of scientific and consumer fraud perpetrated upon an unsuspecting Australian public by an alliance of pet food companies and veterinarians ...**
>
> **Any right-thinking person knows that the slow poisoning of the nation's pets by junk food manufacturers, aided by veterinarians, is against the interests of pets, pet owners and the wider community ...**
>
> **The Australian Veterinary Association (AVA) has financial ties to pet food companies. For ten years the AVA has sought to stifle news of the scandal.**

There appears to have been no real substantive response from the BVS. In Tom Lonsdale's view there are many connections between the BVS and the AVA. Thus, he was not surprised when the AVA took it upon itself to respond to his communication with the BVS. He was, however, somewhat perturbed by the substance of the reply. He received a letter dated 8 January 2004 from Dr Bruce Cartmill, President of the New South Wales division of the AVA. He advised that the AVA had received a complaint that Tom Lonsdale had breached the AVA code of conduct and was bringing the association into disrepute. No complainant was identified so the complaint, from Tom Lonsdale's point of view, was anonymous. The letter from Cartmill made it clear that Lonsdale's email had generated the complaint. The New South Wales division recommended that

Tom Lonsdale's membership of the AVA be cancelled—that is, that he be expelled. This recommendation was referred to the AVA board.

Tom Lonsdale requested full particulars of the allegations against him, but no further information was provided. He was told that he was not allowed legal representation at the AVA board meeting that would consider his expulsion. He then received a letter saying that his membership had been cancelled as of 2 March. Tom Lonsdale was expelled from the AVA on the basis of an anonymous complaint in relation to which further particulars were not provided at a hearing at which he could not have legal representation. The whistleblower was punished. This is the action of a kangaroo court. It is a disgrace. There are two levels of serious public policy concern: Did the BVS refer the matter, either formally or informally, to the AVA? How can the Minister for Primary Industries continue to place reliance upon a group such as the AVA? The practical implication of Tom Lonsdale's expulsion is to silence dissenting voices. He cannot run in elections, and he is prevented from participating in the AVA group discussions. The AVA has decided who can run against it and who cannot.[7]

NSW State Liberal Member of Parliament Kevin Conolly visited my vet practice in August 2018. His incisive, succinct speech to Parliament stated:

> **Animal Welfare**
>
> **Mr KEVIN CONOLLY (Riverstone) (18:57):** I bring to the attention of the House an issue raised with me recently by a Quakers Hill pet owner and which I find has been the passion of an experienced veterinarian from north-western Sydney for many years. I am pleased that the member for Liverpool is in the House because he spoke about this issue many years ago. I will refer to that shortly. The issue begins with identifying what is the most appropriate, healthy diet for dogs and cats, and extends to the influence wielded by large corporations that control the pet food industry. Disturbingly, it brings into question the integrity and ethics of the veterinary profession in New South Wales; of the government and non-government bodies that should be the watchdogs of animal welfare in the State, including the Royal Society for the Prevention of Cruelty to Animals [RSPCA]; and of the tertiary institutions that oversee the education of those in New South Wales aspiring to be veterinarians.
>
> The catalyst for bringing the issue to the fore this year was the decision of an Australian Senate committee to hold an inquiry into regulatory approaches to ensure the safety of pet food. The basic premise drawn to my attention by the local pet owner and by the veterinarian of whom I will speak more in a moment, is that dogs and cats should be fed raw meat on the bone rather than processed

and packaged pet foods. The vet's contention is that this natural diet will give our pets a much greater chance of a healthy life, while a diet based on processed and packaged pet foods will almost inevitably lead to them experiencing chronic ill health, and possibly significant suffering, which of course they are unable to complain about to their owners.

The vet of whom I speak is Dr Tom Lonsdale, who for a number of years ran a veterinary practice at Riverstone but in more recent times has practised in nearby Bligh Park. In 2001 he wrote a book entitled Raw Meaty Bones, in which he both detailed his reasons for supporting a natural diet for dogs and cats and made the criticisms to which I have referred about the stance adopted by those professionals, institutions and authorities to whom we naturally look for direction in the field of animal welfare. It is his contention that these bodies have been hopelessly compromised by their various relationships—often pecuniary relationships—with the pet food industry. Consequently, he asserts, they have not acted to protect the welfare of animals in relation to diet.

It is not a common occurrence for me to refer approvingly to a speech given in this place by the member for Liverpool, but on this occasion, it is appropriate to do so. In 2004 that member delivered a private member's statement highlighting the manner in which Dr Lonsdale was effectively expelled from the New South Wales Division of the Australian Veterinary Association in the wake of publishing his book. It appeared to me, in reading that private member's statement today, that the implications so

> properly identified by the member for Liverpool remain unrefuted and unaddressed in the 14 years since.
>
> But my purpose in speaking today is to focus on the core issue. Are companion animals in New South Wales being forced to endure chronic abuse because of the unwillingness of the veterinary profession, the RSPCA, the regulators and academics to consider seriously the relatively simple questions posed by Dr Lonsdale? Can the lives of our pet animals be made happier and healthier by a change of direction in relation to what they are fed? Can they be spared illness and pain through a simple change of diet? Dr Lonsdale hopes that the Senate committee inquiry, which he tells me has received submissions from all over the world, will lift the lid on this issue at long last. It is my hope that the Department of Primary Industries in New South Wales will undertake the necessary research and investigations to determine whether or not Dr Lonsdale is right and, if he is, will act responsibly to address the issues that he has raised.[8]

Subsequently in 2020 Kevin Conolly agreed to be interviewed for a documentary film. Whether or not the world will see that interview, I don't know. I do know that NSW State MP Kevin Conolly has set a shining example for politicians the world over.

Regulatory capture in plain sight

Regulatory approaches to ensure the safety of pet food

The glimmers of hope brightened for a time. In June 2018 Senator Sterling Griff issued a media release. He was responding to lobbying from dog owners whose dogs had died of an intractable condition—'megaoesophagus'—where the oesophagus becomes limp and flaccid, and food fails to reach the stomach. Ordinarily megaoesophagus is a sporadic disease but in this instance all sufferers had been fed Advance Dermocare products made by Mars.

> **Senate to inquire into problem-plagued pet food industry**
> Centre Alliance Senator Stirling Griff today secured a Senate inquiry into the safety and regulation of the pet food industry in the wake of the most recent contamination case which has left over 100 dogs with debilitating megaesophagus and caused the death of at least 17 pets.
>
> Senator Griff said the death and disability of these valued pets had highlighted to consumers the poor state of regulation and oversight in the industry.
>
> 'It's ridiculous that people can pay up to $50 a kilo for premium pet food, thinking it's the best, and yet they cannot have confidence it's safe for their pet to eat,' Senator Griff said.
>
> 'This is a $4 billion industry and it is self-regulated—it looks after its own compliance and its own recalls. It's hardly a model for transparency and assured good practice.
>
> 'It's the old "Dracula in charge of the blood bank" problem and, frankly, we must do better. People are grieving the death of their pets, or face ongoing costs and guilt because their pets now have to live with an untreat-

> able condition—all from what appears to be dog food purchased in the belief it was one of the better products available on the market.'[9]

There's plenty to like about Senator Griff's media release. He understands the limitations of 'self-regulation'. He wants transparency and assured good practice. His imagery of Dracula makes a decisive point. Unfortunately, he's been swayed by the emotions of those who felt cheated. They had bought what was touted as a 'better product' but incurred costs and lost a pet in gory and immediate circumstances.

Senator Griff's media release seems to suggest that if we just have a closer look, if we tweak some things around the edges, we will once again be able to believe in the 'better products'. Alas, back then Senator Griff did not realise that *all products* give rise to ongoing costs often in respect to untreatable conditions and death. Unfortunately, all other people in the chain of responsibility appear to be under the same set of illusions.

The Senate Inquiry into 'Regulatory approaches to ensure the safety of pet food'[10] invited written submissions and subsequently held public hearings before a panel of senators. All published submissions and all aspects of the public hearings were protected by parliamentary privilege, meaning that contributors could be entirely frank without risking subsequent legal action.

Of the 151 written submissions, 37 were from raw meaty bones feeders who let the senators know the inherent absurdity of attempting to regulate and make safe junk products that give rise to inevitable ill health.[11,12] Sadly, the senators were not listening. They received wordy submissions from Royal Canin, Mars, Nestlé and their incognito proxies. When it came time for the public hearings, the pet owners who had lost dogs to the Mars junk had plenty to say.

When it was Mars's turn to reply, Barry O'Sullivan, general manager, Mars Petcare Australia, addressed the committee·

> We welcome this inquiry. Between me and my colleague Dr Roger Bektash, we have 60 years' experience working with Mars. We thank you for the opportunity to contribute today. As one of Australia's largest pet food manufacturers, millions of Australians put the health of their pets in our hands. This responsibility is the cornerstone of our business and guides the decisions we make. The health of Australian pets is our No. 1 priority. Nowhere is this more evident than in the quality and safety standards that we have as a family-owned business. As a global manufacturer, our standards meet or exceed the most stringent standards in the world. Here I refer to the standards in particular in the United States and the European Union. In fact, the family that own this business insists on that, and they are accredited in every market around the world through a third party, Lloyd's Register Quality Assurance.
>
> We appreciate the committee's concern regarding our voluntary recall of Advance Dermocare dry dog food and the cases of megaesophagus diagnosed in a number of Australian dogs that had consumed our product. The lead investigator, U-Vet, at University of Melbourne, has confirmed upward of 100 cases. All dogs had consumed Advance Dermocare, which clearly indicates diet as a significant risk factor in megaesophagus. Extensive testing has not found a root cause. Till this date, sitting here today, extensive testing has not found a root cause.
>
> Megaesophagus is an incredibly rare condition—one that most vets in Australia will go an entire career with-

> out even seeing a single case. It is usually associated with underlying genetic conditions, not with food, and usually associated with larger dog breeds. There is only one previously recorded instance, as you're aware, where there is an association between the food and this condition, megaesophagus. That was in Latvia in 2015, where 200 dogs were affected. In that case, no root cause was identified.
>
> We feel for every Australian pet owner who has been affected. I can tell you I know what it means to suffer the loss of a loved one, personally. As a pet owner myself, I understand fully what it also means to lose a beloved pet. I'm lucky enough to have been able to adopt a kelpie from the great people at PetRescue. Unlike, probably, most kelpies, she's found at night inside the house—at the end of my daughter's bed. I know the distress it would cause if any harm was to come to that pet. And I feed Lola, my kelpie, on Advance. I feel for those who have lost a much-loved family pet or are living day to day with the burden of this condition. We are speaking with those affected to support them, and we will continue to do so.[13]

With billions at stake, of course Mars welcomed the inquiry. Anything that might help them with their marketing and quality control would, for them, be a good thing. Let setting the standards for processed pet food be a government responsibility. Mars will appear to comply with the rules, especially if they control the committee that writes them. If new rules make for new costs, then no matter, those costs will apply across the board for all manufacturers and be simply passed on to the consumers to pay and pay.

While ostensibly O'Sullivan addressed the committee, we can be sure his carefully chosen words were for the benefit of Mars executives, who you can be sure were watching with interest. If O'Sullivan and the Mars Corporation were a tiny bit sincere about abiding by the statement 'The health of Australian pets is our No. 1 priority', they should close their mass pet poisoning operation at the earliest.

Imagine if the Australian government hearkened to the request for a *robust judicial inquiry*. Imagine the thin end of the wedge being driven into the Mars operation and the subsequent global unravelling with legal, financial and quite possibly jail consequences. Of course Mars welcomed the insipid, lightweight Senate Inquiry.

The transcript of the public hearing records Senator Griff asking me to elaborate.

> Dr Lonsdale, your two main issues appear to be processed food, which you consider to be inappropriate for pets, and a belief that vets are being seriously influenced by pet food companies. They're really the thrust of the two issues that you mentioned.[14]

In part I replied:

> In fact, submission No. 62 is really quite edifying.[15] A lady had two animals treated by us and then decided to change the rest of the household pets to a raw meaty bones diet. Then, in retrospect, she looked back and said, 'I didn't realise just how sick they were.' You can do the experiment yourself. You don't need to go to this so-called scientific literature which, in any event, is totally, totally controlled and constrained by the junk-pet-food industry.
>
> Leading on to that second point about the vets being infiltrated—well, they most definitely are. You see, the vets are effectively the regulators of all things pet. They're

> the self-appointed experts—the authority—that everyone defers to. That's very nice, except that they can't be relied upon. If you go to my website, you'll see all the various freedom of information actions that I've conducted here in this country against the seven veterinary schools. If you go to the UK RMB website, you can see their investigations into the UK schools that are all infiltrated by Mars and Colgate and to a lesser extent Nestlé. If you go to America, you'll find precisely the same.

The final Senate Inquiry written report contained the following passage.[16]

> **Processed pet food**
> 2.56 In addition to the incidents of illness associated with pet food, the committee heard from a number of submitters who opposed commercially produced pet food altogether. These submitters held the view that dogs and cats are essentially carnivores and are not suited to a commercial 'junk food' diet of processed pet food. Instead, they suggested that animals should maintain a diet of 'raw meaty bones' to ensure dental and digestive health. Mrs Jeannine Barnard provided the following assessment of commercial pet foods:
>
> > **Cats are obligate carnivores but are being fed a low protein diet and processed carbohydrates (junk food) and our pets are just not getting enough hydration and proper nutrition from their diets, resulting in ill health and diseases like kidney disease.**

Although dogs are a little bit flexible and may tolerate carbohydrates in small amounts, large amounts can lead to allergies, behaviour problems, upset stomachs, weight gain, bad teeth and health. Still this tolerance for small amounts of carbohydrates, doesn't make them omnivores either.

Sadly, and ironically their diseases are treated by conventional veterinarians prescribing dry food and are mostly the cause thereof.

2.57 Proponents of the 'raw meaty bones' diet argued that they had seen vast improvements in their pets' health after making major changes to their diet. Mr Rolf Hauptmann informed the committee that his cat, once diagnosed with life-threatening diabetes, was put on a diet of raw meat and bones and is now 'disease-free, medication-free, and far healthier than previously'. Another submitter, Ms Christine Lewis, stated that her dog, which had an inflammatory bowel disorder recovered when its diet changed to one of raw meat and bones. She submitted:

It is quite clear that my dog's previous ill health was entirely due to his diet of processed dog food. This is a particularly alarming insight when we take into account the fact that the expensive canned food that I was feeding him was specifically developed for dogs with digestive difficulties.[17]

2.58 Dr Tom Lonsdale, a veterinarian and a prominent advocate of the 'raw meaty bones' diet summarised his view:

> **Conceptually it's impossible to *manufacture* food that is safe for pets. There have never, to my knowledge, been published controlled studies demonstrating that artificial, manufactured products are either suitable or safe for the feeding of domestic carnivores ...**
>
> **...*All* processed pet foods, whether directly or indirectly, injure the health of animals. From time-to-time identifiable additional hazards arise—for instance chemical or bacterial contamination and formulation deficiencies and excesses—that give rise to outbreaks of acute disease and death.**

Those 37 raw meaty bones submitters with a genuine interest in regulatory reform had been heard. We had been permitted a token gesture; part of a pressure release valve designed to placate troublesome, inconvenient voices.

Otherwise, the Senate report started with trivial and absurd recommendations focused on manufactured, packaged products.

> **Recommendation 1**
>
> The committee recommends that the Australian Standard for the Manufacturing and Marketing of Pet Food (AS5812:2017) be made publicly available
>
> **Recommendation 2**
>
> The committee recommends that, as part of its review into the safety and regulation of pet food, the working group focus on mechanisms to mandate pet food standards and labelling requirements in Australia.

Recommendations 3 to 7 were no better. Suffice to say the Senate Inquiry had been largely a waste of effort—not least because the Minister of Agriculture, his apparatchiks at the Department of Agriculture, the pet food manufacturers, Australian Veterinary Association and RSPCA were set to take over.

Pet Food Review Working Group

Even before the Senate committee reported, Agriculture Minister David Littleproud and his apparatchiks at the Department of Agriculture had established a committee, the 'Pet Food Review Working Group', to reassess pet food industry regulations.

I tried, through a Freedom of Information request, to obtain the names and allegiances of the working group members. No names were forthcoming; however, from the redacted email addresses, I gained the impression that Mars, Nestlé, the Australian Veterinary Association and the RSPCA were running the show—with government bureaucrats equipped with rubber stamps in attendance. And so began a paper war with the government bureaucrat responsible for the working group, vet Sally Thomson BVSc MVetClinStud PhD. I wrote to Dr Thomson.

> Senator Griff, in June 2018, when announcing that the Senate was to 'inquire into problem-plagued pet food industry' stated: 'It's the old "Dracula in charge of the blood bank" problem.'
>
> It appears that the Working Group has been captured by Dracula in the guise of the pet-food industry/veterinary/animal welfare alliance. In my supplementary submission to the Senate Pet Food Inquiry, I described the alliance as a 'three party alliance [that] amounts to a massive international white collar criminal conspiracy against

> the interests of pets, people and the planet.'
>
> I note the prominence in the Working Group of the pet-food makers Mars Inc. and Nestlé, the Australian Veterinary Association and RSPCA.
>
> The Working Group veterinary consultant Professor Caroline Mansfield is a known proponent of processed pet food and is mentioned in the April 2018 Melbourne University FOI Enquiry. Speaking on ABC Radio, Professor Mansfield defended processed food and asserted that 'Dogs are omnivores—just like us'. Does the Working Group share Professor Mansfield's views?[18]

Sally Thomson defended the composition of the working group.

> The pet food industry will continue, and dry and tinned pet food will continue to be made so it is important to develop systems and process that will improve the safety and quality of that pet food.

The Pet Food Industry Association of Australia constructed a website where they boasted about 'working in partnership with the Department of Agriculture as a key participant of its Working Group'. Clearly members of the multi-billion-dollar junk pet food industry are not now unduly perturbed. After all, they have a seat at the table and, to my reckoning, they are running the show. Minister Littleproud didn't seem in the least perturbed either. In August 2020 he stated:

> Pet owners have a choice in the type of foods they feed their pets. The aim of the working group is to ensure that,

> when owners choose to feed their pets manufactured pet food, it is safe and meets their pet's nutritional needs. ...
>
> The claims that the working group and veterinarians are compromised by multinational pet food makers and suffer from collusion and regulatory capture are not justified.[19]

What choice? It is a choice between junk or more junk made by Mars, Nestlé and Colgate—the companies with a vice-like grip on the vet 'profession'. David Littleproud was doing what politicians the world over do—shifting responsibility, denying the undeniable and defending the indefensible. He knew that:

- The junk pet food business model involves the production and sale of millions of tons of harmful junk, wrongly, fraudulently advertised and sold as healthy and necessary.
- The veterinary business model depends on ignoring the inherent induced cruelty of junk pet food, engaging in a cover-up and overservicing pets' needs.
- The Australian Competition and Consumer Commission refuses to police the false and misleading advertisements and overservicing.
- Pet owners are massively disadvantaged by the power imbalances.

Notwithstanding these relevant facts, Minister Littleproud suggested owners, the victims, 'have a choice'!

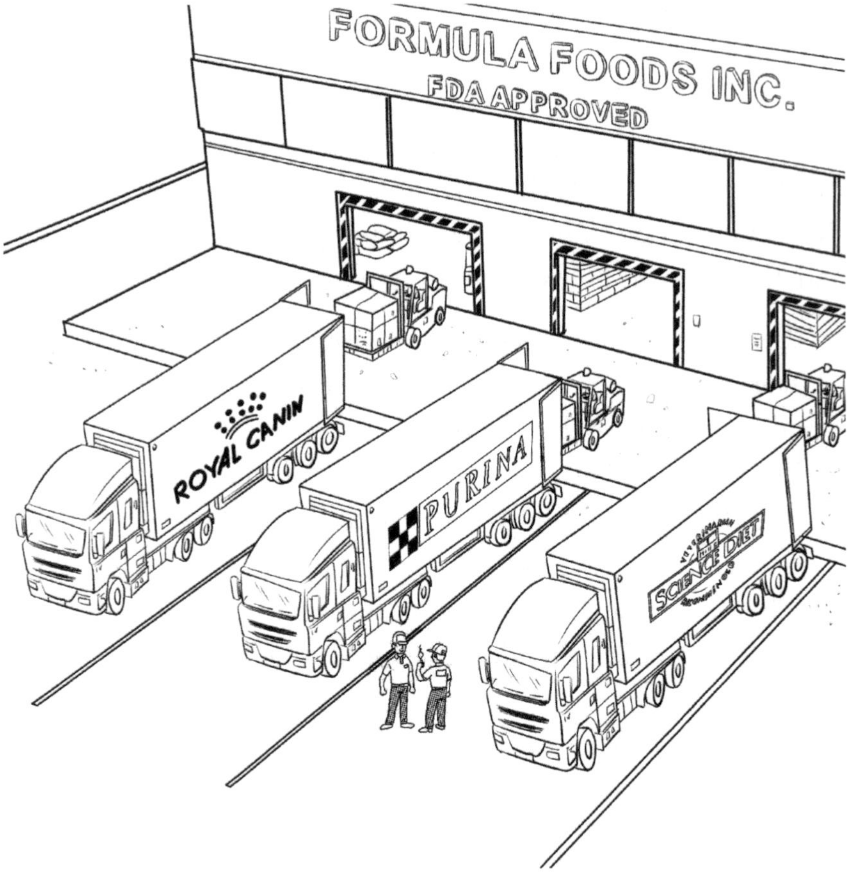
FORMULA FOODS INC.
FDA APPROVED
ROYAL CANIN
PURINA
SCIENCE DIET

PART IV

PRESS ON REGARDLESS

11

THE ART OF WAR

You've read 10 chapters and are suitably appalled by the multi-billion-dollar pet food fraud hiding in plain sight. You want to help improve the situation, but are unsure of how to proceed. In this chapter we explore some of the options for getting started. Doubtless in the chaos of the battles, whether epic or incidental, there will be reason to re-evaluate and reassign priorities. That said, we need to start somewhere. As the great philosopher warrior Sun Tzu, author of *The Art of War*, wrote,

> If you know the enemy and know yourself, you need not fear the result of a hundred battles. If you know yourself but not the enemy, for every victory gained you will also suffer a defeat. If you know neither the enemy nor yourself, you will succumb in every battle.[1]

Clearly, then, our first task is to 'know ourselves'. What led you here? Why are you concerned? When, how and where will you engage with the enemy? Who are the enemy?[2] They are all good questions with plenty of good answers needing regular revision. Your strategies and tactics will vary over time. And to be sure, the pet food war will likely rage for many years into the future.

Here is a list of perceived 'enemies'. Bear in mind that 'enemies' can and indeed need to become our friends. We need to recruit people to our way of thinking in line with the advice of Sun Tzu, who recommends that we endeavour to win without fighting. At the end of every war there are talks where previous sworn enemies sit down to structure the peace. It's the peace we want, but it's the war that we have to have.

Naysayers

Naysayers are everywhere, people who say 'it can't be done', 'it's too big', 'get over it', 'get a life'. They are the people with the glib one-liner that often bends the truth for effect. As the saying goes, 'Truth is the first casualty in war'. Naysayers don't engage in outright lying—that's more the preserve of the junk pet food companies and their allies. Naysayers use pregnant pauses or a raised eyebrow to belittle and disparage your 'truth'.

I say these things in part as a confession, as someone who has uttered the glib phrases. In the war for a better life for pets and pet owners, we need a strategy for dealing with naysayers. On the positive side, naysaying helps communication move along with hints of irony and humour. To that extent, it is worth finding common ground with the naysayer and then, using martial arts techniques, use their momentum to flip them over.

A frequent riposte that I hear is 'It's the same in human diets', referring to McDonald's domination of the junk feeding of humans. To that extent, I agree, but then point out that McDonald's ingredients, at least in the raw form, are recognisable as food types for omnivores—wheat, lettuce, beef, cucumbers. But even McDonald's don't and wouldn't put their breakfasts, lunch and dinner into an enormous mixer, pulverise the contents and then extrude them under intense heat and pressure before drying them in an oven and spraying the surface of the resultant nuggets with fat. It is probable

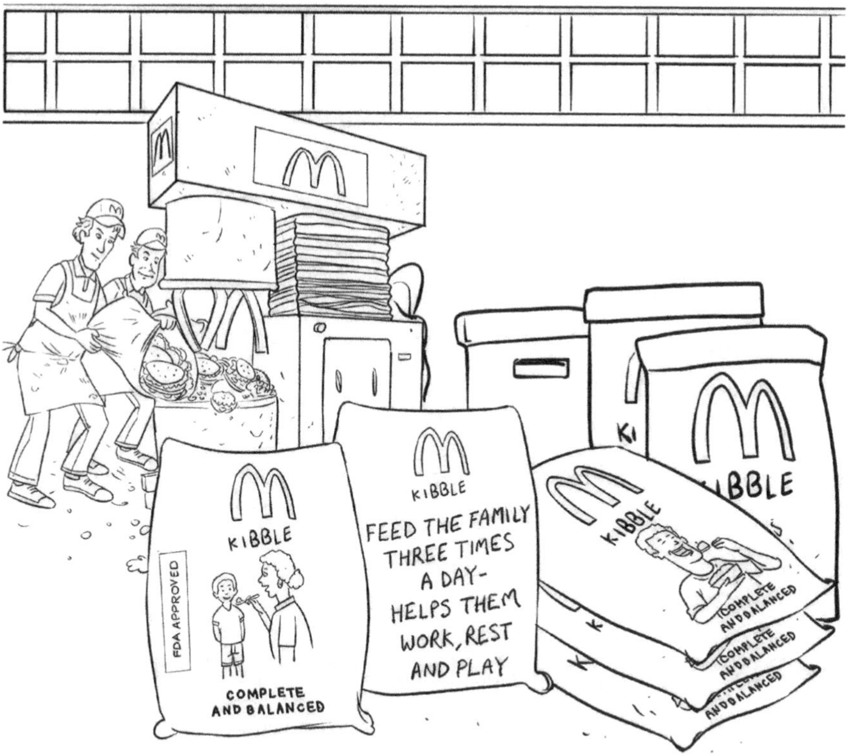

that McDonald's would capitalise on the extended shelf life and marketing reach—if consumers were to play along with the heist. However, humans have a semblance of choice. Pets have no choice except to accept what is on offer.

The doom nuggets are primarily grain-based, with an extended shelf life, giving rise to permanent indigestion. These days I show sceptics and naysayers a video clip of Ruby, the five-month-old miniature poodle puppy that had consumed some Easter chocolate as mentioned in Chapter 3. Almost without exception, those who previously defended the supposed ease, convenience and economy of feeding kibble change their mind on the spot.

Some people tell me that things are the same for human health. They suggest that human doctors are beholden to the pharmaceutical industry, nothing can be done about it and the failings of vets are no worse. I tend to start by agreeing that there are issues with the medical–pharmaceutical professional nexus. However, on the plus side there are the wonders of modern medicine. In any case, there are government departments that regulate some of the unhealthy big pharma excesses. Doctors restrict themselves to the prescription pad and operating theatre. They don't advise their patients on housing, training and diet. And they most certainly don't retail junk food in their waiting rooms with a free sample pack at every consultation.

The aim with naysayers is to win them over—eventually. It may take time, it may take guile, but in the end if you gain a convert, that convert may have the courage of his or her convictions and become a champion advocate for the cause.

BARFers, prey-modellers and assorted cranks

What have carnivorous pet dogs, cats and ferrets done to deserve such punishment? Surely no crime warrants being kept in solitary confinement, denied a toothbrush and obliged to slurp minced meats, finely ground bones, grated vegetables and mineral and vitamin supplements—or elaborately packaged minced meat-and-bone slop. You will not change the minds of the junk raw merchants. Appealing to their better nature would be fine if they had a better nature. On the evidence they, the merchants, get worse as they surreptitiously move consumers over to freeze-dried and canned concoctions with ever more elaborate health-promoting claims.

There is more hope of converting the *followers* of the junk raw scam. But it is a struggle. The term Stockholm syndrome was first coined in 1973 to describe the effects on four bank workers taken hostage during a bank robbery in Stockholm, Sweden. Paradoxically, even when released, the hostages refused to testify against their captors. It is a complex syndrome with many explanations. In the

Righteous And Wrong department, I think we can see a relatively simple explanation for the junk raw followers' resistance.

Perhaps 80 per cent of the health improvement seen in carnivorous pets derives from *stopping* the feeding of cooked, industrial junk from the can and packet. The junk raw merchants basically do two things. First they encourage pet owners to *stop* feeding the Mars, Nestlé, Colgate nasty junk—a significant benefit. Second, they introduce their inadequate minced offerings—expensive and not so beneficial. They then credit *all* the health improvements to their packaged junk. The BARF followers tend not to notice the sleight of hand and become hooked. Many become evangelical, going about promoting the expensive minced pap that costs many times as much as the fully beneficial raw meaty bones.

Educating the BARFer throng about the essential whole carcass or next best raw meaty bones diet would be a welcome step. Unfortunately, those with an evangelical zeal do not usually see the need to look more widely or more deeply. It's a cruel hoax. BARF and prey model zealots swarming over the pet food battlegrounds suck up oxygen and create obstruction, making it all the more difficult to get a direct shot at Mars, Nestlé and Colgate.

BARF, prey model and holistic manufacturers employ 'bait and switch' marketing in their pursuit of prestige and profit. Raw meaty bones are the 'bait'. The 'switch' involves persuading consumers that their ground-up, trademark-protected concoction provides all that an animal needs.

Notice that most of these get-rich-quick merchants employ or hide behind so-called 'holistic' vets who write the bait-and-switch spiel on websites and packaging. Proving that the merchants and their collaborators know about the need for carnivores to rip, tear and chew at every meal should be a relatively easy exercise in a court of law. Then showing that they knowingly and deliberately remove the essential physical texture while lying about the alleged benefits of 'minced chicken and finely ground bone' could serve a useful educational and legal purpose.

Veterinary profession

There are a lot of vets in the world. Approximate numbers are Australia 14,000, UK 27,000 and USA 118,000.[3] On the evidence we must see the vet profession *en masse* as enemy forces ranged up against us. But that is to overlook the individual differences of experience and attitudes of the 150,000 in the three countries mentioned and the many thousands more throughout the world.

In most years when I stood for election to the council of the UK Royal College of Veterinary Surgeons and for president of the Australian Veterinary Association, around 10 per cent of the voters supported the 'radical' raw meaty bones agenda.[4] There is a nucleus of friendly vets ready to break out and lead pets and pet owners to a brighter future. Finding them and encouraging them to stand up and speak out is no easy task.

Humans are imbued with a double dose of cunning—both as predators and prey. Fear and self-preservation are powerful motivators, especially when people have been inducted into a cult. We saw in earlier chapters how the junk pet food monsters' tentacles envelop all aspects of the modern vet practice. We saw how students are brainwashed in the vet schools and emerge blinking into the light as salesmen and women spruiking junk pet food. For most vets interested in the quiet life and making a living, straining at the cultural conditioners that bind them is not part of their plan.

Nonetheless, we need to continue to maintain a dialogue, where possible, with practitioner vets. Truth will out. When the raw meaty bones revolution finally comes, practitioner vets will be swept up in the enthusiasm. Until then we need to chip away, in an attempt to get them first to employ raw meaty bones in the prevention of disease in puppies and kittens and second to incorporate the feeding of raw meaty bones as a first-line treatment in virtually every clinical case before them.

Ultimately, it will be the specialist vets and university lecturers who make an about-face, jettison the junk pet food madcap delusions and come to promote the wonderful, uplifting, health-giving benefits of raw meaty bones. Here and there we see slight stirrings in the hoped-for direction. Back in 1993 I entered a limerick competition. Here are two of the (losing) entries:

1. The demise of a paradigm
   depends upon ideas meeting time,
   ruined reputations faced,
   and of equal distaste,
   that the matter be recorded in rhyme.

2. It's perfectly preposterous
   that those ruling over us
   should shift their position
   in the latest edition
   whilst maintaining it was ever thus.

Understanding the vets and their motivations is an essential first step. Then whether we attempt discussion and education, or more open conflict will depend on circumstances.

These days smartphones and the electronic media enable rapid-fire interactions. You can record images and videos and send them by email or post them on the internet. Try engaging your vet and vet staff in discussions. Ask questions, lots of questions. Try sending them informative articles and video evidence. Stay cool and calm if you can. But if not, consider taking a more robust stance.

If your vet promotes and sells junk food, then you may have a case against her for animal cruelty. If she is knowingly, deliberately avoiding cheap preventative options and instead engaging in repeated, expensive overservicing, a lawyer may be able to help. Yes, I believe that a much greater level of militancy is essential if we are to overcome the junk pet food fraud.

Legal actions

Vets in the UK make an undertaking:

> I PROMISE AND SOLEMNLY DECLARE that I will pursue the work of my profession with integrity and accept my responsibilities to the public, my clients, the profession and the Royal College of Veterinary Surgeons, and that, ABOVE ALL, my constant endeavour will be to ensure the health and welfare of animals committed to my care.[5]

Members of the American Veterinary Medical Association declare:

> Being admitted to the profession of veterinary medicine, I solemnly swear to use my scientific knowledge and skills for the benefit of society through the protection of animal health and welfare, the prevention and relief of animal suffering, the conservation of animal resources, the promotion of public health, and the advancement of medical knowledge.
>
> I will practice my profession conscientiously, with dignity, and in keeping with the principles of veterinary medical ethics.
>
> I accept as a lifelong obligation the continual improvement of my professional knowledge and competence.[6]

Here in New South Wales, Australia vets make the commitment:

> I solemnly swear to practise veterinary science ethically and conscientiously for the benefit of animal welfare, animal and human health, and the community.
>
> I will endeavour to maintain my practice of veterinary science to current professional standards and will strive to improve my skills and knowledge through continuing professional development.
>
> I acknowledge that along with the privilege of acceptance into the veterinary profession comes community and professional responsibility.
>
> I will maintain these principles throughout my professional life.[7]

Can I hear your guffaws? 'ABOVE ALL ... ensure the health and welfare'! 'prevention and relief of animal suffering'! 'benefit of animal welfare'! These are the vets' sworn undertakings from around the world mostly observed in the breach, 'full of sound and fury signifying nothing'.

Add in the various animal cruelty laws and consumer protection (anti-fraud) laws and you would be inclined to think it should be easy to prosecute vets for malpractice in their involvement with the junk food makers. Sad to say, at this juncture getting vets into court or before the disciplinary tribunals and getting convictions has been damnably difficult. In time things may change, especially before independent judges as opposed to tribunals stacked with complicit vets.

Pet owner complaint to Veterinary Surgeons Board

Over a period of three years Ms A was given the run-around by 20 different vets as she sought help for her obese cat. Initially she was prescribed a Mars product, Royal Canin Weight Loss sachets. However, the patient's weight continued to increase, leading to a fatty liver and uncontrolled diabetes. At that point 'specialist' vets switched the diet to Hill's junk. They did not identify or deal with the raging periodontal disease—only recommend more and more tests and higher and higher doses of insulin. At a late stage the 'specialists' recognised the severe mouth disease. But it was too late. The patient developed inoperable mouth cancer and died a miserable death.

Ms A hired a lawyer who wrote a comprehensive letter of complaint regarding the 'negligence in prescribing defective diets'. In support of the complaint, I wrote:

> In my opinion, as a direct result of negligent, cruel and illegal conduct whether independently or collectively those veterinary surgeons either by their actions or failure to perform appropriate actions ensured that B ... would suffer intractable periodontal disease and obesity leading to end stage diabetes and cancer.
>
> In my opinion a higher standard of care is expected of registered specialists than of general practitioners. This expected higher standard of care was not evident from the records produced.

Unfortunately, and as usual, the case turned on whether or not the specialists' conduct met 'current practice standards'. It's the old circular argument: we set the practice standards (feed junk food and treat the resultant maladies); the specialists followed the standards, so they are innocent of any wrongdoing.

In my submission I condemned 'current practice standards' arising from the 'junk pet food saturated environment where veterinary schools prostitute themselves to the companies and young vets are assiduously brainwashed in the dominant junk pet food paradigm.' Instead, I recommended that more dependable practice standards should apply:

1. Basic scientific/biological practice standards

The fundamentals of carnivore biology are well researched and well understood—except perhaps by the most arrogant junk pet-food indoctrinated vets. Yes, there are vets who claim that dogs, only slightly modified wolves, are omnivores.

Otherwise, the vast body of anatomical, physiological, biochemical, ethological and ecological research and teaching sets the practice standards for the feeding of dogs, (modified wolves) and cats.

2. Human medical practice standards

(a) In the medical sciences it is common to employ laboratory animals in researching diseases affecting humans. In respect to human periodontal disease, obesity, diabetes and cancer many lab animals are utilised and the information so gained is extrapolated to the human situation.

(b) Research is also carried out using human subjects for the study of diet, obesity, periodontal disease, diabetes and cancer.

> Since objective study of diet, obesity, periodontal disease and cancer are effectively banned in vet research labs and universities, then the information gained at (a) and (b) must inform the standards applicable to domestic carnivores.

The 'specialist in small animal clinical nutrition' hired by the defence provided an outpouring of indigestible guff that will make you cross-eyed and nauseous. Here are the opening lines.

> It is my opinion that many cats in the feline population can consume a variety of diets without obvious clinical effects for long periods throughout their lives. There are specific cats within the population prone to specific medical conditions, which may benefit from individualized feeding strategies. Unfortunately, we as a profession are not currently very good at identifying these individual pets unless they have a familial history suggestive of development of specific conditions or until they develop specific medical conditions themselves over time. At present we are restricted to a few common pet food options. Commercial dry, canned and semi-moist diets offer many benefits to many pet owners. These include the fact that many have been through feeding trial to ensure digestibility and nutrient balance at least in the short term, they are time-efficient and cost-efficient for many owners, and prolonged storage is possible. There are of course potential negatives to commercial diet, canned or semi-moist diets. These include needing to be selected to ensure the desired nutrient profile and ingredients for individual animals, and that processing may affect nutrient availability.

As you may guess, the vets and vet board closed ranks and the cat owner's complaint was dismissed.

Discovery, losing battles but winning the war

Lawyers can advise you. However, knowing your enemy and choosing when to fight are key elements in a successful legal action. If groups of pet owners join forces and hire specialist lawyers, they may be in stronger position to achieve deep 'discovery'. Discovery is when both sides in a legal action are required to provide to the court the documents and evidence upon which they rely. It is a way of reducing surprises and ensuring that it is the facts that are being adjudicated. As mentioned above, bringing legal actions against the BARFers and their vets may be a shrewd first move. At discovery, what possible justification could they provide for destroying the raw meaty bones medicinal benefits in their calculated pursuit of profit?

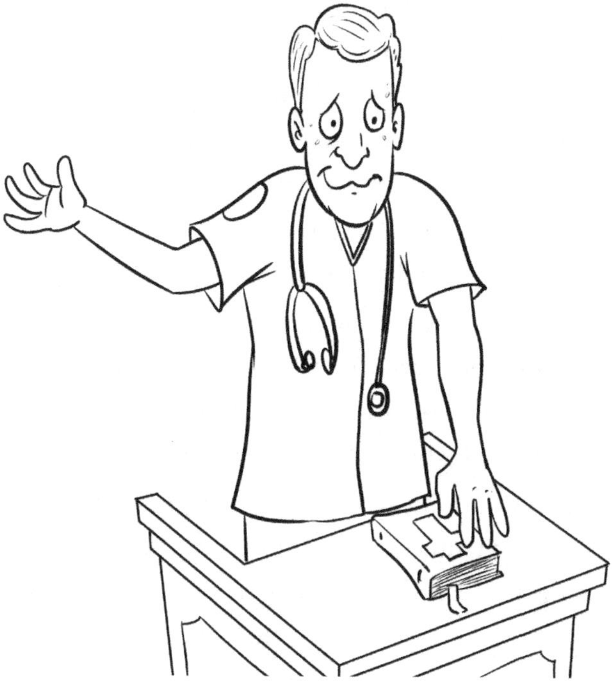

BARFer vet under oath

Going to court and obtaining justice are not one and the same thing. Indeed, in the early rounds of fighting corrupt vets, you will likely lose. However, with each new case, new incriminatory evidence will be provided and more *publicity* given to the cause. A US lawyer compared the raw meaty bones struggles with the spectacular 1925 case, *The State of Tennessee v. John Thomas Scopes* (the Scopes 'monkey trial').

Back in the day Tennessee passed a law prohibiting the teaching of human evolution in schools. The American Civil Liberties Union took umbrage and financed a test case in which John Scopes, a Tennessee high school science teacher, agreed to be tried for violating the law. Wikipedia, drawing on historian Edward J. Larson's 2006 book *Evolution: The Remarkable History of a Scientific Theory* (pp. 211–13), reports on the publicity surrounding the trial.

> 'Like so many archetypal American events, the trial itself began as a publicity stunt.' The press coverage of the 'Monkey Trial' was overwhelming. The front pages of newspapers like the New York Times were dominated by the case for days. More than 200 newspaper reporters from all parts of the country and two from London were in Dayton. Twenty-two telegraphers sent out 165,000 words per day on the trial, over thousands of miles of telegraph wires hung for the purpose; more words were transmitted to Britain about the Scopes trial than for any previous American event. Trained chimpanzees performed on the courthouse lawn. Chicago's WGN radio station broadcast the trial with announcer Quin Ryan via clear-channel broadcasting first on-the-scene coverage of the criminal trial. Two movie cameramen had their film flown out daily in a small plane from a specially prepared airstrip.[8]

William Bryan, counsel for the plaintiff state of Tennessee, complained that evolutionists taught that human beings were descended 'Not even from American monkeys, but from old world monkeys'. *Life* magazine awarded Bryan its 'Brass Medal of the Fourth Class' for having 'successfully demonstrated by the alchemy of ignorance hot air may be transmuted into gold, and that the Bible is infallibly inspired except where it differs with him on the question of wine, women, and wealth'.

At the end of the trial defendant Scopes was found guilty and fined $100—a delicious example of losing the battle but winning the war. Nowadays the theory of evolution is back on the curriculum, even in Tennessee and other southern states of the US.

Perhaps the Scopes trial does set a precedent. Perhaps we can take on the main enemy in highly publicised show trials?

The main enemy

A headline in the business pages tells us the size of the main enemy: 'Pet food market to reach nearly $128B worldwide by 2027'.[9] A further headline tells us who they are: 'Mars Petcare, Nestlé Purina Pet Care and Hill's Pet Nutrition lead the pet food industry into 2026'.[10] They need no introduction. They are household names, bigger and uglier than the headlines suggest. They are the unacceptable face of global capitalism that tramples and exploits wherever it goes—USA, Europe, Africa, South America, Asia. My parents' generation waged war and risked death to defend our freedoms in World War II. Before that my grandparents' generation fought against machine guns in World War I. If they were alive today, they would be appalled to see the monster enemies within who have invaded the peace and occupied by stealth.

Although, in my view, they are massive criminal enterprises, at least the multinational corporations don't fight with live ammunition. As sinister as the Mafia—perhaps more sinister—they nevertheless don't resort to murder of humans ('murder' of pets is another story). They've got an image to protect. Somehow, thanks to many years of public relations spin, they've wheedled their way into the global consciousness as neutral or even beneficial aspects of daily life. For the health and welfare of pets, people and planet we're obliged to expose them and wage war against them.

First be aware of the size and reach of the behemoths. Nestlé is the biggest junk food and baby formula company on the planet. With annual revenue of US$85 billion[11] the company states it is committed to becoming the very best 'Nutrition, Health, and Wellness Company'—which statement appears ludicrous when seen alongside the 'Baby Killer' label affixed to the company[12] as a result of its predatory marketing of artificial breastmilk to third world mothers. In 2017 the *New York Times* carried a headline:

> **How Big Business Got Brazil Hooked on Junk Food**
>
> Children's squeals rang through the muggy morning air as a woman pushed a gleaming white cart along pitted, trash-strewn streets. She was making deliveries to some of the poorest households in this seaside city, bringing pudding, cookies and other packaged foods to the customers on her sales route.
>
> Celene da Silva, 29, is one of thousands of door-to-door vendors for Nestlé, helping the world's largest packaged food conglomerate expand its reach into a quarter-million households in Brazil's farthest-flung corners.
>
> As she dropped off variety packs of Chandelle pudding, Kit-Kats and Mucilon infant cereal, there was something striking about her customers: Many were visibly overweight, even small children.[13]

Mars Corporation revenue is of the order US$33 billion annually. They boast of their family-owned chocolate, chewing gum, junk pet food and vet hospital business.

> Mars has been proudly family owned for over 100 years. It's this independence that gives us the gift of freedom to think in generations, not quarters, so we can invest in the long-term future of our business, our people and the planet ...[14]

Colgate-Palmolive, though smaller than the other two monoliths at US$16 billion annually, can nonetheless leverage its massive research and marketing resources associated with toothpaste, shower gels, deodorants, antiperspirants, shampoos and conditioners, dish-washing liquids, household cleaners and fabric softeners.

With billions at their disposal, the companies have immense defence and forward planning capability. Besides the venal and corrupt veterinary profession providing a protective cordon, they have lawyers, accountants, advertising and marketing people, psychologists and political lobbyists. Besides buying the silence of vets, chances are they tip funds into political campaigns.[15] And of course, the vast advertising revenue buys them a docile media that suppresses bad news and promotes puff pieces. It's the way of the modern world.

As we stand back and observe the commercial empires, we see that they were not built in a day and will not be defeated in a day either. However, we should not be daunted. The weathering of ice, wind and rain can erode a mountain and a falling pebble can trigger an avalanche.

David and Goliath

Speaking of pebbles, the Bible tells us that David slew Goliath with a well-aimed pebble to the temple, Goliath's weak spot. And whether we're thinking of the multinational giants' output or the local BARF supplier, their common weak spot is the *texture* of their junk. Nothing about their junk meets the first three medicinal imperatives as listed in Chapter 3, p. 50.

From a legal perspective the issues revolve around wilful cruelty to animals and consumer fraud, both of which carry criminal penalties if the prosecutions are brought by a government agency. But here's the snag. Police and various regulatory agencies either don't know or don't believe that feeding pets junk food is cruel, or that the advertisements are misleading and false. In the future we can hope the agencies start to take a proper interest in the cruelty and fraud hiding in plain sight. Meanwhile, as aggrieved pet owners, we need to bring civil actions.

Class actions

Lawyers in your locality can advise whether you can bring actions directly against junk food makers and suppliers or against vets and media outlets that publish false and misleading information. Your decision as to whether to proceed will depend on many factors, not least the cost of going to court. In the USA in particular, and increasingly in other countries, the opportunity to join a class action is a favoured way of consumers linking up to bring a lawsuit against manufacturers and suppliers.

Specialist lawyers advertise for business in the wake of consumer goods failings. In 2007 many tonnes of junk food made by Canadian company Menu Foods was found to be the source of melamine toxicity that killed or maimed thousands of pets throughout North America.[16] The company was hit with more than 100 class actions that were finally settled when the company and its insurers agreed to pay US$24 million in damages.

The case was about straightforward toxicity, admitted by Menu Foods. Their supply of wheat gluten from China had been adulterated with melamine, a nitrogen-rich chemical. The original suppliers added melamine in a deliberate effort to make the gluten appear to have extra protein. Of course, we can argue that carnivore foods should not contain wheat gluten and plant protein has poor nutritional value compared to animal protein—matters well understood by junk food manufacturers. But those matters were not the focus of the exercise. The fact that Menu Foods was in the business of duping pet owners about nitrogen content did not matter to the court. Nor did it matter that Menu Foods were duped by their Chinese supplier. What mattered was that Menu Foods fessed up, admitted liability and settled the class action.

Colgate-Palmolive company Hill's settled a $12.5 million[17] class action brought by aggrieved pet owners whose dogs had eaten Hill's canned junk fortified with vitamin D—at levels more than 33 times[18] the recommended safe upper limit. Of course, we can argue that the diets of dogs should not be fortified with artificial vitamins and thus should not be subject to inadvertent error or deliberate fraud. However, for the purposes of the lawsuit it did not matter that the toxic vitamin premix was sourced from an outside company; it was Hill's that paid the price.

So how do we make Hill's, Mars, Nestlé and a host of other junk pet food makers pay the price for their *knowing*, wilful poisoning of the world's pets? How do we show a direct link between the myriad disease outcomes in pets and the junk 'food' their owners have been tricked into feeding? For sure we know that dogs and cats fed junk food have dull, lifeless coats and dull eyes. We know that they often appear depressed, lacking in vigour and subject to bouts of diarrhoea and hard-to-control persistent itching. And after a few years of indifferent health, we know millions of pets succumb to diabetes, cancer, and heart, liver and kidney disease, to name but a few. Knowing these things and proving the junk 'food' connection in court is our problem.

However, in one key area, I reckon we are on a winner against the fraudsters. Stinky bad breath, gingivitis leading to periodontal disease and then periodontitis are the hallmark of junk food diets, whether cooked or raw. Enterprising class action lawyers should be able to gather together a number of pet owners who have sufficient evidence to bring an action. They will need to show that the pets were fed entirely or predominantly the products of one supplier while following the package instructions as to quantity and frequency of feeding.

Photographic, video and written evidence can be obtained. Receipts for the packaged junk can be tendered, as can the veterinary clinical records. In fact, owners who buy most of their junk food from the vet and also have extensive veterinary clinical notes will likely be most able to prove their case. With these things in mind, there are two obvious potential targets: Colgate-Palmolive, makers of Hill's products sold through veterinary hospitals, and Mars, the world's biggest junk pet food maker and owner of Banfield, AniCura, Linnaeus and other vet hospital chains.

Since all dogs, cats and ferrets fed on junk food develop stinky breath and proceed down the periodontal disease path with all the attendant extra problems, it should be possible to bring hundreds of class actions. The success of one should lead to the success of the next, each additional case providing pets and pet owners with restitution for decades of deception.

Potentially, in the USA at least, there may be scope for even bigger actions against the junk pet food makers. In 1970 the Racketeer

Influenced and Corrupt Organizations (RICO) law was passed as a means to prosecuting mobsters for a pattern of racketeering connected to an enterprise as opposed to previous laws that only allowed prosecution of individuals.[19] Of course, junk pet food companies fit the definition of 'enterprise' and we know that they are aware their products inflict immense harm.

Specialist lawyers can advise whether the costs of a civil RICO action may be worthwhile. If you win, apart from striking a huge blow for pets and pet owners, you will receive treble the damages you could otherwise claim. Imagine if a RICO action against Mars, Nestlé and Colgate gained a Scopes Monkey Trial level of publicity with today's electronic media broadcasting to the world.

False friends and pet food recalls

In the fog of war, things tend to get complicated. And friends are indispensable for our wellbeing. Yet recognising what's important and who to trust can be difficult. We need to be cautious and avoid being led astray.

Pet food recalls are a perennial topic guaranteed to light up the internet. Facebook discussions fulminate with rage, generating much heat, venting steam. Of course, recalls are immediately necessary in the event of acute toxicity. The huge melamine scandal and Hill's vitamin D fiasco are clear examples. However, from the point of view of the multi-billion-dollar fraudsters, a few million dollars in payout is just another cost of doing business. The well-known adage 'there's no such thing as bad publicity' is tailor-made for the junk pet food fraud.

If people are raging against melamine and vitamin D, they're not raging against the fundamental problems of junk food diets. In fact, they are consolidating their assumptions that with better regulations or better enforcement of regulations, all would be well.

Assumptions are the great bugbear. People assume that the headlines are relevant, that the intensity of the resultant discussions will somehow make things better. But alas, if we want to deal with the pet food fraud, joining the fervour will not make things better.

A recent dramatic toxicity event in Australia illustrates how the junk pet food industry and its allies pounced on the propaganda opportunity. The story relates to the sickness and death of dogs in Victoria that had consumed large quantities of horse meat. After some days' delay, laboratory testing revealed that the subject meat contained indospicine, a chemical made by plants growing in the arid outback of northern Australia.[20] Apparently, a truckload of horses from the Northern Territory, originally intended for human consumption, was rerouted to a Victorian dog meat plant. Dogs are especially sensitive to indospicine and if fed contaminated meat, for instance from outback camels and horses, in large quantity over a period of days they are liable to succumb to severe liver disease.

Death from liver failure has to be one of the most painful distressing conditions. The Australian Consumers Association circulated a letter calling on the agriculture minister to 'please help us keep our pets safe by introducing new laws to create a mandatory standard for pet food safety'. The RSPCA jumped in on the act with a media release.

> **'Act now to prevent future tragedy': RSPCA says lack of pet food safety regulation is putting Australian pets at risk**
>
> RSPCA Australia has joined forces with the Australian Veterinary Association (AVA) and the Pet Food Industry Association of Australia (PFIAA) in calling for an end to the significant delays in developing and implementing robust pet food regulation, including expediting a mandatory Standard for pet food safety.[21]

Note the unholy alliance of the RSPCA, AVA and PFIAA drawing attention to themselves, making sanctimonious comment—hiding in plain sight. It is an egregious and typical inversion. The PFIAA members are chiefly responsible for the *global* tragedy of diet-induced disease and suffering. The AVA members undertake to 'Hold as a key concern, the health, welfare and respectful treatment of animals'.[22] And the RSPCA mission is to 'prevent cruelty to animals'.[23] Bah, humbug!

Sadly, the conspirators know what works. They know to present themselves as the experts on all things to do with pets and diets. They have had many years' practice pretending to be the friend of animals and the friend of pet owners. First and foremost, they are friends to themselves, their revenue stream and the *status quo* they defend. My advice: don't trust a word they say.

12

SPARKING THE REVOLUTION

The obscure we see eventually. The completely obvious, it seems, takes longer.

Edward R. Murrow

The journey of a thousand miles begins with one step.

Chinese proverb

So, we've identified the *completely obvious* fraud hiding in plain sight and are now beginning to make the *first steps* on the road to sparking the revolution. For nothing short of social, cultural, scientific revolution will begin to compensate for the century-and-a-half of junk pet food industry influence and control. We need friends, lots of them. We need to share our problems and thus to halve them. And by sharing and then resharing we'll reduce our problems to tiny little manageable pieces.

Friends in the making

Almost everyone has been a pawn in the game played by junk pet food companies, vets and animal welfare groups—some more directly than others. At the margin, dead people, who bequeath their estates to the welfare charities, prop up the game. Taxpayers pay for failed laws, hospital emergency centres that treat road accident victims and mauled toddlers, and local pounds holding stray and unwanted pets. Even people who don't pay taxes and don't keep a pet are almost certain to have sat through endless, intrusive junk pet food advertisements. They've progressed from babyhood, through toddlerhood to adulthood accepting junk pet food and the false and misleading advertisements as 'normal'.

Like chess players, the pet food industry uses its pawns strategically and tactically and pawns are often sacrificed for competitive advantage. Vets, animal welfare charity members and pet owners are all manipulated and, where convenient (for the junk food companies), sacrificed and abandoned. Notice how the pet food companies don't defend their defective products; they leave that to the vets, welfare charities and government bureaucrats. The companies know to stay on the front foot, positively promoting their junk but never falling into a defensive position, being called to account.

Our task, then, is to recruit friends to the cause and where necessary encourage people to get off the fence or to switch sides. Here is a non-exhaustive list of people we need to help us in the years ahead. The incentive for us will be the revolution in animal health, with resultant improvements in human and environmental health. Each of our subject groups will gain incentives galore, starting with the pride and passion of joining a worthy cause.

Advertising industry

The advertising industry will eventually, we must hope, be recruited in the service of pets and pet owners. For now, though, it is fully corrupted by the junk pet food makers. If you are like me, you will be disgusted at the artificial bone advertisements concocted on behalf of Mars and Nestlé to offset some of the worst effects of their artificial diets while providing yet another illicit source of income. Now, it seems, we're urged to buy Nestlé Purina 'artificial water'.

Introducing a third bowl as a simple solution

PURINA® PRO PLAN® Veterinary Supplements Hydra Care™ is a complementary supplement that offers a tasty, soft textured jelly that is served on its own, as an extra third bowl. The formula will engage cats to happily lick it up due to its great taste. This revolutionary supplement has been created to help cats increase on average 28% more hydration every day than water alone and increase urine dilution.[1]

Nestlé, Mars and all other kibble producers have a huge, and as yet, unresolved problem. Their dry junk wreaks havoc with cat health, not least by sitting in the intestines drawing precious water out of the cat's circulation. Every year millions of cats suffer painful urinary tract disease. Thousands die an agonising death due to a blocked urethra.[2] The advertising copy writers tell us:

> Water is vital to life and is considered the most important nutrient. It is the predominant component of most body tissues and accounts for approximately 60% of body weight in cats. It serves many physiological functions including transport of nutrients, lubricant, metabolic functions, thermoregulation, and elimination of waste products through the kidneys. Therefore, remaining hydrated is the most important physiological parameter that governs the delivery of key nutrients to the body.
>
> Cats are poor drinkers due to their natural behaviour. Cats have a low thirst stimulus, and consequently, they produce very concentrated urine. These adaptations might trigger long-term health implications, like increased risk of

> suffering Feline Lower Urinary Tract Disease (FLUTD) as urinary stones or Feline Idiopathic Cystitis (FIC). Therefore, increasing cats' liquid intake should be considered as a key factor of reaching a correct level of hydration, together with a healthy diet and proper environmental management. Introducing a third bowl as a simple solution.

Our domestic cats' wild cousins are desert dwellers that depend on their prey for water. For pet cats, when forced into dry junk food addiction, it's a different story. As a trumped-up fanciful solution, we're told that in addition to a bowl of Purina artificial junk, cats need a bowl of real water and now a bowl of 'artificial water'. As to whether the 'artificial water' comes with long-term adverse health consequences, it's too early to say.

Can and will advertising industry executives be persuaded to switch sides and write copy for real food (and its medicinal properties) and real, natural water? That, I suspect, will depend on who's able and willing to pay.

Animal welfare lawyers

Eleven Australian law schools teach animal law. In the USA there are more than 100 schools that teach the subject. Theoretically, then, there's a growing band of lawyers ready to prosecute the cruelty cases arising from the multi-billion-dollar pet food fraud. Unfortunately, in 2022, it remains theoretical because lawyers don't seem to notice the cruelty hiding in plain sight. Things can and will change.

If a few lawyers sniff the breath of animals fed on junk food, they will recoil at the toxic fumes. If they stop to contemplate that the toxic juices from the animals' gums are like sewer water leaching

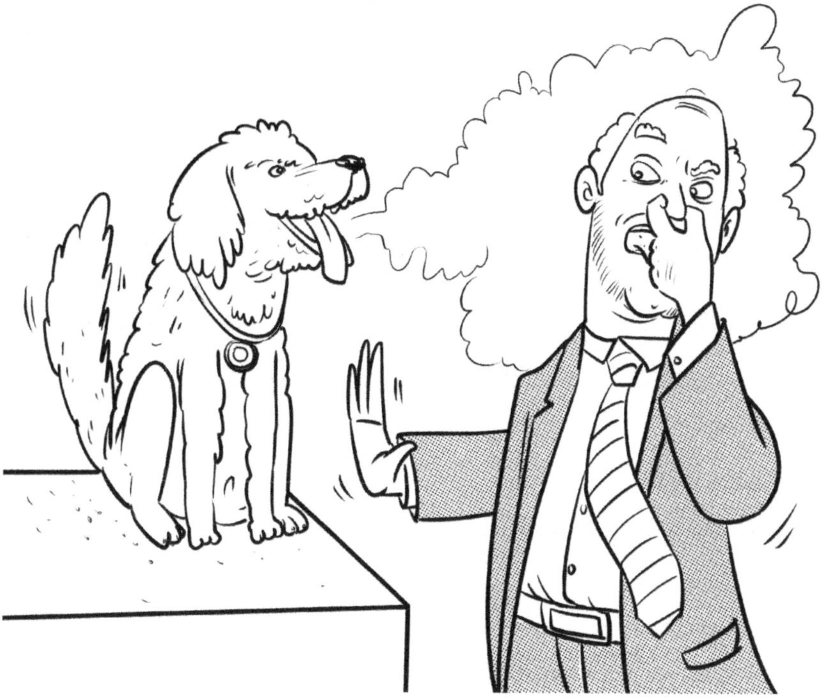

into the capillaries and circulating through the cardiovascular system 24 hours a day, they'll start to understand the gravity of the relentless cruelty induced by junk food. Thus motivated, they can become frontline troops in the pet food conflict.

Archaeologists

Not wishing to be overly pessimistic, we should nonetheless expect the revolution to take ages. The idea that the Earth is round was first understood by the early Greeks about 500 years BC. Unfortunately, the sands of time blew over and buried the idea for around 2000 years. Let's fervently hope that is not to be the fate of the pet food revolution. However, erring on the side of caution, we should recruit archaeologists to the cause early. They can advise us how to store and preserve our information, inscribe on stone tablets and the like, for future discovery and interpretation.

As well as finding a universal language that can be understood by future generations of *Homo sapiens*, archaeologists should consider that aliens from outer space may want to make sense of how we live now. How do you explain to an alien that we domesticated wolves and desert predators and deliberately fed them harmful junk, requiring some of the best and brightest young people to train for five years at university and then spend their working lives deliberately making matters worse? How do you make sense of absurdity?

Bureaucrats

Clever, creative, hard-working bureaucrats ensure the trains run on time, the hospitals stay open 24 hours a day and the aeroplanes land safely at our airports. But where pets are concerned, bureaucrats are deadly. Often vets, but not always, these are the folks who intercept letters to ministers and elected representatives. Or if the minister receives a letter, it will likely be departmental officers who craft a reply.

Over the past 30 years I've accumulated endless responses to my letters signed by ministers but written by their staff. Faceless, nameless and well versed in negotiating the corridors of power, they are adept at telling us why things are just fine and must stay that way. Of course, once the pet food revolution comes, the bureaucrats will switch sides in an instant—their fat salaries depend on it.

In the interim is there anything we can do about the obtuse backroom apparatchiks? Probably not much. We know that they're clever, creative and hard-working. Let's hope they've got a conscience too.

Butchers

Butchers may seem like obvious recruits to the raw meaty bones cause. However, for them, it may not be so easy. They are but one link in the chain with the junk pet food companies controlling both ends of the chain. Abattoir offal and waste go to the rendering plant and thence to the pet food ovens. Waste trim and bones from the retail operations go to the same rendering plant.

Retail butchers have spent many years supplying minced meat to pet owners. And their big, hard meatless bones are sold as 'dog bones' or in modern parlance 'recreational bones'. Butchers have much to 'unlearn' before they can become effective suppliers of raw meaty bones.

Children

Our children are our great hope for the future. When presented with the evidence of junk pet food cruelty they readily grasp the implications. Started early they can (and will) fashion the new revolution. We can rely on them for the future, but for the present they are vulnerable and need protection. The Children's Hospital of Pittsburgh provides facts and figures.

> **Facts & Figures About Dog Attacks**
>
> There are more than 52,000,000 dogs in the United States alone. Approximately one-third of all homes have a dog as a pet. ... According to the Centers for Disease Control (CDC) in Atlanta, Ga., there are approximately 800,000 dog bites each year that require medical attention. Even more amazing is the fact that 334,000 are severe enough to warrant treatment in a hospital. ...
>
> There are 2,400 dog attacks every day, 100 each hour or one every 36 seconds. ...

> More than 50 percent of all dog bite victims are children.
>
> ...
>
> According to the CDC, dog bites are a greater health problem for children than measles, mumps and whooping cough combined. They are more common than injuries from bike accidents, playground injuries, mopeds, skateboards or ATVs. Dog bite treatments cost more than a billion dollars each year. The most common victims are boys ages 5 to 9, and children in general are most frequently bit in the face, neck and head.[3]

Additional disturbing facts concern the role of junk pet food in dog aggression. Carol and Tony O'Herlihy are experienced dog trainers who wrote to the Australian Senate Inquiry into the Safety of Pet Food about dog aggression and a range of unwanted behaviours.

> Even the most severe form of any of the abovementioned [unwanted] behaviours can be solved by the cessation of a refined/manufactured diet and the introduction of a varied diet of raw, meaty bones, supplemented by table scraps. ...
>
> 'Dog behavioural problems' are caused by dogs trying to satisfy their need to eat as a carnivore. Life as a biscuit-a-vore can drive them (and their owners) crazy.[4]

In 1986 Roger Mugford, animal behaviour consultant to the Mars Corporation, told a Mars symposium about aggressive golden retrievers that when switched from commercial junk to home-cooked meals became docile.[5] (He didn't try feeding appropriate carnivore food.) Yes, Mars the biggest junk pet food makers on the planet know the effects of their junk on dogs with the consequent aggression and injury to children.

A professor of paediatric surgery told me how surprised he was to see Mars pet food people at a medical dog bite symposium. I surmised that with billions of dollars at stake, they were probably on a reconnaissance mission, listening for any rumblings from the assembled trauma specialists. If the doctors had made adverse commentary about dog ownership, the Mars people were there to steer the conversation on to more neutral ground. For Mars, commerce must prevail. Trauma surgeons are to be manipulated and children are expendable pawns in the multi-billion-dollar game.

Demoralised, disillusioned and dispirited vets

Vet Practice magazine tells us:

> Vets are four times more likely to die of suicide than the general population and two times more likely than any other healthcare profession. These risks are associated with a high-stress working environment with poor work-life balance due to long hours, demanding work, unsociable hours, and on-call work which form part of the day-to-day work of veterinarians.[6]

'Suicidal ideation, in the absence of another diagnosis, is quintessentially associated with major clinical depression.'[7] Let's be clear, vets are given to self-doubt, even self-loathing, because of perceived failings. We get depressed when, despite our best efforts, pets die. We get depressed when pets with chronic diseases return time and time again. It's like sitting at the sushi train, except that we have no appetite for another unsatisfactory encounter with the frustrated owner of an itchy dog, or arthritic dog or a cat with chronic recurring diarrhoea.

I don't know, I don't have the figures, but it's my guess that once vets subscribe to the wonderful new revolution in pet feeding, the sushi train of diseases will falter and slow down. Instead of a high-stress working environment, it will become a place of solutions and a place of joy.

Doctors, health workers

Many doctors, nurses and allied health professionals keep pets. And it's part of their training to understand the perils of a junk food diet, periodontal disease and obesity for their human patients. But just like the rest of us, they suffer from cognitive dissonance, often believing one thing and doing another.

However, once they recognise the immense benefits of raw meaty bones, they will be able to use the information in varied ways for themselves, their pets and their patients. As frontline counsellors they see the dog bite trauma and financial hardship occasioned by the endless trips to the vet. For older people contemplating the end of their life, counsellors see that an elderly pet fed on junk food creates added depression and anxiety.

The pet food ads and vet associations tell us that pets, in all circumstances, are an inestimable benefit. Doctors see the other side. They can help society strike a better balance between the costs and benefits of owning a pet.

Dog boarding and related industries

Workers on the front line of the pet care industry are in an invidious position. They see the sick and bedraggled pets but are almost powerless to do anything about it. Pet chihuahuas and mastiffs and all sizes in between arrive at the boarding kennels with supplies of brand name junk as their everyday diet, to be fed in measured portions two times a day. The contact details of the pet's regular vet are entered on the admission form. Often a bag of 'essential' heart, skin, thyroid and other medicaments will accompany the pet. Should the kennel-hand bother to look, she will find the stinky breath, tartar-encrusted teeth and flaky dry skin.

During peak season at Christmas and Easter the boarding establishments, doggy day care and groomers will be full to capacity, overflowing with chronically sick dogs and cats. The business owners depend on the revenue, the workers depend on the job. And to stay in business and retain the job it's better to stay mute, to say nothing about the ongoing unfairness of a system that relentlessly exploits pets and their owners.

Eventually, of course, times will change. Meanwhile business owners and workers can plan their strategy for a fairer, healthier future —maybe, cautiously, make changes to the way their business operates.

Dog handlers

Police dogs, army dogs, customs dogs, service dogs all cost lots of money to train. We want them to have long productive lives. At a basic level dogs can only be fit and well if fed as closely as possible to the wild wolf ideal diet. Unfortunately, it's often bureaucrats and vets who decide what the dogs should be fed, with scant regard for the teachings of nature.

An important requirement for tracker dogs, cadaver dogs, bomb detection and drug detection dogs is their sense of smell. When researchers studied the effects of the accumulation of tartar on beagle dogs' teeth, they found a corresponding loss of ability to detect odours. However, within one day of having their teeth cleaned the dogs' odour-detecting abilities returned to normal.[8] Dog handlers form close bonds with their dogs and want good outcomes—especially if finding a lost child or a terrorist bomb depends on a sniffer dog's sense of smell.

Elected representatives

Damned if they do and damned if they don't, the lot of elected representatives is not easy. Hence, they tend to be a profession of fence-sitters, masters of procrastination, seldom leading and if they do, leading from behind.

After 30 years of campaigning, I'm both cynical and somewhat optimistic for the future. A few politicians have given a modicum of help even though there have been no votes in it for them. When, in the future, there are perceived votes, we may see more politicians taking an interest. If so, then the onus is on us, the well-informed, to agitate for change and show how those who support the good pet health, human economy and natural environment cause will get our votes.

Even with thousands marching in the streets, politicians will still be under pressure to preserve the *status quo* and, of course—and this is the bitter truth—pay heed to junk pet food lobbyists. Political lobbying is not illegal and the massively wealthy junk pet food companies, mostly working through their vet proxies, are sure to be doing their utmost to preserve their power and wealth.

Eminent persons

The success of the revolution cannot depend on gaining the attention of eminent persons, but it can help. On the converse side, if they don't know about the issues, then they most certainly can't help. Over the past 30 years I've written to endless eminent persons—mostly without response. However, here are three standout responses.

BUCKINGHAM PALACE

From: The Assistant to The Equerry to H.R.H. The Prince of Wales

6th November, 1992

Dear Mr. Lonsdale,

Thank you for your letter and enclosure.

I shall seek an opportunity to lay these before The Prince of Wales, who I am sure, would wish me to thank you for taking the trouble to write.

Yours sincerely,

Maureen A. Stevens

Maureen A. Stevens

10 DOWNING STREET
LONDON SW1A 2AA

From the Correspondence Secretary 9 December 1992

Dear Mr Lonsdale,

The Prime Minister has asked me to thank you for your recent letter and the enclosure.

Yours sincerely,

Mr T Lonsdale
Tom Lonsdale & Associates
Riverstone Veterinary Hospital
Garfield Road
Riverstone
NEW SOUTH WALES 2765
Australia

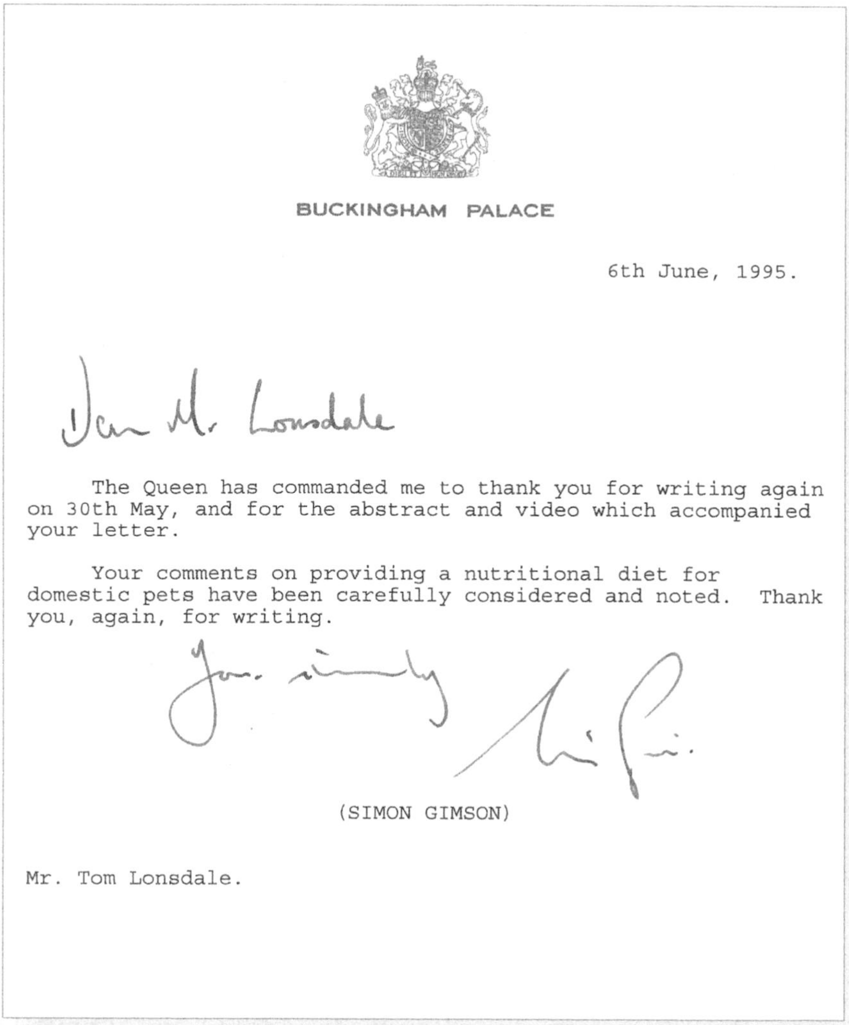

BUCKINGHAM PALACE

6th June, 1995.

Dear Mr Lonsdale

The Queen has commanded me to thank you for writing again on 30th May, and for the abstract and video which accompanied your letter.

Your comments on providing a nutritional diet for domestic pets have been carefully considered and noted. Thank you, again, for writing.

Yours sincerely

(SIMON GIMSON)

Mr. Tom Lonsdale.

At the very least, the letters show the courtesy of the writers despite their very busy lives and enormous responsibilities.

Many celebrities and eminent persons keep pets—Paris Hilton's chihuahuas, dogs in the White House and royal corgis for example—so it's vital they learn how to keep those pets healthy. If enough of us write letters it may start to make waves. Imagine if just one actor at the Oscar's ceremony were to mention the lifesaving, life-enhancing properties of a wolf's natural diet!

Environmentalists

In 2017 Professor Gregory Okin of the University of California Los Angeles published a paper titled 'Environmental impacts of food consumption by dogs and cats'.

> The US has the largest population of pet dogs and cats globally, with an estimated 77.8 million dogs and 85.6 million cats in 2015. The consequences of these animals on wildlife and water quality have been investigated, with studies showing considerable impacts on carbon usage, water quality, disease and wildlife.[9]

Professor Okin's bottom-line calculation revealed:

> The proportion of the dietary energy in the US consumed by dogs and cats was calculated as the sum of the energy consumed by dogs and cats (203 ± 15 PJ y^{-1}) divided by human energy intake (1051 ± 9 PJ y^{-1}), with the result that dogs and cats consume about $19.4 \pm 1.6\%$ of the energy that humans in America do.

Add in the environmental costs of transportation, processing, packaging, the pharmaceutical and pesticide industry and ultimately garbage disposal and we are faced with enormous pet-related environmental costs.

And we need to count the costs, as they affect all inhabitants of our overcrowded planet. Although pets confer numerous benefits on society, the main benefit should not be fattening the bottom line of the junk pet food makers. Environmentalists can provide much needed assistance.

Etymologists and lexicographers

Perhaps etymologists and lexicographers can help us navigate a way out of the misplaced assumptions and false concepts we use every day when speaking about pets and their diets. We know that wolves, knowing what's best for them, run 40 kilometres (25 miles) through deep snow in order to catch and consume prey that constitutes both food *and* medicine. We use the terms 'prey' and 'food' interchangeably without mentioning 'medicine'.

The cat sits patiently for hours at the mousehole, driven by its instincts to seek suitable nourishment. We call the mouse 'food for cats' without so much as a hint at the medicinal value of the mouse. Worse still, we label the harmful stuff in cans and packets piled high on the supermarket shelf not as 'pet poison' but as 'pet food'.

Vets are currently portrayed in a positive light such that the verb 'to vet' means 'to subject to (usually expert) appraisal or correction'. Perhaps that was once true when vets were called in to examine horses offered for sale by unscrupulous horse dealers. Now in the junk pet food age, perhaps our definitions should be updated to match the new reality.

Facebook, Google and Twitter

We know that every word uttered by the junk pet food makers is a lie, or if true then spoken in the service of a lie. For the vet apologists for junk food, the same principles generally apply. Much to my surprise, an advertisement for BARF junk was accompanied by a Google dialogue box asking me if I wished to continue seeing the ad. Without hesitation I ticked 'No' and have not seen the ad since.

The social conscience of the giant social media companies is only now coming to the fore,[10] a dramatic example being the Facebook ban on Donald Trump for 'attempts to incite violence and undermine the democratic process'. Twitter said Trump 'presented a risk to public safety' and permanently banned him from the messaging platform.

Maybe in future years the false and misleading junk pet food ads that undermine pet health and safety will receive similar bans?

Family, friends and neighbours

We all want to be good neighbours and have cordial relations, especially with our family and friends. Unfortunately, adherence to raw meaty bones ideals can split asunder families and friendships. People tell me of the unpleasantness and the struggles sometimes encountered when challenging people's belief in junk food and their faith in vets pushing junk food.

It is embarrassing for anyone to be considered cruel because of their choices. The junk pet food culture, aided and abetted by vets and fake welfare groups, renders almost an entire pet-owning population cruel and dysfunctional. But alas, if you become the messenger, don't expect plaudits; you may well receive the blame. There's no simple answer. However, allow time to work its magic. Plant seeds and lead by example and we will surely win.

Farmers

Farmers can lead by example and feed their working dogs on whole chickens, sheep, goat, pig, fish and rabbit carcasses or, next best, raw meaty bones.

As and when the junk pet food industry goes into decline, enterprising farmers can develop new niche markets for wholesome carnivore food. With the increasing interest in environmentally friendly, organic, free-range and chemical-free farming and the upsurge in farmers' markets, the future for farmers and pet owners could be on an upward trajectory.

General practitioner vets

Regular vets receive much criticism in this book and may feel unfairly treated. A vet's job is to assist and advise society about its use of animals for food and fibre, companionship, recreation and entertainment. From an animal welfare perspective there's plenty not to like about battery cages for egg-laying hens or the overcrowded factory farms with meat chickens or feedlot cattle wandering in tight spaces ankle deep in their own excrement. Consider the Australian range-fed sheep and cattle herded onto a cramped ship and carted off to the Middle East for ritual slaughter—for those that survive the journey through fierce summer heat.[11] Other people take strong exception to performing animals in circuses and wild animal exhibits in zoos. Horse racing and greyhound racing have their share of vocal detractors.

In all the above vets are on hand to advise and assist. They carry rubber stamps; they are not expected to crusade against the industry. So, what's different about pets being fed junk out of the can or packet? I think the *scale* of the problem, the *active involvement of vets* and the *simple available solution*—feeding pets unprocessed raw meaty bones—are key differences.

Hopefully in the coming years most vets will reconsider their previous opposition and welcome a renaissance in vet teaching and practice of inestimable value to pets and their owners.

Historians

We know that 'radical' ideas conflicting with established beliefs often meet a hostile reception. Historians tell us that in 1633 the Catholic Church forced Galileo to recant his theory that the Earth orbits the Sun. A further 359 years passed before the church was prepared to admit that the Earth does indeed rotate around the Sun.[12]

In 1915 when Alfred Wegener proposed his theory of 'continental drift' the scientific community were at first highly sceptical and it took until the 1960s for the idea of the Earth's tectonic plate movement to be accepted.[13]

In 'A study in human incredulity' the author Fred C. Kelly tells us about the world's underwhelming reception to the news of the Wright brothers' invention of powered flight.

> One reason why nearly everyone in the United States was disinclined to swallow the reports about flying with a machine heavier than air was that important scientists had already explained in the public prints why the thing was impossible.[13]

Accordingly, the press missed arguably one of the most important developments of the 20th century because as Kelly tells us:

> Naturally no editor who knew a thing couldn't be done would permit his paper to record the fact that it had been done.[14]

In Chapter 6 we saw that doctors were resistant to the ideas of Semmelweis about childbed fever and to Lister's revolutionary antiseptic surgery, despite both saving lives.

Importantly, none of the above discoveries cut across the commercial interests of global mega-corporations or professions or charities. Admittedly the discoveries may have offended the egos of powerful, self-important people. But the discoveries did not incur the enmity of massively wealthy interest groups with the power, reach and money to suppress the truth. This is the stark reality facing would-be pet food revolutionaries.

With these facts in mind, we need to recruit and inform historians about the struggles so that they can both advise us how to proceed and then to record progress or lack thereof.

Journalists

As we saw in Chapter 10, coverage of the pet food fraud has been a fickle affair. How, then, do we encourage journalists to pay attention and delve deep into this mighty, costly fraud? Eventually I believe some journalists will recognise the importance of the issues—and continue to push for exposure. Tara Parker-Pope, writing in the *Wall Street Journal* in 1997, showed the potential.

> **Colgate Gives Doctors Treats for Plugging its Food Brands**
> Borrowing a page from pharmaceuticals companies, which routinely woo doctors to prescribe their drugs, Hill's has spent a generation cultivating its professional following. ... Since almost everyone asks their vets what to start feeding a new pet, Hill's cleverly has managed to steer billions its way with that all-important early recommendation.
>
> By chasing after the nation's 126 million cats and dogs through the backdoor of vet offices, Hill's has emerged as a crown jewel at Colgate.[15]

In 2007, following the melamine contamination scandal, the *New York Times Magazine* sent Frederick Kaufman to investigate. His article, 'They eat what we are', is a fascinating read told in a neutral voice, but exposing the venality of a disgraceful business.

> I had been told that in the basement of the animal-science laboratory building at the University of Illinois, Dr. George Fahey kept a colony of strange-looking dogs.

> At Fahey's orders, each of the dogs had undergone a surgical procedure to string a length of tubing from its intestinal tract to a clear plastic spout that stuck out its side. Fahey, a professor of animal and nutritional sciences, could open a spout by hand, fill a bag with whatever happened to ooze out and calculate how much the dog had digested before whatever it had not digested could move farther through its body. ...
>
> Piled nearby were stacks and stacks of the commercial pet foods the researchers give to animals in the control groups of their experiments—brands Fahey did not want specified in this article. ...
>
> George Fahey's research spares pet-food manufacturers the negative publicity they might attract if they ran their own experiments on surgically altered dogs.[16]

Unfortunately, both above articles appeared last century. Since then there have been countless articles, puff pieces and general filler describing current fads and culture but seldom or never questioning fundamental values, cruelty and fraud.

Kennel Club

> The Kennel Club, the UK's largest organisation dedicated to the health and welfare of dogs, has announced a new three-year nutritional partnership with Purina PRO Plan. As part of this partnership, The Kennel Club and Purina will support the UK's dog owners and breeders in highlighting the important health role that nutrition plays in all stages of a dog's life.[17]

On 1 October 2021, I wrote to the club with the subject line 'Purina partnership'.

> You may not be aware of my recent videos regarding Purina Supercoat: https://youtu.be/t9JTkQC4lJw and https://www.youtube.com/watch?v=2fTiIjBEhZo
>
> Given the known dangers of manufactured diets for dogs, I wonder what the Kennel Club rationale is for the arrangements with Purina.

Answer pending.

Local municipality

Your local municipal council collects the garbage, operates the parks and gardens, runs (or funds) the local pound and pays the dog wardens to investigate dog attacks and nuisance barking. Clearly the council plays an important role, funded by rates and taxes levied on the community. Unfortunately, there is little awareness that here again we are subject to significant socialising of the *costs* of pet keeping, but privatising the *profits* for Mars, Nestlé and Colgate.

Come the revolution, researchers may help us better understand the interplay of needs and wants, with everyone required to pay their fair share. Let Mars, Nestlé and Colgate bear some costs. Let them pay an environmental levy on their junk. Let them pay for warning labels that should be on the sides of their cans and packets:

- **WARNING:** This product, if fed to your dog over an extended period, will increase its risk of disease and premature death.
- **WARNING:** Dogs fed this product over an extended period are liable to behaviour and health issues requiring veterinary intervention.

Medical researchers

Back in the days of the Cold War, an Iron Curtain divided the Soviet bloc from the West. For the majority of those trapped behind the Iron Curtain, life was a drudge. For the power elites, life was full of benefits. They found ways to amass power, prestige and profit under cover of the oppression and propaganda governing the masses. The Iron Curtain partitioned Europe; the Pet Food Curtain envelops the entire globe. These days, by controlling the flow of information, the pet food and veterinary collaborators maintain a global population in thrall to the contents of the pet food can and bag.

Sadly, in subtle and not so subtle ways, medical researchers, microbiologists and periodontists all fall under the influence of the pet food collaborators. Professionals jealously guard their turf. No matter how ineffectual and dangerous the vet profession, the medical, dental and periodontal researchers are not about to enter veterinary territory. Even when brought face-to-face with vet incompetence, researchers often fail to see the potential research opportunities arising in their own field.

In 2006 I gave a presentation to dental and medical researchers in which I emphasised the wonderful opportunities open for research into periodontal disease given that carnivores live at the extreme end of the nutritional spectrum. Just as oceanographers go to great depths and atmospheric scientists go to great heights, by studying carnivores researchers can obtain a unique perspective. During question time at the end of the lecture, no-one asked about research. All questions were to do with 'my dog' or 'my cat'. Self-interest trumped community interest, once again.

Fred Southwick, Professor of Medicine at the University of Florida, wrote an article titled 'Academia suppresses creativity'.

> By discouraging change, universities are stunting scientific innovation, leadership, and growth.
>
> Creativity enhances life. It enables the great thinkers, artists, and leaders of our world to continually push forward new concepts, new forms of expression and new ways to improve every facet of our existence. The creative impulse is of particular importance to scientific research. Without it, the same obstacles, ailments, and solutions would occur repeatedly because no one stepped back and reflected to gain a new perspective.[18]

Consider that all universities and all researchers function behind the pet food curtain, and you can see why there is urgent, overwhelming need for change.

Moles and sleepers

We need moles and sleepers located within the junk pet food companies and universities—people of good faith who will collect information and leak it to us on the outside. Think of them as resistance fighters acquiring secrets that will weaken an occupying force. And when the day of reckoning comes, informants will be able to supply evidence at any inquiry or trial.

A mole working for Mars at their Wodonga factory in Victoria told me how their research animals received six-monthly dental 'prophies' (prophylactic treatment), dental scaling under general anaesthesia. Let's hope there are more moles, armed with smartphones recording the evidence of the industrial scale fraud.

Nutritionists

Human nutritionists can surely help us. And may I be so bold as to say we can help them?

Some human nutritionists are moving beyond a consideration of ingredients to include consideration of the amount of processing the 'food' undergoes. Professor Mark Lawrence, writing in the *American Journal of Clinical Nutrition*, commented:

> **Ultraprocessed foods and cardiovascular health: it's not just about the nutrients**
>
> In the 2000s, a new paradigm for thinking about a food's nutritional quality began to emerge. The paradigm extended the scope of nutritional quality assessment from a food's nutrient content alone to also include consideration of the processing of the food within which those nutrients are contained.[19]

Some human nutritionists remain trapped in their conventional way of thinking.

Professor Marion Nestle at her blog provides an extract from her book *Feed Your Pet Right*.

> - If you are using commercial foods, make sure they say they are complete and balanced and have been tested at some point
> - If you are cooking for your pet, make sure your recipe includes the needed nutrients (we give generic recipes in the book)
> - Know that no evidence exists that expensive pet foods are better than cheap ones (that research has never been done)

- Vary the products you use. Variety, balance, and moderation work just as well for pets as they do for people
- Most important: do not overfeed. Calories count![20]

Professor Nestle may know how to feed omnivorous humans 'right'. However, in my estimation, she's rather confused about carnivore health and dietary requirements. Unfortunately for pets and their owners, her book is still available in print. *Caveat emptor*, buyer beware!

Periodontists

Potentially periodontists, dentists who specialise in gum disease, hold the keys to a health revolution. Their work focuses on the interplay between dental plaque biofilms and host responses producing the chronic gum disease we call periodontal disease. Increasingly they recognise the interplay of gum disease and human systemic illnesses. These are the connections that I believe can form the core of a new paradigm of medical and veterinary science. However, for best progress periodontists need to acknowledge and incorporate the evidence derived from sick pets.

In April 2021 I wrote to 14 board members of the prestigious *Periodontology 2000* journal acquainting them with the remarkable transformations in health and vitality of domestic pets when treated for periodontal disease. In particular I provided them with copies of *Raw Meaty Bones: Promote Health* and the 1994 *Journal of Veterinary Dentistry* feature article 'Cybernetic hypothesis of periodontal disease in mammalian carnivores'.

Professor Jørgen Slots, co-editor of the *Periodontology* journal, was the only one who responded: 'Personally, I have been a vegetarian (much too much unnecessary killing) for more than 30 years so meaty bones for dogs cannot get me excited. However, I am looking forward to reading your book and learn[ing] about your concepts.'

One year later, in June 2022, the *Periodontology* journal published a review article: 'Interconnection of periodontal disease and comorbidities: evidence, mechanisms, and implications'. Readers are told two sets of important facts:

> Periodontitis is moreover linked epidemiologically with other disorders [comorbidities], including cardiovascular disease, type-2 diabetes, obesity, rheumatoid arthritis (RA), osteoporosis, respiratory infections, inflammatory bowel disease, Alzheimer disease, nonalcoholic fatty liver disease, chronic kidney disease, and certain cancers.
>
> The combined direct and indirect costs (due to loss in productivity) of periodontal disease in the United States and Europe were estimated, respectively, at $154.06 billion and €158.64 billion'.

However, the journal did not tell its readers of the explanatory and predictive power of evidence based on raw meaty bones that has been available for the past 30 years. Instead, the journal advised its readership of specialist, highly trained periodontists that:

> unequivocal evidence that effective treatment of periodontitis can ameliorate the risk or incidence of epidemiologically-linked comorbidities conditions is not currently available.[21]

'Not currently available'?! This statement contradicts verified veterinary information in their possession and the experience of thousands of pet owners whose sick, miserable pets affected by periodontal disease become rejuvenated within days of having their periodontitis treated.

For the future let's hope that there are some open-minded periodontists who will re-evaluate the evidence available to anyone willing to look. A renaissance in medical and veterinary science awaits.

Psychologists

In their brilliant book *Age of Propaganda: The Everyday Use and Abuse of Persuasion*, psychologists Anthony Pratkanis and Elliot Aronson give us an insight into how human psychology renders us easy prey to the confidence tricksters and marketeers.[22] They also describe cognitive dissonance in action, where a person holds mutually conflicting beliefs, or says one thing and does another.

It's the situation very much at play in the veterinary profession and animal welfare communities. Vets say they're well trained and always put the pets' interests first. However, as we know, such statements tend not to withstand scrutiny. Vets pay lip-service to the health care ideal while ignoring the interests of the patient.

Exposing vets to the realities of life for pets forced to consume junk food engenders feelings of dissonance in the vets—which then leads to endless excuses and justifications in an attempt to lessen the dissonance. 'It's too difficult for pet owners', 'bones get stuck and break teeth' or as Colin Harvey, a professor of veterinary dentistry, said, only half joking, raw meaty bones are unacceptable in 'carpeted American living rooms'.[23]

Justice Michael Kirby of the Australian High Court and patron of the RSPCA justified approaching Colgate-Palmolive company Hill's for sponsorship funds because he said 'it's expensive to feed our animals'.[24] These days the RSPCA has cross-promotional ties with Hill's—in my view, hypocrisy on a grand scale.

The endless stream of sick and debilitated pets creates a need for welfare assistance: the animals need feeding. The RSPCA could help turn off the tap of junk pet food abuse, but instead they redirect the flow to their financial advantage. Adept at mining the depths of sentiment in the community, the RSPCA in effect leverages concerns about animal cruelty to gain marketing kudos for the RSPCA and Colgate-Palmolive. There's no nagging dissonance, no troubled conscience for them—the RSPCA simultaneously says and does the *wrong* thing.

It seems to me that there are rich seams of psychological gold to be mined if and when psychologists turn their attention to the anomalies, absurdities and hypocrisy of the alliance between junk pet food makers, vets and fake animal welfare groups.

Spiritual and religious leaders

As we try to find our way out of the junk pet food mire, it's a good idea to take account of the context, our place in the universe. The Earl E. Bakken Center for Spirituality & Healing at the University of Minnesota offers an excellent definition of spirituality.

> Spirituality is a broad concept with room for many perspectives. In general, it includes a sense of connection to something bigger than ourselves, and it typically involves a search for meaning in life. As such, it is a universal human experience—something that touches us all. People may describe a spiritual experience as sacred or transcendent or simply a deep sense of aliveness and interconnectedness.
>
> Some may find that their spiritual life is intricately linked to their association with a church, temple, mosque, or synagogue. Others may pray or find comfort in a personal relationship with God or a higher power. Still others seek meaning through their connections to nature or art. Like your sense of purpose, your personal definition of spirituality may change throughout your life, adapting to your own experiences and relationships.[25]

I hope that you can gain spiritual uplift and satisfaction from getting to know more about the pet food fraud and the simple natural solution to fixing the issues. I know that for me, throughout, it has felt like a spiritual journey. I've gained a deeper appreciation of nature and marvelled at the significance of the pivotal necessity of the carnivores' canine teeth.

The cybernetic hypothesis of periodontal disease in mammalian carnivores came to me in a dream in the early hours of Christmas morning in December 1992.[26] It's a uniting theory of how carnivores are the supreme regulators—or at least were, before humans armed with clubs took control—who themselves need regulating in the scheme of life. It's about balance and the majesty of nature. It's about raw meaty bones being the key to the carnivore code. In nature, as long as predators eat their raw meaty bones they are both fulfilled and are fulfilling their pivotal role.

We can extrapolate to the domestic situation and be spiritually uplifted seeing and hearing our pets' feeding frenzy as they rip, tear and crunch their dinner.

On a formal level, I don't know if religious leaders either can or will teach their flock about the wonders of the interactions among carnivores, herbivores, plants and bacteria. However, in this largely secular world, there are numerous religions all with a faith and trust in nature. One particular religious leader I mention here is Archbishop Desmond Tutu, chairman of the South African Truth and Reconciliation Commission, which was charged with investigating the horrors of the apartheid era. Here's what the commission set out to achieve.

> [The] court like body established by the new South African government in 1995 to help heal the country and bring about a reconciliation of its people by uncovering

> the truth about human rights violations that had occurred during the period of apartheid. Its emphasis was on gathering evidence and uncovering information—from both victims and perpetrators—and not on prosecuting individuals for past crimes.[27]

Here's a magnificent Desmond Tutu quote that we would be well to keep in mind as we seek to atone for the 160 years of hurt inflicted by junk pet food.

> Forgiving and being reconciled to our enemies or our loved ones are not about pretending that things are other than they are. It is not about patting one another on the back and turning a blind eye to the wrong. True reconciliation exposes the awfulness, the abuse, the hurt, the truth. It could even sometimes make things worse. It is a risky undertaking but in the end, it is worthwhile, because in the end only an honest confrontation with reality can bring real healing. Superficial reconciliation can bring only superficial healing.[28]

Stock exchanges

If we want answers, we need to ask questions, lots of questions.

On 7 October 2021 I wrote to the New York, London and Sydney stock exchanges.

> I'm hoping that you can help me find the relevant Stock Exchange rulings regarding listed companies that produce goods known to injure the health of pets, but which goods are promoted as if they are fully beneficial.
>
> If the Stock Exchange becomes aware that listed companies are deliberately misleading consumers and investors, does the Exchange have a system for dealing with such breaches?

No answers have been received. The three stock exchanges remain silent about their part in the multi-billion-dollar pet food fraud. We need to ask again and again until we get answers.

Surely there are people and institutions we can hold accountable. Surely the buck stops somewhere.

Television stations

It's not scientific, but it's maybe instructive to contemplate how many false and misleading television advertisements were broadcast yesterday, last week and last year in your country. How many vet programs and lifestyle programs were aired? Were dogs and cats and junk pet food featured in other television segments that either coincidentally or intentionally promoted the consumption of junk pet food?

I went to the archives to check how many raw meaty bones television segments have, to my knowledge, been broadcast in the English language. See Table 1.

Table 1 Length of television segments discussing raw meaty bones[29]

YEAR	STATION	PROGRAM	LENGTH (IN MINUTES)
Australia			
1993	ABC	The Investigators	6
1993	Channel 9	Ray Martin at Midday	9
1996	Channel 10	Money	3
1997	Channel 7	Today Tonight	5
1997	Channel 7	Today on Saturday	7
2001	Channel 9	A Current Affair	7
2004	Channel 7	Today Tonight	4
New Zealand			
2003	TV One	Holmes Show	5
2003	TV One	Face to face with Kim Hill	26
China			
2006	Southern Television		4
2006	Guangzhou English Channel		29

Perhaps in other countries there have been segments touching on the need for dogs, cats and ferrets to consume their essential food and medicine. Perhaps not! We can be sure of one thing: the equation is massively tipped in favour of the junk pet food alliance.

Let's hope television stations begin to understand the cruelty, fraud and injustice of the current situation, change their policies and help spark the revolution.

US Food and Drug Administration

Imagine if the FDA was a strident antivaxxer during the COVID-19 pandemic. How many millions more people would have died?

Suppose the premier government agency, overly concerned about side effects, cautioned doctors *against* the use of antibiotics. Some argue that due to concerns about adverse effects, penicillin would not be approved today.

As we've seen in previous chapters, raw meaty bones are both the miracle preventative and miracle treatment—the strongest, safest, most gentle, most effective medicine for all domestic carnivores. However, in 2010 the FDA was implacably opposed to the feeding of bones, whether cooked or raw. (See Chapter 3, p 46.) In 2017 they published a revision under the title: 'No bones (or bone treats) about it: reasons not to give your dog bones'.[30] The FDA need to admit error; they need to say 'We were wrong'. They need to give reasons why *you should give your dog bones*. That simple reversal will ripple across the globe, saving the lives of millions of pets, now and into the future.

Veterinary specialists

If veterinary specialists are a large part of the problem, they can and should also become a large part of the solution.

First let's consider the good that they do. They're the folks who devote their professional lives to narrow specialities like ophthalmology, dermatology and neurology. They tend to be the cream of the crop who are both super intelligent, super hard-working and super dedicated to their speciality. They read the latest journals, attend conferences and discuss with their specialist peers. They are at the forefront and in general give freely of their time and expertise to us mere plodders in private veterinary practice. For sure they charge clients hefty fees. But then they do have to pay for years of extra study and usually expensive equipment and systems able to provide the 24-hour service necessary for optimum outcomes.

Given how they excel in so many areas it's both disappointing and frustrating that they refuse to even contemplate that the junk food cult is seriously flawed. The specialists at the Sydney Small Animal Specialist Hospital recommend Mars and Hill's junk. The hospital is in alliance with Royal Canin, their 'nutrition partner'.[31] The Sydney Animal Referral Hospital issues invoices to clients with the prominent statement 'ARH thanks Hills Pet Nutrition for providing quality nutrition for the patients at our hospital'.

When the Australian Pet Food Review Working Group wanted a consultant's report they commissioned Professor Caroline Mansfield of the University of Melbourne.[32] When speaking on the radio she told listeners to 'feed a diet that has been verified to be nutritionally complete' and that 'dogs are omnivores, like us'.[33] As for the so-called nutritional specialists in the USA, see Professor Sandra Scarr's caustic remarks in Appendix E.

Will the veterinary specialists eventually see the 'completely obvious', turn through 180 degrees and start the journey of the future, one step at a time?

Veterinary students

Caught on the horns of a dilemma, what are they to do? For veterinary students the pressure to conform to the dominant paradigm (the junk pet food cult) is enormous, no matter how much common sense tells them that a staple diet of junk food must be inimical to good health.

Challenging university lecturers, telling them they're engaged in a cruel conspiracy to defraud pet owners and trusting vet students is not, in the short term, a winning strategy. However, we're engaged in a long-term struggle for the better health of pets and better tuition of veterinary students. Courage is required, risks must be taken. Here are some questions requiring answers. To all veterinary students and recent veterinary graduates, is your veterinary school—

- in receipt of artificial pet food company funds?
- suppressing information about the impact of artificial pet foods on pet health?
- failing to provide complete and balanced information regarding the so-called 'complete and balanced' pet foods?
- failing to provide proper training in diets ordained by nature?
- training you in dental treatment, not dental disease prevention?
- suggesting you advise your clients to brush their carnivores' teeth?

Are your veterinary teachers—

- in receipt of artificial pet food company funds?
- assisting pet food companies to cover up deficiencies in their products?
- encouraging you to recommend or feed unsuitable or unsafe products to your patients?
- teaching 'nutrition' without declaring any conflict of interest?
- teaching medicine and surgery without declaring any conflicts of interest?
- teaching you to perform treatments when disease prevention would be a better option?

And does this conduct by your school or teachers—

- make you a laughing-stock?
- disadvantage your clients and the patients under your care?
- leave you in professional and financial jeopardy?

Depending on the answers, some well-organised, well-motivated veterinary students can be champions of the revolution. They can document the evidence in written, photographic and video form. They can band together to seek legal and other remedies. Students of today are the heads of veterinary schools and research establishments tomorrow—and tomorrow is a new day.

Zookeepers

Many years ago, I took my two young sons to the Western Plains Zoo in Dubbo, NSW, Australia. We were having a splendid time riding our bikes from enclosure to enclosure, reading the inscriptions describing the geographical range and habitat of the species on display.

However, as we approached the cheetah enclosure, we were confronted with an A-frame sign.

Alas, after John Mars's visit to the zoo a deal had been struck to use the cheetahs and the white tiger in a promotion for Mars liquid junk. Whiskas dry and canned junk does nothing for the good dental and general health of cats whether little or large. Past weaning, milk should not be a feature of any cat's diet. But for the zoo and Mars such pesky considerations do not appear to have been part of the conversation.

I mention the Whiskas Milk Plus story for it reveals the potential zoos have for educating the public. If information is accurate then incrementally over the years they can do much good. If they have wolves or dingoes on display, they can easily refer to them as ancestors and cousins of German shepherds and chihuahuas and all breeds in between. If they display small wild cats, they can mention how the biology and diet of domestic cats should follow suit. Indeed, zoos could invite visitors to view the ripping and tearing of appropriate prey—quail, pigeons, fish, rats and mice—at feeding time. The same pertains if the zoo exhibits 'Mustelidae, the largest family within Carnivora', which is 'comprised of 56 species in 22 genera'. Ferrets, evolved from polecats, are domestic members of the Mustelidae family, with the biology and needs of their wild cousins.

These days zoos encounter criticism for confining wild animals in enclosures. I think that criticism, although valid, could be somewhat softened if zoos were to help with sparking the revolution in pet feeding.

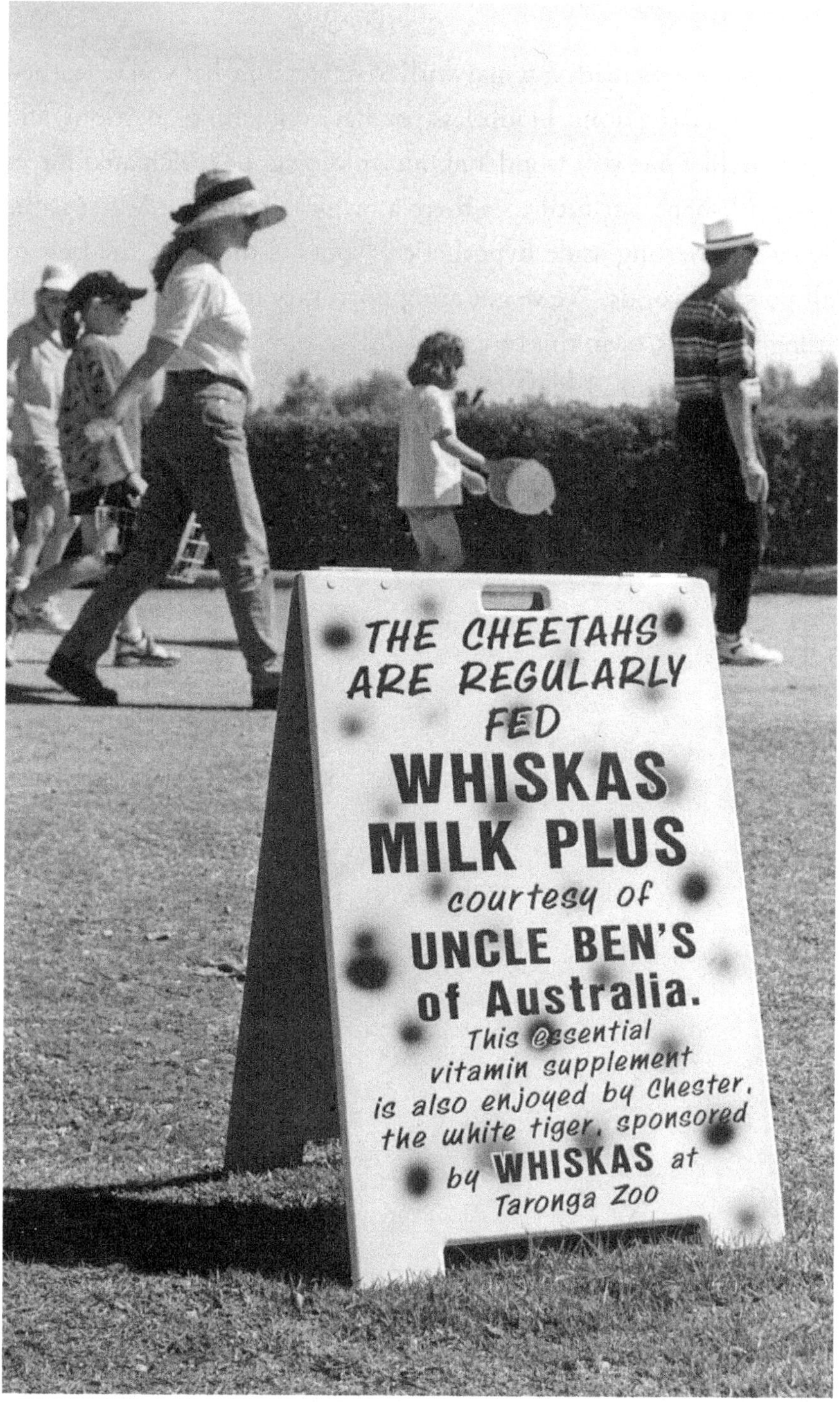
THE CHEETAHS
ARE REGULARLY
FED
WHISKAS
MILK PLUS
courtesy of
UNCLE BEN'S
of Australia.
This essential
vitamin supplement
is also enjoyed by Chester,
the white tiger, sponsored
by WHISKAS at
Taronga Zoo

What next?

Now after a long read, you may wish to reflect on what you've learned and what's to be done. Doubtless you have remaining questions, and if you're like me, you wonder about unknown, unanticipated forces that will shape our future. Is there a magical X factor? What is the X factor? Setting aside hypotheticals, ours is the only, the best of all possible worlds. We've got an opportunity to make it better still using the tools, or in this case the words at our disposal.

I wish you good luck, good fun, good progress and leave you with the inspirational words of Victor Hugo: 'There is one thing stronger than all the armies in the world, and that is an idea whose time has come'.

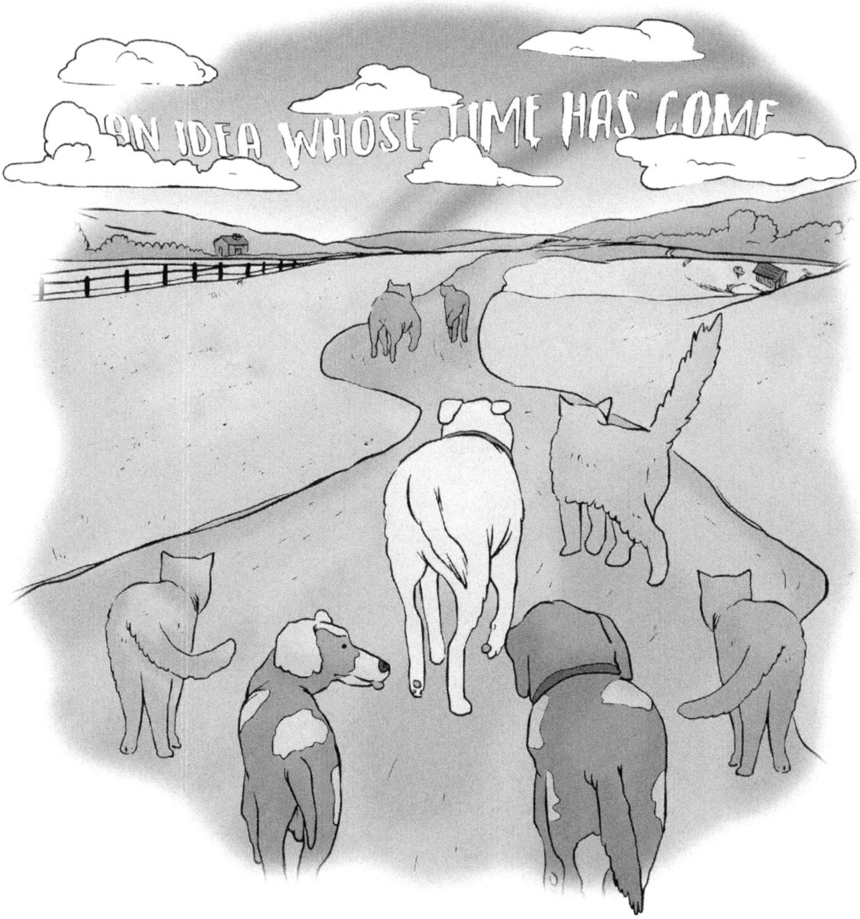
AN IDEA WHOSE TIME HAS COME

APPENDIX A

Regulatory approaches to ensure the safety of pet food
Submission 62

Melanie Christie

Executive summary

- A cat's serious digestive issues could not be solved by multiple trained vets over a period of seven years, leading to dire illness.
- Within 1 week of switching to a diet of Raw Meaty Bones, the digestion began to function properly. The remaining issues involving skin, fur, teeth and demeanour have consistently improved to the point where he is finally healthy, 2 years later.
- Other pets housed at the same address which were switched for convenience have all shown markedly improved health—all unlooked-for, all noticed after the fact.
- Vet bills have dropped dramatically.
- I will never have any of my pets eat commercial food again.

Initially, as with almost all other pet owners, I believed that the best way to feed my pets was by using the commercially available canned and packet products. I tried to do this, choosing 'premium' brands over those at cheaper price points.

However, one of my cats developed digestive problems which persisted for seven years resulting in constant 'cow pat' style faeces tinged with blood (a very bad sign), weight loss and bone-dry fur which began falling out in clumps. During this time multiple vets were consulted and thousands of dollars spent on tests and different foods (from home concoctions from the internet to multiple Vet-recommended prescription diets to BARF (Bones and Raw Food) mush) in an attempt to solve the problem. All the medical tests yielded negative results and became more and more invasive. With no guarantee of finding a reason, let alone a cure, I baulked at the removal of a piece of his bowel for inspection.

It was at this point I stumbled over a news article[1] and found others[2,3] recounting how the manufacturers of Hill's Science Diet deliver lectures for animal nutrition and provide branded goods at the University of Sydney's School of Veterinary Sciences. Through these articles I discovered the web site www.rawmeatybones.com and, knowing my cat at this point was seriously ill, with nothing to lose, I decided to see Dr Tom Lonsdale at Bligh Park Pet Health Centre.

His recommendation was to switch my cat's diet to Raw Meaty Bones. This was the only change to his daily routine.

Within 1 week of feeding Raw Meaty Bones to my then ten-year-old cat, I knew this was the correct diet for him. The bloodied 'cow pat' faeces, which had plagued his life for seven years, disappeared in a matter of days.

Within 1 month, his whole demeanour had changed and he was starting to 'talk'—purr and chirrup—to me again.

Within 1 year, his skin and fur had vastly improved—the former no longer flaking and scaly and the latter no longer bone dry or falling out at the slightest touch. His vocalisations had returned to normal.

After the initial success of the first week I decided to switch all my pets onto Raw Meaty Bones. I thought they were in reasonable health and only did it for convenience. However, it was only when I took them all to my local vet for their annual check-up (nine months later) did I see the transformations that had taken place under my nose.

PET	COMMERCIAL DIET	RAW MEATY BONES (AFTER 9 MONTHS FEEDING)
Cat #1 (11 years)	• 'Cow pats', huge volumes of stinking faeces • Dry skin with scaly patches • Thin, low density coat, dry and dull • Bad breath • Plaque on teeth and irritated gums • Animal extremely ill, with no interest in life. No communication.	• Firm, small, species-appropriate faeces, with significantly lowered odour • Skin is not dry or scaly • Improving coat—ceased to fall out and was less dry • Breath is odourless • Teeth and gums require no veterinary intervention† • Has recovered his joy in living. Communicates and behaves as prior to his long, steady decline.
Cat #2 (6 years)	• Bad breath • Plaque on teeth and irritated gums • 'Normal' fur, only realising afterwards that 'normal' was nothing like what it should be	• Breath is odourless • Teeth and gums require no veterinary intervention • Fur is beautifully thick, glossy and kitten-soft.§ Could do shampoo ads—no need for soap.
Dog #1 (11 years)	• Bad breath • Near-constant ear infections involving unpleasant ear drops • Thick, mucous-like saliva which was difficult to clean off plates • Plaque on teeth and irritated gums	• Breath is odourless • Not a single ear infection, even during hot and humid seasons • Saliva removal from surfaces no longer requires industrial strength dishwashing liquid • Teeth and gums require no veterinary intervention
Dog #2 (8 years)	• Bad breath • Ear infections, requiring painful administration of ear drops • Huge human-sounding burps post eating. Amusing at the time. • Plaque on teeth and irritated gums	• Breath is odourless • No ear infections, even during hot and humid seasons • Post-prandial burping has disappeared. • Teeth and gums require no veterinary intervention

§ I had always assumed that a cat's fur became rougher with age. I realise now it is the feeding of a commercial diet which causes the deterioration that I had observed in previous pets.

† My local vet, who doesn't advocate a raw meaty bone diet (but is completely supportive of my choice), at my animals' most recent check-up said that she 'couldn't even sell me a teeth clean' for any of my pets (at this staged aged 12, 12, 9 and 7).

Watching my cat suffer for years, along with the dramatic transformations of all my pets upon shifting to Raw Meaty Bones made me aware that the commercial products were harmful, as opposed to 'well-balanced' or 'nutritionally complete'. This parallels the earliest infant formula preparations where the infants consuming these blends failed to thrive due to ignorance of the basic requirements of human nutrition. We still have not produced an infant formula near the quality of breast milk. Our knowledge of animal nutrition, as shown by my experience, lags much further behind.

All the vets I dealt with over the years were caring and professional, and I believe truly wished to see my cat become healthy.

Unfortunately, the training they received (from different Veterinary Schools and a wide generational sampling) did not enable them to assist and their attempts only furthered his torment.

I believe the current veterinary training is so influenced by the commercial pet food industry that a student entering First Year would find it almost impossible to develop their own ideas about nutrition. A student, keen to help animals, with so much to learn so quickly is constantly bombarded with advertising and even lectures from commercial enterprises. How can they resist this when their ideas about pet nutrition are placed in their heads before they are even aware of it? How can they not sell commercial pet food when the usual business model for a veterinary practice is supported by such sales? How, when an animal-loving future vet goes to the RSPCA to pick a pet sees commercial food sales[4] and that this is constantly reinforced through online, TV and other media advertisements?

Specifically:

- Advertising and respected institutions such as the RSPCA push commercial food.

- Vets, due to their training, lifelong influences and how veterinary practices are set up, push commercial food.
- I, as an owner of an ill animal, desperate to 'make him better', took the advice of my (multiple) veterinarians and tried the prescription brands, despite the hideous, stinking results.
- I tried commercial minced raw products, hoping that would work. It was relatively shortlived: even the dogs refused to eat that stuff and only the ill cat ploughed on, getting sicker by the day.
- It was only when I started feeding whole carcasses and raw meaty bones that all my pets underwent a miraculous transformation.
- I read the books *Work Wonders* and *Raw Meaty Bones* by Dr Tom Lonsdale.
- There is no need for fake teeth cleaning products[5] (more expenditure) or 'oral care' foods[6] when my carnivores clean their teeth at every meal, as is done in the wild. See Dr Lonsdale's latest article published by Sydney University: 'Raw meaty bones essentials'.[7]

I now provide my responses under the Committee's Headings:

Possible regulatory approaches to ensure the safety of pet food, including both the domestic manufacture and importation of pet food

- I believe the current concerns have arisen from the megaesophagus outbreak in police dogs as reported in the media and the presence of plastic particles in dry dog 'food'. There is a general belief amongst consumers that if it is for sale in Australia, then it is safe. This is reflective of the confidence people have in the Australian Government and I am aware how hard public servants work to ensure this is so.

- Unfortunately there are two issues with pet food safety. The first is in the attempt itself to *manufacture* food that is safe for pets. There have never been controlled studies demonstrating that any of these products are either suitable or safe for the feeding of domestic carnivores.
- The second is that as there is now a market for pet foods, how to ensure the safety of these 'foods', and what is meant by safety? There is acute toxicity, which grabs headline and kills pets relatively quickly. Then there is chronic toxicity which lowers the overall health of the animal, killing them slowly over years with the path to cancer and renal failure paved with skin and ear complaints, bad breath and rotten teeth. This, coupled with humans being ill equipped to read signs of pain and suffering in non-human animals, can result in years of pain and suffering, most obviously for the animals, but also for humans who care for those animals; one example being humans in therapy who have companion animals.
- Regulation for acute toxicity should be of a quality and effectiveness such that the death of a pet becomes as rare as the death of a human. As a pet owner, I would like to see as much information about manufactured pet food on the label as I see for my own food.
- Regulation for chronic toxicity will require that all manufactured pet foods come with labels warning that the food is not the ideal choice for the feeding of domestic carnivores. Raw meaty bones options should be promoted as the preferred method, whilst acknowledging this might not be possible for all owners, much like breastfeeding is the acknowledged preferred method for infant feeding over infant formulas.
- Please see how systematic failures affect the veterinary educational and regulatory mechanisms as per the Freedom of Information pages.[8]

a) The uptake, compliance and efficacy of the Australian Standard for the Manufacturing & Marketing of Pet Food (AS5812:2017)

- AS5812:2017 is available for $100+ or $200+, depending on the format.[9] It's a creation of the Pet Food Industry Association of Australia Inc. (PFIAA). Their website clearly states that the purpose of this 'standard' is 'to promote prepared pet food as the preferred method of pet nutrition reinforced through the establishment and self regulation of industry standards'.[10] Although the 'standard' does not intend to result in bringing harm against pets, there is nothing in the 'standard' that protects against the deleterious effects of adopting a diet for pets consisting of prepared pet food. It is worth noting that self-regulation by industry is generally not the preferred approach when the industry may have objectives (e.g. profit) that don't align with those of the public (e.g. animal welfare).
- Besides the PFIAA, the following were involved in the development of the document:
  - Australian Quarantine and Inspection Service (Commonwealth)
  - Department of Agriculture, Fisheries and Forestry (Commonwealth)
  - Department of Primary Industries, Victoria
  - RSPCA Australia.
  - Australian Veterinary Association
- The two Departments and the PFIAA are bodies which are interested in increasing trade and sales of products. AVA members and the RSPCA rely on the sale of prepared pet foods as part of their business models. Where increasing sales is paramount, quality will suffer. A Pet Food Standard which deliberately sets out to ignore pet health outcomes is not one which should be in use.

b) The labelling and nutritional requirements for domestically manufactured pet food

- Unfortunately, the labelling and nutritional requirements of manufactured pet 'food' cannot meet fundamental biological standards.
- I am aware that manufactured pet foods will be on shelves for many years to come and therefore believe that consumer education about species-appropriate diets is important and should be promoted in the community. This information is easily obtained from zoos as they do not feed canned and packaged products.
- However, it cannot be left to consumer education alone. Regulating the claims which can be made by pet food companies on their products and attaching warning labels about the chronic toxicity when feeding manufactured foods should be mandatory.

c) The management, efficacy and promotion of the AVA-PFIAA administered PetFAST tracking system

- The PetFAST[11] system is designed to provide the vet/pet-food alliance with early warning of acute toxicity and bacterial contamination issues. The onerous veterinary checklist[12] ensures plenty of scope for the industry to increase doubt and shift blame to pet owners. As detailed in Senator Stirling Griff's media release[13] it took three months for Mars to initiate a voluntary recall. It is an utter failure. I agree with Senator Griff regarding Dracula in charge of the blood bank.
- Most importantly, this system does nothing to address the chronic debilitating ill-health arising from long-term use of these 'food-like' products.

d) The feasibility of an independent body to regulate pet food standards, or an extension of Food Standards Australia New Zealand's remit

- I believe an independent, properly informed body needs to oversee pet food standards. No industry which wishes to make money will succeed with voluntary regulation as concern over being bested by the competition leads to improving the bottom line by the quickest method i.e., cut costs. This behaviour can be combated by an independent body backed by practical legislation and effective penalties, levelling the playing field for all.

e) The voluntary and/or mandatory recall framework of pet food products

- The current voluntary recall framework of pet food products has proved to be a failure (see point (c) above). Even when issues have been identified, potentially harmful products remain on the shelves: for example in the 2008 irradiated cat food case,[14] whilst irradiated cat food was banned, irradiated dog food was not, ignoring the very high possibility of cats accessing dog food.

f) The interaction of state, territory and federal legislation

- I support the investigation of the above interactions. This would enable the drawing together of all the disparate pieces of legislation affecting consumer safety, animal cruelty, vet education, dangerous dog legislation, labelling, etc. Until these interactions are understood, it will be difficult to draft effective and practical legislation.

g) Comparisons with international approaches to the regulation of pet food

- A similar situation prevails in the United States where pet food manufacturers assist in writing suitable laws, governments are given conflicting remits[15] and there is little in the way of enforceable deterrents for bad behaviour.
- It is unsurprising that Mars Petcare has announced its support of Australian pet food regulation.[16] This is straight from the playbook of any large industry that sniffs the slightest threat to their current business model—get on the front foot, pretend to care, get a seat at the table, and ensure they 'help' to draft the 'solution'—one that will not affect their bottom line in any way.

h) Any other related matters

- The fundamental issue is that the agriculture and meat industries generate enormous amounts of excess product and waste which need to be disposed of. Selling these waste materials as 'food' and promoting them as healthier than a natural diet has been the method of choice.
- I am not against people turning waste streams into money. On the contrary, it is vital money is made somehow otherwise the system we currently have will remain.
- Abattoirs could send species-appropriate carcasses and offal to pet food retailers. We could kill more of our animals here, keeping more jobs in Australia, rather than send them for live export, and innovate ways of becoming the source of raw meaty bones for the world's pet carnivores. Ill animals, such as 'downers' (those that are too sick to walk to the kill floor) and inedible parts (*e.g.* chicken feathers) should be repurposed for the manufacture of fertiliser, biogas, soap, or burned to generate energy, amongst other uses.

- Farms with excess grain products need to be assisted and encouraged to open markets in additional areas including innovative plastics manufacture, ethanol production, compost and others.
- People are incredibly smart at inventing useful products and spotting good opportunities to make money. If they think they will be crushed by giant pet food manufacturers before even getting started, this needs to be addressed.
- Raw Meat Diets are deliberately targeted as 'potentially dangerous'—food which these animals have been designed to eat. This is similar tactics to the targeting of women to believe that infant formula is 'safer' and 'more nutritious' than breast-feeding. It has, at its source, the same problem. Infant formula and manufactured pet foods make billions of dollars. Breast feeding and buying carcasses from the local butcher do not. Both infant formula and pet foods have a place, but they should not be promoted over breast feeding and natural diets. However, if it is economically advantageous to do so, industry will find a way to fill the gap created by changes to the prepared pet food industry.

APPENDIX B

Regulatory approaches to ensure the safety of pet food
Submission 109

Tafline Gillespie
Attn: Committee Secretary
Senate Standing Committees on Rural and Regional Affairs and Transport

As a pet owner and competitive dog trainer for dogsports I was very glad to hear about the Senate Inquiry to ensure the safety of pet food.

I have owned dogs and cats all my life but only within the last 8 years did I learn how to feed them for maximum health and performance. I initially looked into how to properly feed my pets after my dog got very sick on Hills Science Diet.

Every dog lover is familiar with:

- That wet dog smell after a dog has been in the rain or for a swim
- The doggy breath when getting some doggie kisses
- Huge mushy stinking dog feces that don't easily deteriorate naturally in sun, rain or hail

We are all familiar with this and more but none of it is normal in a healthy dog. Unfortunately we are all just so used to it because we all seem to have forgotten how to feed dogs and cats properly.

Feeding dogs processed food is so much worse than a human trying to live on a diet of fast food.

Since switching my dogs to raw food I have been horrified at what I used to consider normal levels of health in my dogs.

Many people believe the marketing lie that your dog or cat can't get all the goodness they need unless you buy the complex concoctions they have put together in their processed foods. This is a lie that puts one in mind of the marketing lies many years back that stated cigarettes were good for you or at the very least wouldn't cause any harm. People are also scared of their dogs and cats possibly choking on raw chicken or fish bones. This is outrageous, dogs and cats were made to eat raw meaty bones, one quick look at those wolfish teeth that even the little ones have can tell you that. They were not made to eat grains.

People are scared NOT to feed commercial pet foods because of these huge lies. In fact it's very simple to feed a dog or cat the best food there is. There is no complex formula required and you can buy the food from your supermarket for a fraction of the cost of what is touted to be the very best of the commercial foods.

The very best you can do for a dog or cat is feed it raw meat and bones. If you have access to a wide range of these that's great. You could include raw whole fish, raw chicken frames, raw lamb or goat necks, raw offal, raw kangaroo, raw rabbit etc. etc. the list is endless. However, even if the only raw meat and bones you can buy is chicken frames, chicken necks or chicken wings you can easily feed your dog and cat this every single day of its life and it will be outrageously healthy. It will have clean teeth, no dog breath, no wet dog smell, and it's poo literally won't stink and won't hang around like radioactive waste with a half life of forever.

I train dogs in the competitive sport of IPO and Mondio Ring. These sports emulate the tasks that police dogs are required to do such as tracking, obedience and bite work. These sports are very taxing physically and mentally on dogs so my dogs must be at peak health mentally and physically to train and compete and therefore I never feed them anything other than raw meaty bones. They are outrageously healthy physically and mentally.

I could go on but Doctor Tom Lonsdale has books, videos and more that prove that raw meaty bones are by far the best way to feed dogs and cats. He is an incredible advocate for dogs and cats that tells the truth unlike the majority of the industry that scares people into doing the wrong thing with terrible lies.

I hope that your enquiry helps open people's eyes to the fact that this industry makes its profits from the suffering of pets and their owners and there is a better way to feed dogs and cats.

Best Regards,
Tafline Gillespie

I agree to the publication of this submission on the internet.
Please find some examples of my experiences below.

This is a video of me and one of my competition dogs competing in a long obedience routine that shows the physical stamina and ability to concentrate that feeding raw unprocessed meat and bones contributes to: **https://www.youtube.com/watch?v=q-ije6782bI**

Below are some of my dogs and cats and the differences I found after feeding them what they were created to eat.

Princess—toy poodle 3 years old

4.5 kilos

Before eating raw food Princess had:

- Terrible breath
- Burps that smelt like sewerage
- Upset tummy with sticky poos

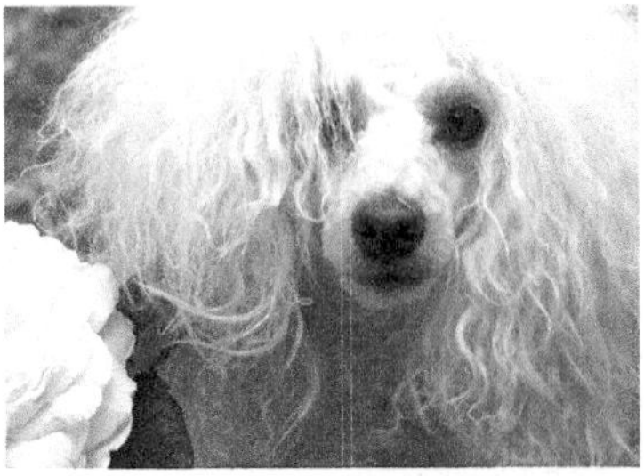

Now Princess only eats raw food and has:

- Fresh odorless breath
- No burping
- Happy tummy with firm low odor poos

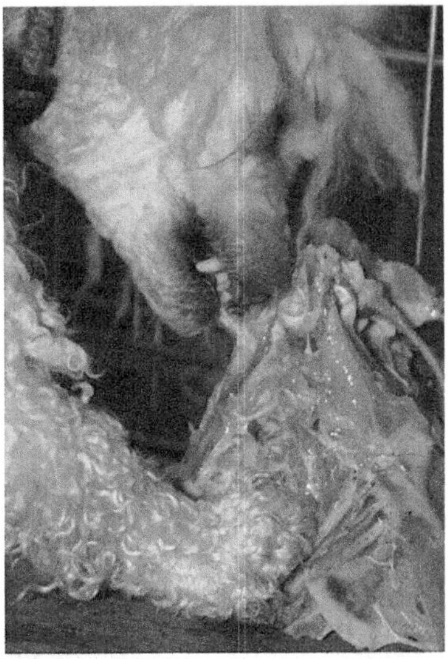

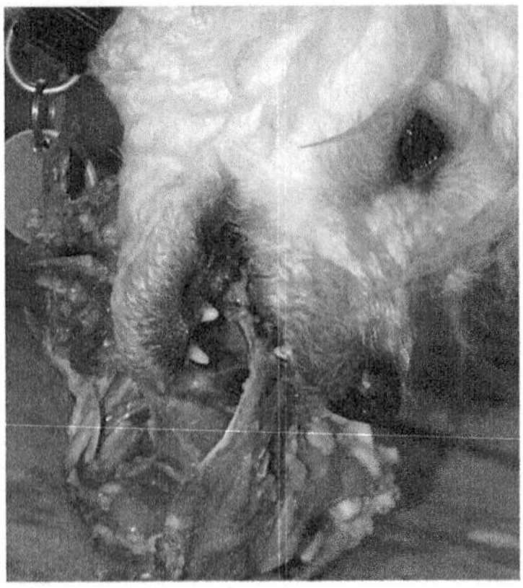

Teddy—Pekingese 5 years old

<u>Before</u> eating raw food Teddy was:

- Always hungry
- Overweight
- Anal glands irritated and needing regular expressing by the vet

<u>Now</u> Teddy only eats raw food and is:

- Satisfied not hungry all the time
- The right weight
- Firm poos meaning less expressing of anal glands needed

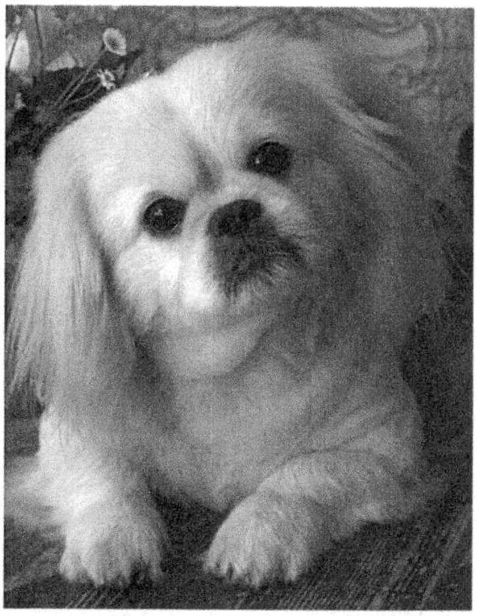

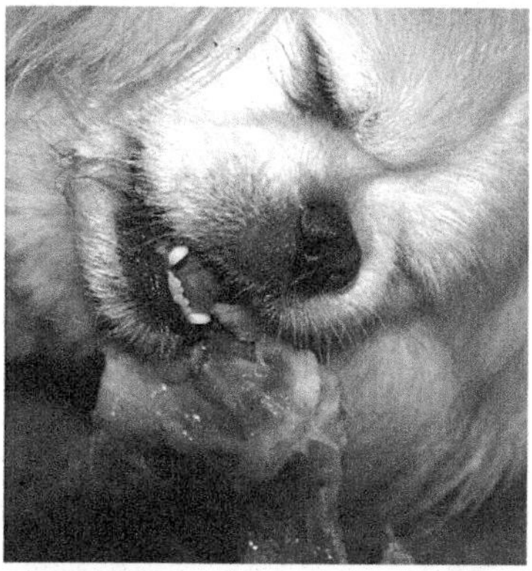

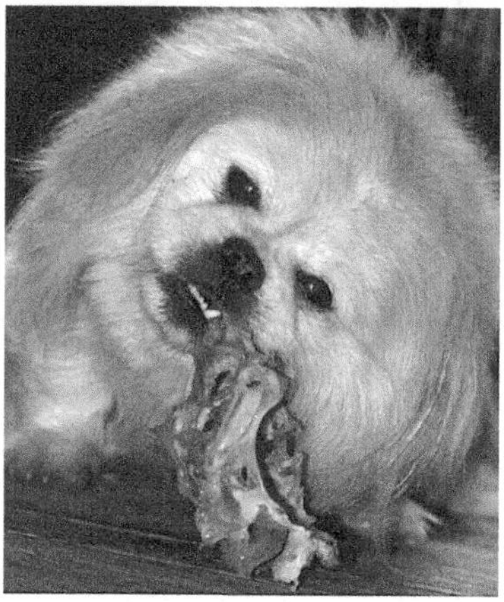

Blacky—German Shepherd, 18 months

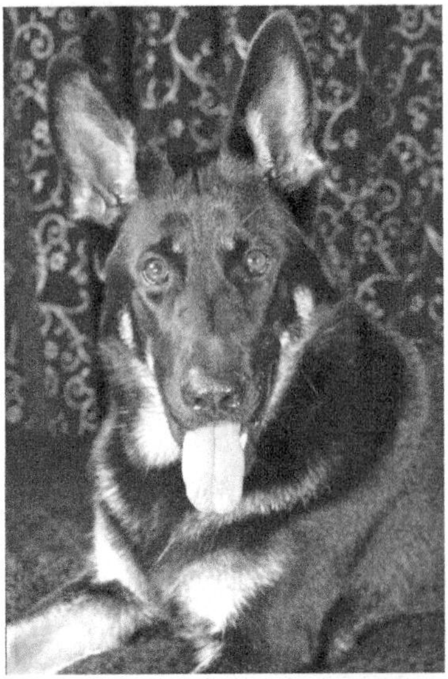

Blacky has eaten raw food since a puppy.

She is:

- Very bright and easy to train
- Lots of energy
- Shiniest coat on the block
- Very clean teeth
- Perfectly fresh breath
- Firm low odor poos

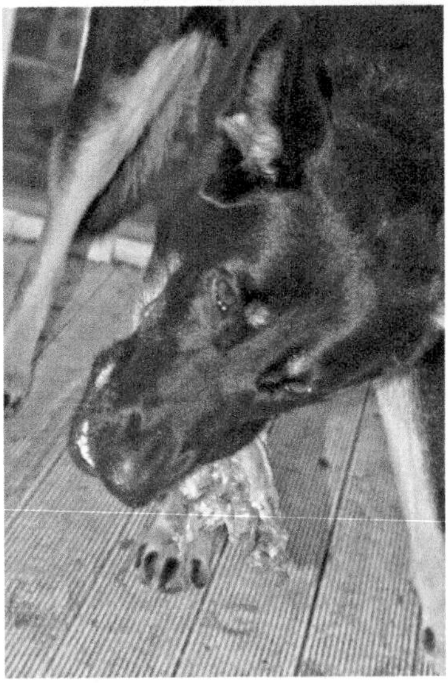

Blacky's staple diet is chicken carcasses and once a week she enjoys a sheep head, goat head, goat neck, turkey neck, fish frames or any other yummy raw meaty bone. She also loves her 1 kilo chunk of liver, ox heart or green tripe every Friday night.

Tiger—Cornish Rex, 7 years old

<u>Before</u> eating raw Tiger had:

- Smelly breath
- Dirty bottom
- Hair loss
- Very fussy eater
- Very whingy

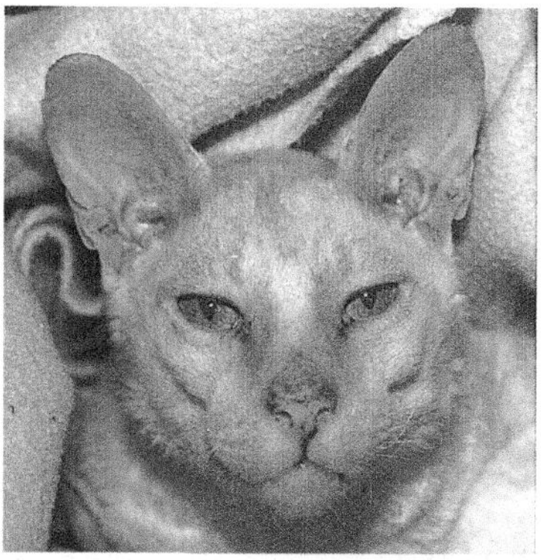

Dr. Lonsdale cleaned Tiger's teeth and after about 2 weeks Tiger got over his processed food addiction and onto raw food. Tiger loves quail carcass, chicken frames, ox heart, lamb heart, kidneys, liver and fish offcuts.

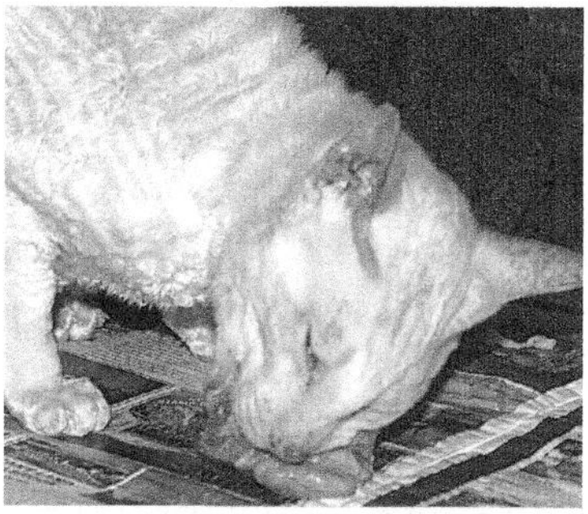

<u>Now</u> Tiger only eats raw food and has:

- Fresh breath
- Clean bottom
- Thick coat with no more bald spots
- Satisfied and not whingy
- Much more loving and content

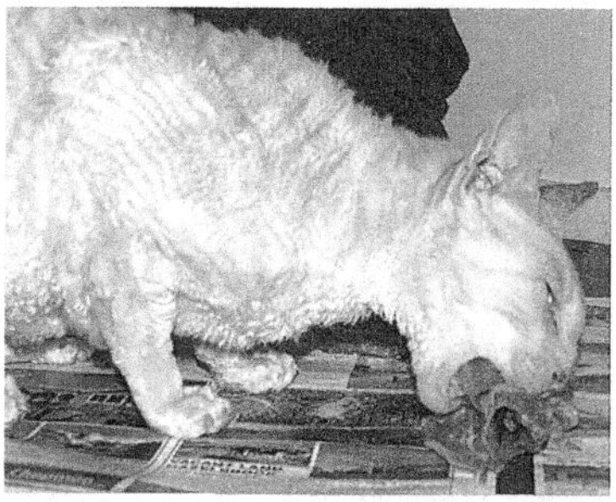

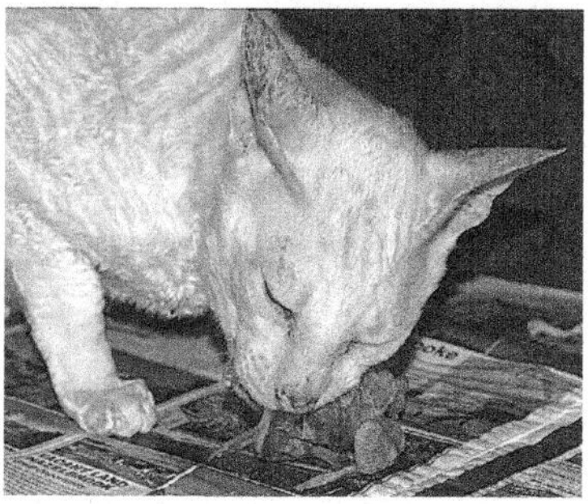

APPENDIX C

Regulatory approaches to ensure the safety of pet food
Submission 134

J Vale

My focus is on how feeding commercially produced cat foods has damaged the health of my cats and how the promotion of these foods is both misleading to pet owners and detrimental to pet health.

I have two cats. Their health was damaged due to feeding them commercially produced cat food. Their health improved when their diet was changed to a carnivore appropriate raw meaty bones diet.

Cat A

- was adopted from the RSPCA at 4–5 months of age
- is now approx 2 years old
- was raised by the RSPCA on Hills Pet Nutrition dry biscuits

Hills pet food is the staple diet fed by the RSPCA. Hills Pet Nutrition is the RSPCA's major sponsor.

At one year old Cat A was diagnosed at two different veterinary practices with dental tartar/gingivitis. On both occasions I was advised to wait until the condition had worsened enough to require a surgical clean and scale by a vet. This would have incurred considerable cost and, in isolation, would not have resolved the condition. Rather it would have formed the basis of ongoing annual management of the condition over the life of the cat—as well as providing guaranteed ongoing income for the vet.

No other options were offered. No explanation of why the problem existed was tendered.

Cat B

- was adopted from a rescue organisation
- is now approx 18 months old
- was raised on Royal Canin kitten food as advised by both veterinarians and also the original rescue organisation

At approx 6 months of age Cat B was exhibiting dental/health problems

- two vet practices and four examining vets later the default for treatment remained repeated and ineffective prescriptions of antibiotics
- no diagnosis, other treatment or testing was offered
- in desperation I consulted a third vet and was referred to SASH Small Animal Specialist Hospital
- SASH performed extensive testing and determined Cat B was suffering from Feline Gingivostomatitis. This is considered to be an autoimmune disease that ultimately requires the extraction of all of the cat's teeth as the only means of potentially, not definitively, resolving the condition. Long term management is also an option.
- Despite this definitive diagnosis obtained at the cost of almost six thousand dollars I was advised to wait and to bring the cat back at a later date 'to reassess'. This would have been at further expense to me.
- Vet advice from SASH on feeding Cat B was that commercially produced cat food was the best option; that pet food manufacturers would not have spent so much on their products to 'get it wrong'; that the feeding of raw meat is not a

good option because, among other issues of concern, it carries a risk of causing toxoplasmosis.

I continued to feed both cats commercial cat foods due to my ignorance in trusting commercial pet food advertising, the advice of RSPCA staff, the rescue organisation and veterinarians.

At the same time, being both confused and frustrated as to why my cats had these issues and the standard vet default was to advise waiting instead of treating their respective conditions I searched elsewhere for help. I found that:-

- commercially produced pet foods are a 'lucky dip' where the 'prizes' for the pet can range from poor health to illness and/or death
- overall commercially produced pet foods do not contain the necessary ingredients that cats require to maintain optimum health
- pet food labelling is complex and confusing and is also misleading, if not downright dishonest, with regard to the ingredients and stated benefits
- the pet food industry is, at best and worst, self-regulated and lacking accountability
- corporate pet food manufacturers are significantly involved with the education of vet students and with sponsorship of vets, animal welfare organisations/charities and with the marketing of their products through vet practices.
- that within this industry there appears to be a dishonesty that contributes to ill health for pets and for which uninformed pet owners pay the price of pet suffering and death—as well as through stress, financial outlay and grief.

My perception of why the vets did not proactively treat my cats includes any or all of the following:

- lack of interest, care or concern
- by delaying while the cats' health further deteriorated vet treatment would be more extensive and so provide the vet with more income
- these vets lack education in, and understanding of, appropriate animal nutrition and so were ignorant of the fact that the commercial food was the major contributor to the dental issues of these cats
- the vets were fully aware of the cause of my cats' issues but it would have been counterproductive for them to address this with me.

Treatment—finally

I found the website www.rawmeatybones.com which led me to consult the author of the site, veterinarian Dr. Tom Lonsdale.

Dr. Lonsdale was proactive in treating my cats:

- he performed surgical dental procedures on each cat. Cat A had a clean and scale. Cat B was in such a bad state that there was a need for gum excisions and the extraction of some teeth.
- Dr. Lonsdale advised I cease feeding commercial cat food and prescribed feeding both cats an appropriate raw meaty bones diet, explaining that carnivores clean their teeth through the process of ripping, tearing and chewing raw meaty bones.

Positive progress

Within weeks of switching both cats to a raw meaty bones diet I witnessed the following positive changes in both of them:

- significantly improved moods and energy levels
- more alert
- shiny coats
- soft fur

- loss of excess weight
- healthy looking pink gums
- non-odorous breath
- clean teeth
- less odorous urine and faeces
- improved hydration
- better formed stools

Both cats continue to be fed a raw meaty bones diet and to maintain the positives on this list.

Diet is the common denominator with regard to the dental issues that each cat experienced. Both cats were sick, and getting sicker, while eating a commercially produced cat food diet.

My conclusions

- my cats' experiences attest to the fact that feeding commercial cat food, at the *absolute minimum*, facilitates the creation of dental disease
- dental and gum disease in general in domestic cats and dogs is directly linked to, and exacerbated by, the feeding of commercial pet food diets
- the alliances and sponsorships between the commercial pet food manufacturers, veterinarians and organisations directly involved with the care and welfare of animals in Australia represents a gross conflict of interest and of which the public is mostly unaware
- it is obviously not in the financial interests of the commercial pet food manufacturers nor the veterinary industry to promote the feeding of an appropriate, healthy raw food diet to domestic carnivore pets

- if the appropriate raw food diet was fed to domestic pets dental diseases would either not occur or would be drastically reduced overall

General points for this submission

Pets are the victims

- Cats are obligate carnivores. Almost all commercially produced cat foods contains sugars, starches and carbohydrates which are not necessary for cats, cannot be digested by them and are damaging to their health when fed long term. Therefore these do not form an appropriate diet for cats. Why then are these ingredients included? Is it because they are cost effective?
- Maintaining cat health does not appear to be a motivation for the producers of commercial cat food or the vets since long term feeding of commercially produced cat food commonly leads to chronic ill health requiring vet interventions. Many vets promote and sell commercial cat foods, which creates a cycle of pet illness and vet income.
- The RSPCA feeds the cats and dogs in their care Hills Pet food because Hills is their major sponsor. Again, this is a conflict of interest and is damaging to the health of these animals.
- Further, RSPCA staff advises pet owners/adopters to feed Hills pet food. I volunteer for the RSPCA and witness this happening ongoing. This disadvantages pet owners who have no idea of appropriate feeding and who trust the RSPCA to give them accurate information.

At the very least these practices seem to me to be unethical. At worst pets are knowingly victimized for profits.

Costs

Commercial cat food is commonly prohibitively expensive. For example:

- Royal Canin Kitten food pouches with gravy @ 85g and priced at over $2 per pouch x 3 pouches per day incurs an outlay of more than $180 per month per kitten
- Hills Science Diet Kitten Liver & Chicken Entree Wet Cat Food 156g, priced at over $3 per can x 3 cans per day incurs an outlay of $270 per month per kitten
- A 2kg bag of Hills Science Diet Feline Care (which is emblazoned with 'Veterinarian Recommended' on the packet) costs a minimum of $32.95 depending upon the retailer.

Additionally, each of these products contains ingredients that cats do not need in their diets.

In contrast, I spend around $30 per month per cat to feed an appropriate raw food diet.

Dental disease

Most current day veterinary literature concerning the dental health of domestic cats and dogs states that these animals will exhibit dental issues by three years of age and will require ongoing dental care through veterinary intervention.

I submit that this would not be the case if pet carnivores were fed a more biologically appropriate raw meaty bones diet.

Raw feeding is not new news

Raw feeding is not new news but it is ignored and regularly demonized by the commercial pet food industry and veterinarians. See: http://www.rawmeatybones.com/pdf/Vet%20Dentistry%201993.pdf (See paragraph: Understanding the Mechanisms. Page 235) It can be seen here that the existence of periodontal disease and the relationship to diet has been known and documented since pre 1950.

These facts remain unchanged so:

Why are the facts being ignored?
Who benefits from this?

Dental Health Month—how is this NOT a conflict of interest? The Australian Veterinary Association promotes August as 'Pet Dental Health Month'. This is sponsored by Hills Pet Nutrition.

So the process can be seen as:

- unsuspecting owners feed diets of commercially produced pet food on the basis of advertising and advice from the trusted 'experts' such as the vets, RSPCA, Animal Welfare organisations and Charities.
- this leads to pet health issues where commonly the first visible signs are dental diseases.
- Vets, via Hills sponsorship for this promotion, provide a free dental health check where any existing dental issues will be identified and owners will be encouraged to seek further vet treatments, thus generating revenue for the vets.
- It is very unlikely that pet owners will be advised by these 'experts' that commercial pet food is a major reason for why their pet is suffering dental disease.
- If the subject of non-commercial raw feeding arises at all, it is common practice for vets to warn against it, citing reasons that range from the sublime to the ridiculous.

*I have friends whose dog has a dental clean and scale performed *every six months*. The dog is exclusively fed commercial pet food.

I would still be feeding commercial pet foods and be engaged in this toxic cycle had I not done my own research.

I have been subjected to vets promoting commercial food while also demonizing raw food. At this time my cats have been raw fed for approximately one year. Neither cat has ever become ill from raw feeding. In fact both cats have demonstrated significant improvements in overall health.

Zoo animals

Carnivores in zoos are not fed commercially produced pet food. They are fed appropriate raw food which includes meat chunks, carcasses and whole prey. What is the incidence of dental disease for these zoo animals by comparison to domestic carnivore pets that are exclusively fed a commercial diet?

Further information:

Some sources of information available via a Google search that may be of interest to the inquiry:

- Raw Meaty Bones—Dr Tom Lonsdale www.rawmeatybones.com
- The Dog Risk Project in Helsinki, Finland—a research programme about nutritional, environmental and genetic factors behind canine diseases as well as cancer detection in dogs. This research has been ongoing for many years. A review of the findings would likely prove useful for this inquiry.
- The video series The Truth About Pet Cancer.
- The Australian Animal Cancer Foundation
- Video: Pet Fooled—it is beyond horrifying to know what is allowed to be incorporated into a commercially produced pet food diet! It is criminal that this has been allowed to go on, unregulated, throughout the years.
- Three Ways Pet Food Companies are Lying to You

- Pet Food Reviews—Australia
- Feline Nutrition Foundation—provides a wealth of information https://felinehttps://feline-nutrition.org/nutritionorg/
- Specifically for raw feeding: https://feline-nutrition.org/the-blogs/falling-off-thehttps://feline-nutrition.org/the-blogs/falling-off-the-recipe-cliffrecipe-cliff
- Pottenger's Cats—Dr Francis Pottenger https://vetsallnatural.com.au/pottengers-cat-study/ Although this study 1932–1942 predates the knowledge of the importance of amino acids, etc to cat health the findings just on feeding raw vs cooked meat remain valid.

In conclusion

Domestic pets have no control over what they are fed. Pet owners have no control over the selective information and dishonesty of pet food advertising.

The pet food industry needs to be strictly regulated and monitored by an independent body where:

- there can be no possibility of any conflict of interest
- the health and safety of pets is the guaranteed focus and the production of all commercial pet foods is subjected to thorough scrutiny and the highest standards available
- the producers are subject to the highest standard of the law

Sincerely,
J. Vale

APPENDIX D

The following article on preventative dentistry was part of the proceedings for a refresher course for veterinarians given at the University of Sydney in association with the Australian Veterinary Dental Society, 14–17 June 1993. The proceedings were published by the Post Graduate Committee in Veterinary Science, University of Sydney.

Preventative dentistry

Tom Lonsdale BVetMed MRCVS

Summing the effects of tooth brushing, flossing and fluoridation has transformed human dentistry. Logarithmic improvement in the health of companion animals can be expected from the adoption of natural prevention strategies. Veterinary dentistry will be relegated to a minor role and profound changes will overtake veterinary science.

Understanding the mechanisms

How can such a turnaround be effected when 'more than 85% of dogs and cats over the age of three years are suffering from periodontal disease to a degree that would benefit from treatment' Waltham International Focus, Vol 1, No 3, 1991. The answer is hidden in the literature and a few quotes will point the way.

> The test confirmed the feasibility of preventing the accumulation of dental calculus in experimental beagle dogs by regular weekly feeding of oxtails. Brown and Park 1968.

> The dogs affected with paradontal disease are those fed on soft, pappy food; those fed on a diet which necessitates the use of their teeth for the grinding of their food are free from the disease. Sir Frank Colyer, 1947.

> Uncooked bones had the most marked effect followed by rawhide chews and super hard baked biscuits. It is imperative that in addition to this basic commercial diet bones, preferably or rawhide chews or super hard baked biscuits be added to it so that periodontal disease can be prevented. PC Higgins, 1987.

Overcoming existing prejudices

Reaching a level of enlightenment, in retrospect, has been relatively straightforward. Much like the solving of a Rubic's cube it was necessary to purposefully adopt 'wrong positions' in order to finally lock into place the coherent pattern.

Initial surprise at the 85% figure led to anger that we could allow such widespread, slow torture. Even for me, advancing years produces a softening of attitudes and this was the required key to unravelling the mystery. The softening attitude allowed the intellectually sound approach of assuming the opposite. If 85% were affected then perhaps periodontal disease was either a (a) trivial or (b) desirable feature of small carnivore biology.

Trivial

Indications were that this was far from trivial.

> 'What's more, research indicates that dogs with periodontal disease may develop further problems in the heart, liver, kidneys or bones marrow.' (Upjohn Company Poster 1992).

> 'Veterinarians have long suspected and research supports the fact that periodontal disease can become systemic and can predispose the animal to problems such as right-side heart failure, hepatic compromise, renal failure and bone marrow depression. This anachoretic effect can have drastic repercussions on the overall health of the pet and presents one of the greatest challenges facing small animal practitioners today.' G Beard 1991.

But wait a minute. Doesn't it usually start with relatively minor gum disorder before progressing to the major entity? Isn't this gum disorder readily fixed by massage?

> 'Gingivitis can be cured in about four or five days. The secret is actually to clean the bleeding gums more, not less. This tends to run counter to normal medical advice for other bleeding areas of the body. However, gums are different.' 'On the first day, the gums will bleed and feel sore. The second day the gums will bleed more and feel even sorer. The same thing will happen on the third day, by which stage you may be saying that the whole treatment is madness and you may be thinking of giving up. Do not! By about the fourth to fifth day the gums will start

> to feel better and become firm and healthier. This will be noticeable by the virtual absence of bleeding. A day or so later the gums will not bleed at all upon brushing.'
>
> Produced by the Dental Health Foundation—Australia, The University of Sydney, NSW 2006.

So, nature has arranged the cure to be simple cleaning and massage taking place at each natural feeding session. Indeed, a trivial matter if attended to early in the piece.

We still have the problem of:

Desirable

Accepting that the disease was trivial required some effort. Accepting that a severe disease with devastating consequences was desirable would require a somersault. Or alternatively one could question the validity of this seemingly absurd enquiry. Garbage in, garbage out. Ask the wrong question and obtain a lie. The semantics might be getting in the way here.

Until breakthrough ...

In the immortal words of Arthur Lee, it is desirable that 'all that lives is gonna die'. Periodontal disease might prove to be the desirable means to secure this outcome.

A quick reference back to the 'trivial' side of the equation and we can now see that coupled together we have a balanced statement.

Ingesting natural foodstuffs at natural intervals will control impending gingivitis.

Failure of the feeding function allows the accumulation of plaque, the development of gingivitis and progressive periodontal disease.

The expanded cybernetic hypothesis of periodontal disease says that it is an essential link in carnivore population dynamics.

Periodontal disease is the dependable disease which modulates the effects of starvation in wild carnivore population dynamics.

- A feedback loop ensures daily chewing of raw meaty bones sanitises the oral cavity of the successful carnivore.
- Failure of the feedback loop facilitates multiplication of pathogenic bacteria within plaque and development of periodontal disease.
- Incremental losses of carnivores and herbivores are thereby facilitated.
- The populations of herbivores, carnivores and bacteria are maintained in dynamic equilibrium.

Unpublished work, T Lonsdale, December, 1992.

You may accept the logic so far but still remain unsure of the drift so let us adopt a couple of different perspectives.

> 'Day and night the Carnivora are playing their appointed part in keeping down numbers. They themselves are without visible foes yet have a mysterious check on over-multiplication. All the flesh-eaters are more numerous at birth than the herb-eaters. But an unseen agency takes off cubs from every nursery, or the flesh-eaters would be too numerous, and would destroy all herb-eaters. Check and countercheck are constantly at work to maintain the balance and for the terrors of it all—they hardly exist!'
>
> *Children's Encyclopedia*. Editor Arthur Mee

This lyrical passage of uncontested fact sets the carnivores in their ecological niche at the top of the food chain.

In the natural ecology things are infinitely varied and finely tuned. If we were to make a generalisation, the cats are hunters preferring their food warm and, on the hoof, or wing. The canines as a family being more content with an opportunist hunter and scavenger role.

A vital subset of the niche function is the consumption of bone. As humans we make a point of separating our meat from the bone. Carnivores consume virtually everything. Thus, we can see they perform a vital function converting herbivore bones to powder prior to return to the soil in readiness for the cycle to start over again.

The requirement for bone is so great that it translates into characteristic behaviour patterns. Aesop's Fables tell of the dog dropping the bone in the water when he stopped to threaten his reflection in the mirror-like pool. Tom Hungerford remarks:

> 'Rightly or wrongly, I regard the feeding of raw bones daily as being one critical factor in the health of dogs. Why is this? The crunching of the bones may clean the teeth. The enormous dental pressures of crunching bones may cause great circulatory changes in the jaws and gums. The primitive euphoria generated by the crunching of bones is obvious. To tease my dogs and take away their food is nothing, but to tease them and take away the bones causes a very definite reaction. The canine joy of crunching up bones is a daily feature of exhilaration and well-being which may have a bearing upon their immuno-competence and their immune system. Bones may have a nutritional effect (don't overlook trace minerals).'

In 1968, the Royal Veterinary College Expedition to East Africa reported a parasite cyst of hyenas tucked away in the pelvic bones of wildebeest. The hyena target species have the jaws and digestive tract perfectly suited for digesting the hardest bones. That the parasite/

host relationship was so well-defined points to a long evolutionary process.

Setting aside how the environment has needs which are met by the carnivores let us look at the needs of the carnivore satisfied by its food source.

This passage from The Australian Veterinary Practitioner establishes the ground rules.

We must then make the further assumption that the quality, quantity, and frequency of feeding are the prime determinants.

Quality—chemical and physical

a) Chemicals Carbohydrates, proteins etc including the trendy taurines, arachidonic acid, Ca:P ratio etc suited to physiological needs of the animal.
b) Physical Texture/temperature to ensure correct masticatory through to defaecatory process. Equally important physiological needs.

Quantity—chemical and physical

Our principal concern here is for the amount of cleaning that takes place in the oral cavity. Clearly one tough mouthful will not be sufficient quantity of chewy food to ensure a clean mouth. In dogs, experience shows that if raw meaty bones approximate to half the diet, then other sticky foodstuffs will be adequately compensated. In the case of cats, the obligate carnivores, our experience indicates that almost every meal must consist of chewy, raw meaty bones.

Naturally the quantity of chemicals, absolute and relative, should occupy that zone between too much and too little.

Frequency of chemical uptake and physical stimulation
Clearly there is trade-off again in this area between frequency, quantity, and quality. Most carnivores can survive if fed once a week in large quantity and good quality. This is not an optimum and frequency of feeding probably differs between cats and dogs. Certainly, frequency of gum massage and teeth cleaning needs to be at least once per day. This corresponds with the mineralisation of plaque beginning within 24–48 hours of deposition.

We can see that it is morphology and behaviour which serves to differentiate species. All species have roughly equivalent needs for the chemicals; carbohydrates, proteins, etc. To take two taxonomically different species which both eat trees we can cite termites and elephants. They both need trees for the chemical and physical constituents.

It would be a cruel hoax to fortify a heat-treated pile of sawdust with vitamins and minerals and then suggest that either the elephant or the termite could thereby sustain life.

Such an absurd proposition has now so insinuated itself into our way of thinking that we readily accept it for dogs and cats. Natural and unnatural ingredients are pulverised, blended, heat-treated and fortified with vitamins and minerals and placed before cats and dogs as their total requirements for life.

Making the transition

From an early age we have been inculcated with the idea that domestic cats' and dogs' dietary needs can be met from the can or packet. By the time we get to university the subject is firmly in the hands of the biochemists who calculate the chemical formula.

Of course it is a trifle unnerving to have one's icons smashed with all in disarray and absence of familiar landmarks. A veterinary surgeon raised the following objections to feeding raw bones.

OBJECTIONS	VERDICT	REBUTTAL
1. It is impractical.	False	Modern distribution and refrigeration make natural feeding easy.
2. Previous dietary imbalance problems will arise.	False	Imbalance problems exist today as before. Better education and better access to people will enable us to eliminate imbalances.
3. It costs more.	False	It costs much less.
4. Some processed foods assist with dental hygiene	Misplaced emphasis	Raw bone diet far outstrips biscuits and raw hide chews for dogs. Dry food exacerbates cat dental problems. (Higgins 1987)
5. Only a couple of bones need to be given weekly.	False	Consumption of bones is a powerful cleanser of teeth. Plaque and calculus are active between times.
6. Brachycephalic breeds cannot handle bones	False	Started from a young age they soon learn. Given their predisposition to dental disease their need for prevention is greater. Brachycephalics are in the minority—why hinge any argument on the minority case.
7. Physically impossible for some breeds	False	The raw bones and vegetable—carrot, apple etc can be selected according to circumstances. The brachycephalic breeds were genetically selected over hundreds of years of natural food feeding.
8. Little research has been done to justify natural feeding	False	Evolution is an ongoing experiment. Sir Frank Colyer and Peter Higgins list experimental and survey work.
9. Dogs live longer and have higher pedigree and therefore cannot cope.	Misplaced emphasis	Old pedigree dogs surviving a lifetime without bones become addicted to the wrong food and usually suffer painful mouth conditions making chewing difficult. There may be breed dispositions to problems but none documented.
10. Bones get stuck in the teeth.	Misplaced emphasis	An animal practised in handling the correct style of bone has little difficulty.
11. Teeth get broken.	Misplaced emphasis	Any system in use can become damaged. All systems require suitable exercise. Inappropriate e.g. ox marrow bone most likely to inflict damage.
12. Constipation is a problem.	Misplaced emphasis	Dogs habituated to bones have regular, firm stools of powdered bone. Bones fed once a week in large quantity can give rise to excessively dry stools. It is cooked, sharp, indigestible bones which are mostly associated with bowel problems.

13. Complete diet is impossible. (Meaning complete chemical)	False	Natural diets readily achieve complete physical and chemical needs.
14. Nutritional disease will become common.	False	Removing animals processed complete diets and putting them on natural diets has always resulted in increased health.
15. Deficiencies are bound to show up.	Unlikely	Processed foods have been implicated in most direct deficiency states, e.g. Taurine, arachidonic acid. In the hypothetical event that a deficiency is detected then appropriate action can be taken.
16. Excess nutrient disorders will occur.	Unlikely	Carnivores can process limitless quantities of bone. Many processed foods have excess salt and protein as judged by their own standards. (Cowgill, 1991)
17. Table scraps are no better than canned or dried food.	Misplaced emphasis	Scraps are cheap (free to user). Less highly processed, even raw. It is true they do not massage teeth and gums.
18. Raw bones and scraps not viable alternative.	False	They are available—cheap and health-giving.
19. Legal implications of advising raw bones.	False	Nonsensical that recommending natural diet would carry legal penalties. Advising processed food giving rise to dental and systemic disease much more likely to invite legal action.

Even if you withstand the onslaught designed to obstruct or impede your progress it still remains a tricky problem putting into practice the injunction 'feed a natural diet'.

Getting started

Psychologists advise that your behaviour package is made up of four components:

- How you act
- How you think
- How you feel
- Your body's workings (Physiology)

Taking on difficult tasks is best performed by doing the act and the other functions will line up. For instance getting out of bed on cold mornings is not much helped by thinking about it. Best, 1) is to do it 2) become aware that it is happening 3) feel positive about accepting the challenge 4) notice the limbs beginning to free up.

Unfortunately as a practitioner making a cultural change there are so many cerebral and practical changes that need to be wrought. Then this whole package has to be sold to unwilling/unreceptive clients (often people who have received contrary advice from you in the past). The consequence of this is that no simple act will get you underway. Instead, you will need to think through the process with all the attendant props.

Thinking through the process is not enough unless you conceive of a goal for the endeavour. I leave this goal to you but suggest you might see yourself playing an instrumental role in bringing widespread health to animals, cost savings to people and easing the burden on the environment. ...

Once you have thought through your props, strategy and goals you need to do some simulation exercises. Ideally you should be up to speed before tackling the real thing—just like a fighter pilot going through the flight simulator or the down-hill skier thinking through his descent.

Equipment, visual aids, educational material

The assumption I start with is that you have a general small animal practice with the usual facilities and equipment. If your practice is like ours then greater than 85% of patients have active periodontal disease and all of them need to eat food which is conducive to health, not a recipe for disease.

The chances are that your clients hold pet dental hygiene in low priority, are attending the clinic for reasons quite separate from dietary and dental health concerns. The trick is to shift the owner's focus away from the ostensible reason for the visit, vaccination, de-sex, skin rash etc and on to dietary and oral hygiene concerns.

Sales trainers tell you that 'you need to believe in your product'. Initially you may be a little sceptical that all health concerns can be overshadowed by diet and oral hygiene. Please let me reassure you that once underway you will develop a fierce conviction. Skilful use of equipment and visual aids will see you on your way.

In the waiting room

Arrange posters on dental disease, have a photo album of past cases and displays of faecal material. We have a pot of cooked bone fragments removed from constipated dogs. Normal faeces from bone-fed dogs is dry, firm and off-white. We soak our specimens in alcohol for 24 hours, then dry them before putting them in the specimen jars.

In the consulting room

At every treatment station where we may examine an animal there are a range of instruments including thermometer, stethoscope etc. An indispensable tool is the claw and spoon dental scaler which is used to point out particular problems in the mouth and perform immediate supra-gingival scaling. Testimonial letters are kept in a loose-leaf binder. Posters are used for illustration and the ubiquitous 'poo pots' abound. Periodontal disease survey forms and a highlighter pen complete the picture.

Treatment room/wash stand

Apart from the usual anaesthetic equipment the chief requirements are:

a) Fluid therapy equipment, and
b) Dental hand instruments.

A selection of Smith-Baxter gags are to hand and a series of champagne corks for gagging cats and small dogs. A polaroid camera is kept at the ready for recording events, both educational and litigation inspired.

Ward/preparation area

Extra freezer space is required for consignments of chicken carcasses and lamb bones. A microwave oven can be used for defrosting otherwise overnight retention in the refrigerator suffices.

Other supporting material

Local newspaper coverage makes excellent material for the waiting room noticeboard. Be sure to laminate any permanent display. A diet sheet is essential. Keep it simple and practical in orientation. Of course, it must meet chemical needs of the animal and just as importantly the physical needs.

Our diet sheet is reproduced here. It is acknowledged that we may need to make amendments in the light of advancing knowledge. (*Nullius in verba*. The Royal Society of London's motto adopted in 1660 means 'No man's word shall be final'.) For the moment we can affirm that all patients switched from well-known canned/dry/table-scrap diets have shown a marked increase in well-being. Puppies and kittens have thrived from the outset.

We rather assume that animals are free to eat soil, faeces and grass as part of the normal ingesta of carnivores. We allow that in the long run hyper- or hypo-conditions could arise, and which could be corrected by dietary modification or in the extreme by the administration of supplements. We are content that the processed industry's mass destruction of taurine and arachidonic acid will not befall this diet. An encouraging rider: it seems almost impossible to feed too many bones. As one would expect of nature's bone recyclers; the more the merrier.

Do not forget to locate cheap sources of chicken carcasses, whole rabbits, kangaroo tails, lamb flaps, oxtails, chicken necks etc. You will need these products for your in-patients and your clients will appreciate the information.

Protocols and morale building

Include the staff in all aspects. Lay staff will be forgetful and need constant reminding. Professional staff will be dubious and resisting. Provide a few successes, establish guidelines and the troops will soon be smiling.

Our nurses are eager to provide clients with our updated literature with a covering: 'Please take our material on diet and dentistry. We have found it to be important. The vet will explain when he sees you.'

Regardless of the reason for the visit every animal must have its mouth examined. To encourage a closer involvement of both vet and client the survey is frequently filled. Much information can be obtained. Above all it gets vets and clients to start taking account of halitosis. (You will have no doubt as to the prevalence of oral disease and the correlation with processed food once you complete a few forms.)

One huge drawback of conducting the holistic approach is that it takes time. Clients come in to get their pet's flea dermatitis fixed up and we launch into a long, free discussion.

Raw bones to treat fleas!

> **'One very important concept we have learnt is that animals eating a healthy diet and leading a healthy life-style have a healthy immune system. A healthy immune system can usually cope with average flea numbers.**
>
> **Raw meaty bones daily keep mouths healthy, immune systems healthy and keep flea allergy dermatitis at bay.'**
>
> Extract from client information sheet.

There is no opportunity to charge for the time because the clients do not ask for the service. The certain knowledge that animals will be back in a couple of years requiring dental work and heart, liver and kidney treatments unless we do provide renders us honour bound to give advance, preventative advice.

A few *bon mots* enable me to convey the message in a picturesque way. I stress the need for:

- Fresh air—we can live three minutes without it.
- Fresh water—we can live three days without it.
- Fresh food—we can live three weeks without it.

This enables clients to focus on what supports life.

But evolution provided a niche for each species and detailed the fresh food of the carnivore contrasted with sheep, cows, elephants and termites.

I stress that dogs and cats use their mouths as tools of trade for carrying out a diverse range of tasks. The delicate function of carrying the cubs contrasts with ingesting bone and cleaning the anus. Just as the carpenter can only expect to gain a decent living if he maintains his equipment then the same applies to carnivores. This maintenance function is simply achieved by chewing bones, not merely as a chewing aid but as the very food itself.

Failure to chew bones results in the accumulation of plaque, necrotic gum, pus, putrefying food and faecal material. The equivalent of 'suffering silently, sipping sewerage seven days a week'. No one relishes that thought even for five minutes.

Above all I stress the need for the immune system and its regulatory role in the body. Not the constant vain attempt to sanitise a septic mouth where the physical chewing system has failed.

Artificial teeth cleaning is discussed. Clients readily relate to the difficulties they experience finding the time or mastering the technique. They are then invited to imagine a cooperative family member needing a teeth clean and finally the family pet. Laughter usually follows.

We do acknowledge the exceptions. Canine teeth may benefit from brushing since the killing and dismembering function seldom occurs in domestication. Brushing may be the only option in some brachycephalic animals, those with missing teeth and those unaccustomed to bones.

Common things are common

Puppy and kitten first vaccinations

The emphasis is placed squarely on prevention to ensure a lifetime of health. Mention is made that the animals are particularly vulnerable to gum disease at teething. Owners are encouraged to smell the breath of their new pet. Frequently it stinks at six weeks of age.

Chicken necks and wings are the recommended food together with whole, raw fish. It is mentioned that fish can be associated with hypo-vitaminosis B1 but never seen by us. That in truth chicken is too large a bird for kittens and that smashing the wing with a mallet helps.

We recommend that the whole wing be put through the mincer for younger kittens and pups.

Clients usually exclaim that 'I thought that chicken bones were harmful'. We explain the persistent myth dating from when chicken was a delicacy, and the only available bones were cooked. How, in fact, ground-nesting birds are virtually a free meal for wandering carnivores. They do not even need to give chase.

Second and third vaccinations

All the preceding material is reiterated. Clients usually report on the success of the venture although some slip back into old habits. If pups or kittens have been processed food fed, there is frequently visible calculus build-up. We show clients how to hold the forelegs of the pet, pressing the body between their forearms. It is then an easy matter to scrape off the supra-gingival calculus. We acknowledge to the client that this is an imperfect job but not to worry. The emphasis is placed on on-going management. That chewing the bones removes the vestiges of supra-gingival calculus but more importantly scrubs the sub-gingival plaque.

De-sex at six months of age

The mouths of surgical patients are often putrid. During teething and in the absence of bones, a stagnant mess prevails. We advise accordingly.

Cats with moderate calculus presenting for any problem

Naturally the presenting problem is diagnosed and treated. Cats usually submit to scaling. They are suitably overwhelmed by the surroundings. Dietary changes are initiated and the client asked to return in one to two months for reassessment.

Dogs with moderate calculus presenting for any problem

It is mentioned that the 'silent disease' is frequently only fully assessed by examination under anaesthesia. If the animal needs an anaesthetic for the presenting complaint, then dentistry is offered at a further charge.

If anaesthesia is not required then dietary changes are recommended and a return inspection recommended in one to two months.

Cats and dogs presenting for any problem with concurrent moderate to severe periodontitis

The inter-relationship of all disease processes is stressed. A treatment protocol is devised including dentistry under anaesthesia. The owner is advised that pain relief and restoration of function should be our guiding principles. Consequently, we shall likely remove a number of teeth. From the outset we advise that the patient has probably become addicted to harmful foodstuffs not unlike the nicotine, alcohol or heroin dependent person. Changing the dietary habits may prove difficult and that they may prefer to board the animal with ourselves until dietary change is achieved.

Blood tests prove a useful adjunct in the treatment of these patients. A baseline of values is established and can be compared with results at follow-up in a couple of months time. The research benefit of having lab results is considerable both for in-house demonstration to clients and also for contributions to professional journals. Blood tests are always read against 'normal' values. We do not know the source of these values but suspect they have been obtained from colonies of research animals. Research colonies are usually processed food fed, and therefore suffer periodontal disease. There can be noticeable blood changes in animals suffering periodontal disease thus rendering the so-called 'normals' invalid.

Periodontal disease diagnosis and treatment is discussed elsewhere. Measurement of pocket depth is notoriously unreliable as a means of assessing the severity of the problem. Cats in particular often show little or no pocketing. The tell-tale sign for us is the bulging gums over the roots of the canines. If these teeth are squeezed together between thumb and forefinger a characteristic pain response is elicited. Removal of these teeth is usually easy and produces a tooth with severe apical resorption. Subsequent attitude/behaviour changes confirm that we have done the patient a huge favour.

When extractions have occurred it is stressed that the normal scissor action is lost and accordingly remaining teeth will lack appropriate massage. Tooth brushing may be necessary to prevent the disease progressing. Immediate follow-up appointments are arranged. A six-month recall reminder is inserted in the record system in order to keep the patient under constant review.

Following dental surgery we frequently advise raw meaty bones and water only for the first week. Contrary to expectation pain does not seem to be a problem for our patients. Rather they appear more content without the periodontal disease-affected teeth and tear into their first post-operative meal with gusto. By keeping dental patients in hospital for a couple of days you will gain experience and thereby confidence.

Special groups—Persian cats, pugs, Pekingese and chihuahuas

These breeds are predisposed to dental disease due to malocclusion, mouth breathing and the propensity of owners to treat them differently. We stress that they have the physiology of the carnivore with an increased need for preventative dental hygiene. These animals do just fine on raw chicken necks, rabbits and whole fish.

Bulldogs

I heard of one bulldog that could not breathe and chew a bone simultaneously. Our experience is that chicken carcasses, carrots and apples are handled easily.

Boarding animals

We board a few 'healthy' animals. In every instance we know that gum disease will be underway unless the owners have had exposure to the new ideas. It is always a delicate business recommending dental care to these owners. They frequently deny a problem exists and suspect our motives. Usually, the bad smell coupled with the written material serves to convince them.

Cautionary tales

Murphy's law prevails and not unexpectedly any system in use can experience setbacks and deviations from the norm. The moral here is not to be complacent but be eternally vigilant and on the lookout for the unexpected. Do take care not to translate valid concerns into rash action. To risk a cliché—'Do not throw out the baby with the bathwater'.

Early in my career I was lucky enough to attend the animals in the local safari park. At any one time there were twenty to thirty lions and perhaps a dozen tigers. One day each week the animals were fasted and frequently vomited on that day. Most days the food consisted of half a cow's head. One tigress vomited mucus for a couple of days and went off her food. A presumptive diagnosis of small intestinal impaction with bone was subsequently confirmed at surgery. Her recovery was complete. After a first meal of whole rabbit her usual diet was reinstituted. The owners were certainly not agitating for a change to mushy canned food.

Recently a ten-week-old Rough Collie puppy was presented with rectal impaction of chicken vertebrae. The puppy belongs to two friends who own 22 adult and 26 Rough Collie pups. Despite this incident they are both delighted with their new natural feeding regime. The cost saving of $150 per week is a factor but otherwise 'feeding time is halved', 'my dogs adored the diet from day one'. 'We are spreading the word'.

The comments I would make are that:

a) Bolting chicken necks without proper mastication before a litter mate gains advantage could be a factor. Lamb flaps could be a better proposition for this particular litter.
b) Some animals may have a problem with bone digestion just as some human babies cannot digest breastmilk.
c) The inability may be genetic in origin. If generations have been fed exclusively on mushy food, it will be quite possible for a defective gene to persist to the present.
d) Penetrating the fable of the tiger and the collie dog may bring us into contact with a fundamental fact of evolutionary biology. That carnivores are highly specialised animals which, if conditions are right, will thrive. Small perturbations at the margins bringing about dramatic outcomes e.g. tiger with bowel impaction. Domestic dogs are derived from specialist feeders and are further specialised. Tantamount to making modifications to a Ferrari. In the case of the collie breed, it is known that Collie Eye Anomaly and Blood Brain Barrier/ Ivomectin toxicity problems exist.

Possibly the breed modification predisposes to digestive upset such that even minor perturbations of little consequence to the parent species will have a major impact on the modified genotype.

> 'Specialised organisms thrive when conditions are optimum but experience considerable pressure to adapt or perish when the conditions change. Relatively undifferentiated organisms can accommodate change with relative ease.' Adaptation of C Darwin

This proposition needs testing. It will be a most alarming indictment if we have so modified dogs that they are condemned to acute bone impaction if they consume natural food or condemned to chronic periodontal disease if they do not.

It is well known that dogs jealously guard bones and will engage in savage fights to protect them. This natural behaviour can alarm owners as can the habit of burying bones surplus to need. Do not be deterred. Dogs can be separated at feeding times and bones just sufficient for need can be supplied.

When one client was pressed for complaints about bone feeding, she mentioned that she would be more readily convinced if we published the constituent parts. My answer was that fresh human food, meat, bread, vegetables etc. do not carry lists of ingredients. It is only packages of processed foods that display a list of contents. As we all know a table of contents does not guarantee suitability for purpose.

Sparring with clients is counterproductive and, appealing to intellect is frequently unrewarding. The current level of cultural conditioning is such that it may take years before sanity returns. One firm resolution arising out of this encounter was the need for a good colour histological diagram of bones. Clients think of bone as solid inert material instead of the intricate organic and inorganic structure.

Periodontal disease consequences

The objective problem here is whether all disease states can be traced to the diseased mouth. Lacking a control group of naturally fed animals, which at no stage have suffered periodontal disease, we have an intellectual problem. Put another way, all animals presenting with a disease either have, or have had, significant periodontal disease during their history.

It is axiomatic that correlation does not imply causation. There is, however, sufficient evidence from Chaos theory (about interconnectivity) through to a knowledge of immune pathways to suggest that periodontal disease plays a significant/dominant role. (As a digression, let me say, that causation is a vexatious concept plagued with as many problems as it solves. It needs to be used sparingly and with caution)

From a practical standpoint we find making the assumption that periodontal disease is an integral part of all disease processes provides us with a powerful, predictive and explanatory tool.

Bacteraemias and viraemias

An inflamed mouth presents a widened portal of entry to the capillaries and lymphatics. By contrast, intact mucosae and skin is impenetrable to most organisms.

Hyper-immune conditions

We have case histories of eosinophilic granuloma and plasma cell pododermatitis responding to dentistry and diet change. This supports the view that hyper-immune conditions develop due to the over reactivity of the system when seeking to sanitise a foul mouth.

Autoimmune conditions

It is well known that over reactivity can lead to autoimmune conditions. It is interesting to note that the periodontal ligament is collagenous. That the pododermatitis of cats affects the highly collagenous digital pads. All ruptured cruciate cases treated by us have a foul mouth.

Hypo-immune conditions

We have an extensive line of cases demonstrating leucopaenia. These animals, once the periodontal disease is brought under control and commenced on a raw bone diet, gain:

a) an increase in health status and
b) an increase in leucocyte count.

This is a ready and objective test that you can conduct yourself. (Depending on the stage of the disease you may see an inflammatory profile or no change at all.)

Multicomponent immune disease

In our population of aging pets nothing is ever tightly defined as a single problem. It is common to see flaccid, elderly animals with foul mouth and heart, kidney, joint, skin and cancerous conditions attributable to the preceding four immunological disasters. We used to depend on antibiotics to kill bacteria and cortico-steroids to suppress the immune response. Now we clean up the mouth and change the diet.

Treatment failures

Some cases of plasmocytic-lymphocytic stomatitis of cats have not responded to dental care and diet change. This has been disappointing considering the rapid improvement of the eosinophilic granuloma and plasma cell pododermatitis cases. One long-standing case is 'stable' on a raw, rabbit-leg diet with periodic prednisolone therapy.

Of course we are aware that once immune disease is underway the simple removal of the excitatory cause will not necessarily bring about cessation of the disease process.

As we increase the numbers of cats reared and maintained on a natural food diet, we gain an opportunity to observe if the plasmacytic-lymphocytic stomatitis will arise spontaneously. Little doubt exists in my mind but the statisticians will require numbers.

Things to avoid

Avoid losing focus on the goal you have established. Along the way some will induce you to recommend feeding bones once or twice weekly instead of every day. Do not feel compelled as if you need to prove your reasonableness and willingness to compromise. Just remember that the enemy never rests.

> 'Microbial plaque is a structural, resilient, yellow-greyish substance that adheres tenaciously to teeth. It is comprised of bacteria in a matrix of salivary glycoproteins and extra-cellular polysaccharides like glucans (e.g. dextrans, mutans) and fructans (e.g. levan). This matrix makes it impossible to rinse plaque away with water; it must be removed mechanically ... Plaque is not a food residue. Supra-gingival plaque forms more rapidly during sleep when no food is ingested than following meals. The consistency of diet also affects the rate of plaque formation and pathology is increased in soft diets.' M Tholen 1987.

Do not invest heavily in a dental workstation to achieve shiny white ivories on one occasion each six months. Keep the focus on daily chewing and spend the money on a freezer instead.

> 'Manual removal of calculus was not required when dogs were fed one-half or one whole oxtail per week.' Brown et al 1968.

By the time you have read this far you will be aware that selling processed pet food is taboo. This includes the so-called prescription diets which simply retain the physical form but alter the chemical formula.

By now you will be thinking pro-actively and with prevention uppermost in your mind. Make long-term estimations for your pharmaceutical needs and ultimately your cash flow.

This paper was written with practitioners in mind. The legal ramifications are a recurring concern for anyone in business. My NSW-based solicitor was asked for an opinion, and he advised that the following matters may become issues of relevance in the future.

1. Potential claims by pet owners under various pieces of consumer legislation throughout the States and Territories of Australia.
2. In the federal sphere potential Trade Practices Act claims for false or misleading claims may be made either in relation to advertising or promotional material or labels.
3. The new Truth in Labelling activities instituted by the Federal Government.
4. Potential problems or claims under the recently introduced Product Liability provisions in Part V of the Trade Practices Act.
5. The, as yet, unknown effect of class actions which have been lawful in Australia since the 5th day of March 1992 which may tend to overcome the existing drawbacks to actions brought by individual pet owners, namely the high cost of litigation and claims which may amount to only several hundreds of dollars in relation to an individual pet.

The foregoing relates to potential claims against manufacturers, distributors and possibly even retailers of processed pet food. Query what may be the legal problems of veterinarians who fail to consider the issues in this paper or fail to address those issues in advising pet owners who make known to the veterinarian that they rely wholly and solely on processed pet food to supply their pets' diet. Is it too much to suggest that, as pet owners, in common with everyone else in the community become more litigious, veterinarians may someday share top billing on a Writ?

Epilogue

Since Lister (1827–1912) antiseptics, Pasteur (1822–1895) discovery of microbes and Fleming (1881–1955) discovery of penicillin we have been obsessed with microbes and conquering them with 'magic bullets'. Despite the evident successes there seemed to be evermore requirement for magic bullets and practitioners to fire the shots.

A number of veterinarians and most clients find the old chauvinist approach has lost its appeal. Although hard to specify why. How much better this newfound holism providing comfort and harmony?

For me each day is greeted with eager anticipation; as an opportunity to spread the message. Fast tracking to redundancy may seem a trifle odd; nevertheless, I cheerfully predict that you will enjoy it too.

Acknowledgements

Thanks to Bruce Duff of Macquarie Pathology Service for Laboratory Support.

References providing inspiration or fact

Altman, E G. and Wendon, K H Preventative Periodontics 1974 Dental Health Education and Research Foundation University of Sydney

Bawden, R Agpack SU-141 Sustainable Agriculture—Hawkesbury's Position University of Western Sydney

Billinghurst, I Canine Nutrition—A Point of View Sydney University PGCVS Nutrition Conference

Brown and Park Control of Dental Calculus in Experimental Beagles Lab Animal Care Vol 18 No. 5, 1968

Colyer, Sir Frank Dental Disease in Animals Vol LXXXII January 17, 1947

Dental seminar AVDS July 1991 PGCVS UNI SYD Proc No 169

Edney ATB Editor The Waltham Book of Dog and Cat Nutrition 2nd Edition. Pergamon Press 1988

Gleick, J Chaos, Making A New Science Cardinal 1987

Higgins P C Proceedings No 100. TeethOpen Wide (Dentistry in Dogs and Cats) 1 10–14 August, 1987

Hungerford, T Control and Therapy 169 PGCVS University of Sydney

Klenk, V Understanding Symbolic Logic 2nd Edition Prentice Hall Learning Performance Aust P/L 1990

Lonsdale, T Plasma Cell Pododermatitis of Cats Control & Therapy 168 No 3270 PGCVS

Lonsdale, T Feline Eosinophilic Granuloma Complex Control and Therapy 168 No 3271 PGCVS

Lonsdale, T Raw Meaty Bones Promotes Health Control & Therapy 169 PGCVS University of Sydney

Lonsdale, T Pandemic of Periodontal Disease A Malodorous Condition Monograph 20/8/92

Lonsdale, T Cybernetic Hypothesis of Periodontal Disease Unpublished Work Dec 1992

Lonsdale, T Professional Point of View Australian Veterinary Practitioner 1993

Lovelock, J Gaia—A New Look at Life on Earth, OUP 1979

Nutrient Requirements of Dogs 1985 NRC National Academy Press

Nutrient Requirements of Cats 1986 NRC National Academy Press

Pack Tries New Tricks But Pal Remains Top Dog Business Review Weekly April 5, 1991

Pieroni, P The Greening of Medicine Gollancz 1991

Uncle Ben's of Australia Feeding the Dog and Cat

Uncle Ben's of Australia Feeding the Dog and Cat 1990

Veterinary Dentistry 1990 AVDS Proceeding of the First Annual Conference Melbourne PGCVS University of Sydney Proc No 145

Waltham World Authority on Pet Care and Nutrition Waltham International Focus VOL 1 No 3 1991

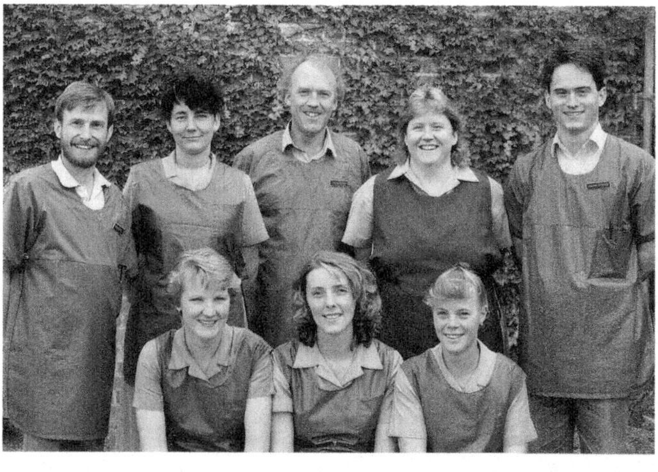

Riverstone Veterinary Hospital team in early 1990s during dynamic period of pet dentistry research and application.

APPENDIX E

Blog of Professor Emerita Sandra Scarr
Raw Meaty Bones for Healthy Pets

My passion is to expose and eliminate the unholy alliance between pet food companies and veterinarians. Pet food companies fund and control veterinary education, research, and practice, keeping pets on a harmful, starchy diet they did not evolve to eat. Feeding RMB keeps our carnivorous pets healthy for their lifetimes.

As breeder of Labrador retrievers for twelve years, I have tried kibble, BARF and Raw-Meaty-Bones diets with my dogs and puppies. Before retiring to breed Labs and to grow Kona coffee in Hawaii, I was Commonwealth Professor of Psychology at the University of Virginia and an award-winning researcher in behavioral genetics and developmental psychology. You can find my biography in Who's Who in the World, Who's Who in America, Who's Who in Science and Technology, and in Wikipedia.

My scientific background is relevant to the topic of pet diets, because I can evaluate the research purporting to support bad pet feeding practices. I can also point out the obvious gaps in pet nutritional research, gaps caused by pet food companies' control of what studies are funded. The unholy alliance of pet food companies, veterinarians, and animal welfare groups (who also depend on pet food funding) is costing pet owners worldwide billions of dollars in diet-caused illnesses and causing unmeasurable suffering and premature deaths for hundreds of millions of pets. This money-driven cabal has to be exposed and stopped.

Wednesday, June 9, 2010

How to feed pets—as taught by Hill's Pet Nutrition

To understand why veterinarians recommend and sell cooked, processed starches as 'food' for meat-eating cats and dogs, one must delve into relationships between veterinary medicine and pet food corporations. Hill's Pet Nutrition (Science Diet and prescription products) were the pioneers in corrupting veterinary medicine.

Mark Morris founded Hill's Pet Nutrition in his garage in 1948. Morris was a veterinarian, whose son also trained as a veterinarian. Mark Morris's son carried on the family business. Their products, Science Diet and Hill's prescription diets, expanded into factories and ultimately were sold to Colgate-Palmolive for several billions of dollars in 2003.

From the outset, Mark Morris believed that convincing veterinarians to believe in Science Diet and Hill's prescription products was the key to the company's success. He was absolutely right. Hill's Pet Nutrition invested heavily in veterinary education, pet nutrition research, and helping new graduates to set up small animal practices with Hill's products on the shelves.

Hill's representatives infiltrated veterinary schools, aiding students with donated pet foods, teaching pet nutrition courses, giving research grants supporting commercial pet foods, providing funds for student activities, summer internships, and many other initiatives. Morris enjoyed a three-decade lead over other pet food companies in corrupting the veterinary profession.

By contrast to other pet food companies, such as Mars and Nestlé-Purina, Hill's Pet Nutrition spends a pittance on advertising to pet owners and focuses their funds on veterinarians. Once purchased by Colgate-Palmolive, however, advertising of Hill's pet products accelerated, but their focus is still on controlling veterinary medicine. Hill's investment in controlling pet nutrition teaching, research, and practice has paid off very handsomely for the company, which is now a high-profit unit of global Colgate-Palmolive.

Rich from the sale of the family business to Colgate-Palmolive, Morris's son endowed the Mark Morris Institute in his father's honor. What does the Institute support? Teaching small animal nutrition in veterinary schools, of course!

- They write the textbook (Small Animal Clinical Nutrition, 5th Edition) that is used in nearly every pet nutrition course in every veterinary school.
- They teach the pet nutrition course.
- The Mark Morris Institute pays a dozen veterinarians, whom they send, free of charge, to veterinary schools to teach pet nutrition and to consult with veterinary students about setting up successful pet practices.
- Most Mark Morris Institute Fellows are current and/or former employees of Hills Pet Nutrition and the Morris Animal Foundation. They speak about nutrients, not food, and teach vet students to believe that commercial formulations are the best nutrition Father Manufacture can concoct. Mother Nature is nowhere to be found.

Mark Morris Sr. and Jr., with hundreds of millions of Hill's dollars behind them, also founded an interlocking set of self-congratulatory professional associations in veterinary nutrition and internal medicine. By controlling memberships, they bestow Diplomate status and honors on each other and exclude those who do not pledge allegiance to commercial pet foods.

The Mark Morris Institute (MMI), Morris Animal Foundation, and Hill's Pet Nutrition have interlocking directorates. One can easily see the lines of communication and conspiracy in the faculty biographies below. Even more alarming is the extensive penetration of these pet food entities into leading veterinary schools.

Although lengthy, the evidence is worth reviewing in detail. You can find information on the Mark Morris Institute says about its University Teaching Program and the faculty who carry their message at www.markmorrisinstitute.org.

Have a look at the Hired Guns the Mark Morris Institute sends (free of charge) to veterinary schools to teach pet nutrition. I highlighted their pet food positions, but please note their positions in leading veterinary schools and professional associations.

Debbie Davenport DVM, MS, DACVIM

Dr. Davenport received her DVM from Auburn University in 1981. She completed an internship at Louisiana State University and a medical residency and master's degree at The Ohio State University.

Dr. Davenport was an Assistant Professor in the Department of Small Animal Clinical Sciences at the Virginia-Maryland Regional College of Veterinary Medicine where she was the recipient of the University Teaching Award for instructional excellence. **She is currently the Director of Professional Education at Hill's Pet Nutrition and the Executive Director of the Mark Morris Institute.** In addition, she holds an adjunct professorship at the Kansas State University College of Veterinary Medicine and serves as a **Trustee and Scientific Liaison for the Morris Animal Foundation.**

Dr. Davenport is a Diplomate of the American College of Veterinary Internal Medicine. Her major professional interests are gastroenterology, oncology and clinical nutrition.

S. Dru Forrester DVM, MS, DACVIM

Dr. Forrester received her DVM from Auburn University in 1985. She completed an internship and residency in internal medicine, and received a Master of Science degree at Texas A&M University.

Dr. Forrester was a faculty member in the Department of Small Animal Clinical Sciences at the Virginia-Maryland Regional College of Veterinary Medicine for 13 years and a professor at the Western University College of Veterinary Medicine in southern California for 2 years. She has received many awards in recognition of teaching excellence, including the national Carl Norden/Pfizer Distinguished Teacher Award in 2004.

Dr. Forrester's professional interests include urology and nephrology. She joined **Hill's Pet Nutrition in 2005 in the Department of Scientific Affairs and is a Mark Morris Institute Fellow.**

David Hammond DVM, MS, DACVIM

Dr. Hammond received his DVM degree from Washington State University in 1980. After owning and operating a mixed-animal veterinary practice, he returned to academia where he completed a medicine residency at Mississippi State University.

Dr. Hammond was a faculty member at the University of Pennsylvania before joining **Hill's Pet Nutrition as a Veterinary Affairs Manager**. He is currently the owner of Horizon Veterinary Services, Inc.

Dr. Hammond is a Diplomate of the American College of Veterinary Internal Medicine. His major interests are endocrinology and clinical nutrition. He is an adjunct professor at Colorado State University, the University of Minnesota, and Washington State University as well as a **Mark Morris Institute Fellow**.

Michael S. Hand DVM, PhD, DACVN

Dr. Hand received his DVM from Colorado State University in 1968. After ten years of private practice in Wyoming, he returned to Colorado State University where he received a PhD in nutritional physiology.

Dr. Hand was a faculty member at the School of Veterinary Medicine at North Carolina State University for three years before joining **Mark Morris Institute in 1985. He was the Vice President of Research at Hill's Pet Nutrition Center** until his retirement in 2000.

Dr. Hand is a Diplomate of the American College of Veterinary Nutrition. He has authored over 60 research publications and book chapters and holds two patents. He is a **co-author of the textbook, Small Animal Clinical Nutrition III and editor of Small Animal Clinical Nutrition, 4th Edition.** He is an adjunct professor at North Carolina State and Kansas State Universities and **Chair of the Board of Directors of Mark Morris Institute**.

Claudia Kirk DVM, PhD, DACVIM, DACVN

Dr. Kirk received her DVM degree from the University of California-Davis in 1986. She completed an internship at the Animal Medical Center in New York City and medicine residency at University of California-Davis. She remained at the University of California-Davis as a Hill's Fellow in Clinical Nutrition where she also completed a Ph.D. in Nutrition.

Dr. Kirk joined **Hill's Pet Nutrition as a Veterinary Clinical Nutritionist** in 1994. She is a Diplomate of the American College of Veterinary Nutrition and the American College of Veterinary Internal Medicine. Dr. Kirk is currently Associate Professor of Medicine and Nutrition and acting Department Chair of Small Animal Clinical Sciences of the University of Tennessee College of Veterinary Medicine.

Dr. Kirk's major professional interest is small animal clinical nutrition, with special interests in feline nutrition, lower urinary tract disease, geriatrics, and endocrinology. She is a **Mark Morris Institute Fellow**. She has served as president of the American

College of Veterinary Nutrition. Dr. Kirk is currently Associate Professor of Medicine and Nutrition and acting Department Chair of Small Animal Clinical Sciences of the University of Tennessee College of Veterinary Medicine.

Ellen Logan DVM, PhD

Dr. Logan received her DVM degree from Kansas State University in 1988. She spent five years as the University Veterinarian for Kansas State University providing veterinary care to a wide range of animal species. She also instructed students, inspected university laboratory animal facilities, and provided consultation to university researchers. She completed a Ph.D. in oral pathology in 1994.

Dr. Logan joined **Hill's Pet Nutrition as a Veterinary Scientist in 1994. She is currently the manager of the Veterinary Consultation Service.** Dr. Logan's major professional interests are pathology, dentistry, and clinical nutrition. She is an adjunct associate research professor at the University of Kansas, an adjunct assistant clinical professor at Kansas State University, and a **Mark Morris Institute Fellow**. She has served as president of the American Veterinary Dental Society and national spokesperson for Pet Dental Health Month.

Chris L. Ludlow DVM, MS, DACVIM

Dr. Ludlow earned his DVM from Kansas State University in 1986. He worked in general practice in southern California for five years. He then completed a combined internal medicine/small animal clinical nutrition residency and masters degree at Kansas State University.

Dr. Ludlow was a faculty member at Kansas State University for one and half years before joining Veterinary Information Network in internal medicine and nutrition.

Dr. Ludlow is a Diplomate of the American Veterinary College of Veterinary Internal Medicine. His professional interests include gastroenterology, endocrinology, cardiology, and clinical nutrition. He is a consultant for the Veterinary Information Network in internal medicine and nutrition, and a **Fellow for Mark Morris Institute**.

Richard C. Nap DVM, PhD, DECVS & DECVCN

Dr. Richard Nap received his DVM from Utrecht University (NL) in 1979. After graduation he worked in both small and large animal practice (2 yrs), at Utrecht University (13 yrs) and in a corporate environment (11 yrs). Since 2005, Dr. Nap has owned an independent private consulting firm, Uppertunity Consultants. He is also co-owner of Vetstart International Ltd. His special areas of interest are Clinical Nutrition, Orthopedic Medicine & Surgery, Practice Management, and international student programs.

Dr. Nap is a Diplomate of the European Colleges of Veterinary Surgery (ECVS) and of Veterinary and Comparative Nutrition (ECVCN). As consultant he supports international companies around the world. Dr. Nap has a passion for supporting veterinary students around the world by providing support during the transition from student to practitioner.

Dr. Nap is the chairman of the international specialist group on hip dysplasia that advises the scientific committee of the FCI (international kennel club) on the hip dysplasia screening protocol. He is also a member of AO-Vet and ESVOT.

Phil Roudebush DVM, DACVIM

Dr. Roudebush received his DVM degree from Purdue University in 1975. After two years in a private small animal practice in Denver, he completed a medical residency at the University of Missouri.

Dr. Roudebush remained at the University of Missouri for two years as a faculty member before joining the College of Veterinary Medicine at Mississippi State University. He was a faculty member at Mississippi State for eight years before joining **Mark MMI** in 1989. While at Mississippi State, he served as Chairman, Department of Clinical Sciences, for three years and received three college or university awards for teaching excellence. He is currently a **Director of Scientific Affairs at Hills Pet Nutrition, Inc.**

Dr. Roudebush is a Diplomate of the American College of Veterinary Internal Medicine. His major professional interests are clinical nutrition, veterinary education, cardiopulmonary disease, and dermatology. He is an adjunct professor at Kansas State University and a **Mark Morris Institute Fellow.**

Meri Stratton-Phelps DVM, MPVM, DACVIM (LA), DACVN
Dr. Stratton-Phelps graduated from the University of California, Davis with her DVM in 1996, and completed her MPVM degree in 1999. After working as an intern at San Luis Rey Equine Hospital, Dr. Stratton-Phelps returned to U.C. Davis for an equine emphasis large animal medicine residency. She proceeded to complete a nutrition residency and PhD at U.C. Davis. Her research interests include the dietary management of small ruminant urolithiasis, equine enteral nutrition, and the effect of dietary management on the microbial profile of the equine gastrointestinal tract.

Dr. Stratton-Phelps was a Clinical Assistant Professor in the Department of Large Animal Medicine at the University of Georgia from 2005-2006, and remains an adjunct professor in the Department. In 2004 she started a clinical nutrition consulting business, and currently works full time as a multi-species clinical nutritionist. She is a **Mark Morris Institute Fellow.**

Dr. Phil Toll DVM, MS

Dr. Toll received his DVM degree from Kansas State University in 1986. He spent two years in private practice working with large animals and racing greyhounds.

Dr. Toll returned to Kansas State University and completed an M.S. in physiology in 1990. He remained in the Department of Anatomy and Physiology for another year as a research associate before joining **Hill's Pet Nutrition in 1991. He is currently an Associate Medical Director.**

Dr. Toll's major professional interests are exercise physiology, metabolism, acid-base balance, and clinical nutrition. He is an adjunct assistant professor at Kansas State University, past president of the American Canine Sports Medicine Association, and a **Mark Morris Institute Fellow.**

Todd Towell DVM, MS, DACVIM

Dr. Todd Towell received her veterinary degree in 1990 from the Virginia-Maryland Regional College of Veterinary Medicine. She completed an internship in small animal medicine and surgery at North Carolina State University in 1991 and a residency in small animal medicine at the Virginia-Maryland in 1994. Dr. Towell also received a Masters degree in Veterinary Medical Science from Virginia Maryland in 1994.

Dr. Towell practiced as in internist in both referral specialty and general practices for 5 years. In 1999, Dr. Towell became a clinical trial coordinator for Heska Corporation. She joined **Hill's Pet Nutrition, Inc. in 2002 as a Veterinary Affairs Manager and is currently a Scientific Spokesperson.**

Dr. Towell is a diplomate of the American College of Veterinary Internal Medicine. In 1996, she received the Jersey Shore Veterinary Medical Association's Veterinarian of the Year Award and received the Colorado Veterinary Medical Association's Up and Coming Veterinarian Award in 2000. In 2005, Dr. Towell served as President of the CVMA.

Dr. Steve Zicker DVM, PhD, DACVIM, DACVN

Dr. Zicker received his M.S. in biochemistry from the University of Wisconsin-Madison in 1982, his DVM degree from the University of California-Davis in 1986, and his Ph.D. in Nutrition from the University of California-Davis in 1993.

Dr. Zicker also served an internship in medicine and surgery at Texas A&M University and a residency in medicine at the University of California-Davis.

Following his graduate education, Dr. Zicker spent one year as a lecturer and postgraduate researcher at the University of California-Davis and 18 months in private practice in Colorado Springs, Colorado. He joined Hill's Pet Nutrition in 1996. He is currently a Principal Nutrition Scientist in the Department of Advanced Research at the Hill's Pet Nutrition Center. In 2007, Dr Zicker received a Fulbright award to teach Veterinary Medicine in Ethiopia.

Dr. Zicker is a Diplomate of the American College of Veterinary Internal Medicine and the American College of Veterinary Nutrition. His major professional interests are protein and amino acid nutrition, neonatal nutrition, nutrition and behavior interactions, and general comparative nutrition. He is a Mark Morris Institute Fellow.

This who's-who list of credentialed, veterinary nutritional professionals [redacted] many are university faculty or consultants, that so many have Diplomate status in professional associations, that so many have held office in professional associations—is breathtaking.

Surely, the close, financial relationships of university faculty with commercial interests deserves more public and legislative scrutiny. Given the extent of interlocking university-professional-commercial entities, an outside investigation is essential. No veterinary group could begin to conduct an independent inquiry, because too many leading members are involved in the corruption.

Before doing this research, I would not have believed that veterinary medicine was so [redacted] pet food interests. Now, there can be no doubt.

Thursday, June 10, 2010

Why is there no outrage or adjudication of veterinary corruption? In the last post, I documented the use of pet food dollars to hire credentialed professionals to teach veterinary students Commercial Pet Food 101, rather than an unbiased course on the evolution of pet species and natural diets of carnivorous pets. These same professionals hold offices in veterinary associations, hold faculty positions at veterinary schools, and populate regulatory commissions dealing with pet foods.

In sum, pet-food dollars buy biased instruction in veterinary schools, favorable treatment in professional associations, and toothless pet food regulations. The scope of pet-food corruption in veterinary medicine is breath-taking. Pet-food companies completely control those aspects of veterinary medicine that concern them—pet nutrition, internal medicine, and research on diseases associated with bad diets.

Pet-food money is not seen as tainted, of course, because veterinary authorities are on the take. Pet-food endowed chairs in university departments seem legitimate, until one looks at the control pet-food companies retain over the selection and activities of the chair-holder. Endowed buildings and research programs look legitimate until one sees that the scope of activities is defined by pet-food donors. There's no free lunch in pet-food/veterinary relations—although pet-food companies do often sponsor 'free' luncheons and dinners for their hired hands.

Veterinary schools and professional associations thank their pet-food donors for their generous support, which sums to tens of millions of dollars per year. Pet-food companies reap billions of dollars in profits from the veterinary endorsements they purchased for about ten-cents-on-the-dollar.

Why is there no outrage about pet-food companies' control of pet nutrition and associated health issues in veterinary medicine? In recent correspondence, Australian Tom Lonsdale, DVM likened corruption in veterinary medicine to crooked police:

> Currently there's a TV program on here about the Wood Royal Commission. Basically all the cops were corrupt and engaged in massive scams, rape, murder and etc. The Commissioners got a corrupt detective to roll over and film his colleagues in corrupt activity.
>
> It would be good if we found either a champion or [redacted] in the system who would help this along.

There are [redacted] quite openly on the payroll of pet-food interests, paid to promote commercial pet foods, while holding office in professional associations and faculty positions at universities. For US examples please see the last blog post.

Why authorities don't see this cozy arrangement as conflict of interest, at the least, or bribery is baffling. How can a faculty member at a veterinary school be permitted take payments from a pet-food company or pet-food front to teach pet nutrition to veterinary students?

The ongoing scandal in medical schools is faculty members at leading universities taking large fees from pharmaceutical companies to promote off-label use of drugs in their lectures and appearances. That's shocking and undermines public trust in physicians. Authorities—professional and legal—are looking into the matter.

We can identify plenty [redacted] and authorities seem not to care.

Here's why: Commercial pet food is the unchallenged right-way to feed pets, so no-one sees the harm in allowing pet-food companies to pay faculty, support research, and provide income to vets in practice. It's not corruption or biased instruction, until other theories/concepts of pet nutrition are seen as valid options.

Thus, we need, first, to define pet-food payments to veterinary faculty as corruption, because there are valid pet-feeding options that are omitted from their biased courses. Second, we need to persuade the public and authorities to accept this definition of corruption. Otherwise, no-one is outraged, except those of us who believe that small animal nutrition ought not to be taught as Commercial Pet Food 101.

Imagine if the only 'vegetable' served in school lunch programs was ketchup. (Ronald Regan once agreed that ketchup could be considered a vegetable in school lunches.) Suppose that Heinz and Del Monte, the largest ketchup manufacturers, funded instruction for school nutrition programs, endowed chairs and buildings in human nutrition programs, and hired a cadre of nutritionists to promote ketchup as the only vegetable children need for a complete and balanced diet (sound familiar?).

If ketchup companies spread enough dollars and bought enough expertise, they probably could have ketchup enshrined as the only vegetable in school lunch programs. Anyone who suggested kids need green and yellow vegetables and unprocessed tomatoes would be confronted by research showing ketchup has sufficient nutrients (ah, the key word) to replace all other vegetables. Ketchup would flow through the nation's school lunch rooms, while ketchup dollars bought all the professional support they need. All it takes is money.

Why is no-one within the veterinary medical establishment publicly blowing the whistle on commercial pet-food corruption? There are dissident voices, but they remain largely anonymous, for fear of professional reprisals. At the very least they would be excluded from honors and offices in professional associations and could lose their livelihood. An inquiry into pet-food corruption must come from outside, because virtually no-one inside the veterinary establishment has clean hands. They are all on the take in one manner or another.

Motivation for reform is lacking within grassroots veterinary medicine, for economically understandable reasons. Vet students are taught Commercial Pet-Food 101. After graduation, they establish pet practices in which sales of junk pet foods contribute up to 40% of their incomes.

Even better, commercial pet foods create periodontal problems that require expensive veterinary treatment and chronic diseases that generate lots of income for vets. Laboratory tests, according to Idexx—the leading veterinary laboratory—are the most profitable revenue stream in veterinary practice. Chronically-ill pets require lots of lab tests. Prescription drugs, dispensed by vets, are marked up by hundreds of percents, generating enormous profits. Chronically ill pets require lots of medications.

Commercial pet foods are the gift that keeps giving. By undermining pets' health, kibbles and canned mush not only generate profits from their sales but their exclusive use as pet diets creates patients that need extensive and expensive veterinary treatments. Why would veterinarians voluntarily surrender such a gift?

...

Owners of sick pets are wising up to the junk pet-food–illness connection. Against veterinary advice, many are switching pets to raw diets and marvelling at the pet's improved health. Even if the sick pet dies, they vow never to feed junk foods to the next pet. By promoting junk pet foods, veterinarians are losing credibility in pet owners' minds.

When the public recognizes the stranglehold pet-food companies have on small animal veterinary medicine, there will be reform. Pet owners are the most likely force to push authorities to inquire into pet-food funding and control of veterinary medicine and to demand change. Disseminating information on appropriate diets for carnivorous pets is beginning to change the world.

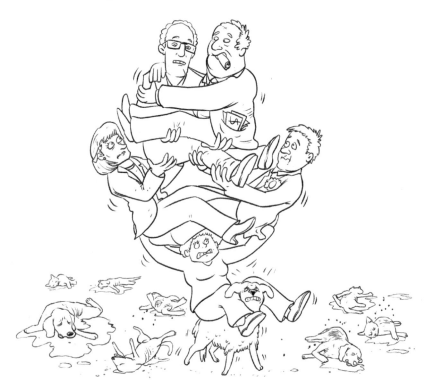

APPENDIX F

Correspondence with NSW Minister of Agriculture, all Members of the NSW Parliament and copied to NSW Veterinary Practitioners Board regarding correspondence with Sydney Small Animal Specialist Hospital (SASH)

Email A: 30 May 2021
To: ElectorateOffice NorthernTablelands <ElectorateOffice.NorthernTablelands@parliament.nsw.gov.au>
Subject: Junk pet-food scandal

Dear Minister,

Please see Small Animal Specialist Hospital (SASH)[1] correspondence below, supporting videos and books concerning the devastating effects of the junk pet-food/vet 'partnership'.

It's a multi-level governmental failure with the Australian Veterinary Association (AVA) controlled NSW Vet Board[2] at the core. (Note: AVA Platinum sponsors Colgate (Hill's) and gold sponsors Mars (Royal Canin[3]).)

Please investigate and reassert parliamentary control.
Thank you for your consideration.

Yours faithfully,
Tom Lonsdale (veterinarian)

PO Box 6096
Windsor DC NSW 2756
Mob: 0437 292 800
Email: tom@rawmeatybones.com
Web: www.rawmeatybones.com

Email B: 31 May 2021
ElectorateOffice NorthernTablelands wrote:
Your email has been redirected to the Ministerial office.

Email C: 5 August 2021
To: ElectorateOffice NorthernTablelands
<ElectorateOffice.NorthernTablelands@parliament.nsw.gov.au>
Cc: ElectorateOffice Monaro
<ElectorateOffice.Monaro@parliament.nsw.gov.au>;
Barnaby.Joyce.MP@aph.gov.au
Subject: Re: FW: Junk pet-food scandal

Dear Electorate Office,

Thank you for directing my 30 May enquiry to the Ministerial Office.

Several NSW State Ministers and MPs have confirmed that they have referred the matter to Minister Marshall.

Please indicate when a reply will be forthcoming.

Thanking you in advance.

Best wishes,
Tom Lonsdale

[No reply has been received either from Minister Marshall or the NSW Veterinary Practitioners Board.]

Correspondence with Small Animal Specialist Hospital (SASH), Sydney

Email 1: 25 March 2021

To: thopkins@sashvets.com
From: Tom Lonsdale <tom@rawmeatybones.com>
Subject: Feedback?
Cc: Clinic <clinic@bpphc.com>, Mei Yam <dr.mei@bpphc.com>

Hi Tim,
Following up after your fact-finding visit.
How are you?
I hope you've had chance to look at the reading material.
Mei Yam the new owner of the practice and I were discussing your visit and the need for dialogue.
Do you have any comments from you personally or from SASH?

Best wishes,
Tom

Email 2: 1 April 2021

To: thopkins@sashvets.com
From: Tom Lonsdale <tom@rawmeatybones.com>
Subject: Reminder
Cc: Clinic <clinic@bpphc.com>, Mei Yam <dr.mei@bpphc.com>

Hi Tim,

Sending this again in case you missed it.
Looking forward to your comments.

Happy Easter,
Tom

Email 3: 10 May 2021

From: Tom Lonsdale <tom@rawmeatybones.com >
To: Tim Hopkins <thopkins@sashvets.com>; Info <info@sashvets.com>
Cc: Mei Yam <dr.mei@bpphc.com>; Clinic <clinic@bpphc.com>; jbaguley@vpb.nsw.gov.au <jbaguley@vpb.nsw.gov.au >; admin@vpb.nsw.gov.au <admin@vpb.nsw.gov.au>
Subject: Fwd: Reminder

Hi Tim,

After leaving messages with your switch board and now a third email, I still await your response.

You may remember that on 17 February 2021 you visited the Bligh Park Pet Health Centre on a fact finding and diplomatic mission. Head nurse Sandra Sultana and I commented on the SASH conduct in respect to the endorsement and promotion of junk pet food, animal welfare and over-servicing issues. You viewed the video Feline gingivostomatitis[4] and took away some written material and copies of the two books attached.

You assured me that you would talk with SASH management and get back to me.

Naturally the issues raised cannot simply be ignored. By any objective measure, they need to be elevated to the appropriate level and pursued to a conclusion.

I have copied this email to the NSW Board of Veterinary Surgeons so that they may be informed that an attempt is being made to help resolve perceptions.

I look forward to hearing from you soon.

Best wishes,
Tom

Email 4: 11 May 2021
Tim Hopkins <thopkins@sashvets.com> wrote:

Hi Tom,

Thanks for your email and apologies for the lateness of my reply.

Following our discussion at Bligh Park Pet Health Centre I met with members of our Internal Medicine team, who I believe are best placed to comment on the issues you raised. We had a good discussion at that point but I have been remiss in following up with them to give you a proper response.

I will do so this week and get back to you by COB Friday.

Best wishes,
Tim

Email 5: 14 May 2021
Timothy Hopkins wrote:

Hi Tom,

Thanks for bearing with me on this one.

As you say below, you have raised issues that require a conclusion. While I don't see this email as conclusive, I hope it will help to explain our current position on these issues.

Having spoken with several members of the Internal Medicine team, we agree that we do not have suitably qualified staff members to comment on these issues. In the past, where clients or clinicians have broached similar issues, we have consulted with animal nutritionists from various entities, including but not limited to, Massey University and private nutritionists such as the Vet Nutrition Group and dentistry vets such as Sydney Pet Dentistry. As a specialist referral centre, we believe it is our duty to outsource these questions in the absence of specific nutrition or dentistry qualified staff members.

Given our approach, we feel that your concerns are best addressed by these entities, who are external to SASH. Naturally, we would be interested to hear the outcome of such discussions and would change our practices accordingly.

With best wishes,
Tim

Timothy Hopkins
Veterinary Relationship Manager
BVSc(Hons I) MSc MRCVS N8553
www.sashvets.com
T: (02) 9002 7290

Email 6: 30 May 2021
To: Timothy Hopkins <thopkins@sashvets.com>, info@sashvets.com
From: Tom Lonsdale <tom@rawmeatybones.com>
Subject: RE: Reminder
Cc: jbaguley@vpb.nsw.gov.au, admin@vpb.nsw.gov.au

Hi Tim,

Thanks for your 14 May 2021 reply which, as you say, does not reach a conclusion.

Your current position, as you seek to portray it, is in my opinion unsatisfactory. I believe that you need to either defend your conduct with robust evidence or admit error and demonstrate a willingness to change. Pretending it's someone else's problem is, I believe, untenable.

At your visit on 17 February 2021 you noted the evidence that the junk pet-food industry, in cahoots with the veterinary profession, is engaged in the mass poisoning* of animals. You indicated that you would seek the advice of the SASH team and return for further discussions.

This is an important public issue for all vets: feeding pets the wrong foods injures their health and in my view amounts to cruelty to animals (a criminal offence).

Further, failing to alert pet owners to the consequences of harmful diets and then proceeding to provide elaborate and costly treatments, should be viewed as over-servicing, and should be viewed as representing a further level of fraud.

My concerns therefore include that any diagnosis and treatment of animals that fails to address diet is deeply unsatisfactory, and that it is also a cause for alarm for any veterinary practice (including SASH) to conduct lectures and webinars 'in partnership' with Mars Inc.[5] (see first 7 mins) and Colgate-Palmolive—notable makers of harmful junk pet food.

So that there can be no misunderstanding about the subjects under discussion I reattach the two books and refer you to the following videos:

Nestlé Assault on Pets Part 1[6] (3.58)
Nestlé Assault on Pets Part 2[7] (4.00)
Main Coon cats[8] (7.16) This video shows a 12 year old cat rescued from the ravages of junk pet food, vet incompetence and over-servicing. The owner's submission to the Senate Inquiry into the Safety of Pet Food is here.[9]

Stop the Mass Poisoning of Pets by Vets[10] (17.53) Eight year old dog undergoing total mouth extraction. Dog previously fed junk product 'My Dog' made by SASH 'nutrition partner' Mars Inc.[11]

Avenging Kitty[12] (6.24)

Feline gingivostomatitis: Nature's best medicine—raw meaty bones —to the rescue.[4] (15.16) SASH report reveals that 6 month old kitten 'was examined by several specialists' leading to no effective treatment, no preventative strategy and $5,600 bill. See owner's submission to Senate Inquiry into the Safety of Pet Food here[13] [Appendix C].

I am copying this email to decision makers and other interested parties, all of whom should have an interest in these important matters of public concern.

Please get back to me at the earliest so that we can move towards a resolution of significant problems.

Best wishes,
Tom

CC: Decision makers and interested parties
* poisons impair health and/or bring about premature death

[No further reply has been received either from SASH or the NSW Veterinary Practitioners Board.]

APPENDIX G

Correspondence with Colin Harvey, BVSc, FRCVS, DipACS, AVDC, EVDC
Professor Emeritus of Surgery and Dentistry
School of Veterinary Medicine, University of Pennsylvania

-----Original Message-----
From: Tom Lonsdale <tom@rawmeatybones.com>
Sent: Thursday, November 11, 2021 10:29 PM
To: Colin@ColinHarvey.info; Colin Comcast <colin.harvey@comcast.net>
Subject: Hello again

Hi Colin,

How have you been these past decades? How is life treating you?

Maybe extraordinary, but I think of you often and very much miss our chats.

I hope I'm not being overly melodramatic when I say our divergent paths is one of my greatest regrets. I believe we had a meeting of the minds—that was and is, for me, very rare and very sad to let it go.

These days age has caught up with me. I'm 72, a bit younger than you, I think.

As a last hurrah, I'm writing a third book—part autobiography, part text book and very much a criticism of the junk pet food/vet/fake animal welfare alliance.

Of course, you feature in the book and I'm struggling with how to describe your involvement. On the one hand I very much appreciated your 1993 help and indeed friendship. On the other hand, I choked on your decision to stay within the confines of the vet establishment.

Is there a third dimension of the aging Colin?

You did say that: 'Our different styles and directions for pursuing this issue will, one day I am sure, be seen to be complimentary rather than at odds.'

Where does the truth lie?

Here's hoping this finds you well and enjoying life.

Best wishes for Christmas and the New Year,

Tom

At 12:24 AM 13/11/2021, colin.harvey@comcast.net wrote:
Hi Tom:

Interesting to read your note.

I am 77. I retired from the University of Pennsylvania in 2013. Since then, I continued as Director of the Veterinary Oral Health Council (www.VOHC.org) until 2019, and still participate as a consultant in some periodontal research projects.

Ours has been an interesting relationship, and the dichotomy mentioned in your note is pretty accurate. There is much that we agree on (some commercial pet foods, particularly canned food, are a contributing cause to development of periodontal disease), but you go rather further than I do in considering the significance of commercial foods. Where you see it as a somewhat black and white issue, I see is as much more nuanced. I have not come out as a vocal supporter of your point of view for several reasons.

1. Feeding a raw food diet is not a convenient option for most dog or cat owners, because of the mess that such a diet may cause in the house (most North American owners are not interested in having to feed their pets outside, and many do not have an outside space that can be used to feed the pet anyway), and because the prolonged shelf-life of commercial foods does not result in smell or take up refrigerator space. Like it or not, modern dog and cat owners want something that fits their life-style, and commercial pet foods fill that need.

2. The commercial pet food companies have done or supported significant research in the nutritional needs of dogs and cats, and carry that information over to the sourcing and manufacture of commercial foods to ensure that the nutrient profile is optimal. A raw food diet is not optimal from a nutritional profile perspective, and pet owners are largely not interested in having to figure out how to ensure that the micronutrients are included, or obtain and feed viscera that would meet that need.

3. There are ways to off-set the plaque and calculus accumulation on canine and feline teeth that can enhance the pet–owner relationship—in addition to the oral hygiene benefit, feeding chew treats provides a positive opportunity for owner and pet to enjoy some time together.

I don't know if this will help you in figuring out how to handle mention of me and my point of view in your book, but it is the best I can do.

Colin

From: Tom Lonsdale <tom@rawmeatybones.com>
Sent: Sunday, November 14, 2021 1:28 AM
To: Colin.harvey@comcast.net
Subject: RE: Hello again

Hi Colin,

Delighted to hear from you—though I fear our views are now more polarised.

Thanks for providing suggested reasons for supporting the feeding of artificial 'foods' and the use of artificial teeth cleaning aids. Seems to me your three categories are heavy on commercial marketing aspects and light on the veterinary and health imperatives.

Are you aware of how harmful the dry junk is from the time it's ingested? A recent video has my clients sworn off the junk[1] the moment they watch it.

In the new book I'll speak about the Australian Parliamentary Inquiry into the Safety of Pet Foods[2] and in particular the following links.

Melanie Christie [Appendix A] wrote about her experiences with the health of her dogs. Tafline Gillespie illustrated her submission [Appendix B]. Her father David Gillespie filmed me removing all 42 teeth of a junk food fed eight year old Maltese terrier.[3]

J Vale wrote about her cat [Appendix C] Jiminy and we also made a video.[4] George the diabetic cat's story is here[5] [Chap. 4, p 72] and subsequent video here.[6]

Notice how Australian pet owners do not share your concerns. It's the same for USA pet owners that make contact with me. They've lived the unpleasant experience arising from junk 'foods' and junk teeth cleaning aids. They've made the comparison with *nature's food and medicine*—raw meaty bones—and can confirm that junk 'foods' and junk cleaning aids are neither suitable nor safe for their intended purpose. Has the University of Pennsylvania and the Veterinary Oral Health Council or any other institution made similar comparisons?

What were the findings? Please let me know and I'll endeavour to include the findings in the book.

I seem to recall that your 1993 plans for a longitudinal study comparing processed diets with a more natural raw meaty bones-based diet was not supported. Can you reveal the reasons and what's happened in the 28 years since?

With your consent I'll publish our discussions for public consumption leading, I hope, to a more enlightened populace and healthier pets.

Have fun, best wishes,
Tom

At 04:14 AM 15/11/2021, colin.harvey@comcast.net wrote:

Hi Tom:

The project that I was seeking financial support for in 1993 would have been a life-long study starting with litters of dogs at the time of weaning (similar to the life-long study conducted by Ralston-Purina reported a decade or so ago in which litters of puppies were randomly separated at weaning into two groups; one group was allowed ad-lib access to a commercial dry food diet every day, the other group was allowed daily access to only 75% of the amount of food consumed by the ad-lib group). The limited food group live longer and had fewer orthopedic and arthritic problems than the ad-lib group.

In my proposed study, there would be several groups:

1) Fed a commercial canned food diet.
2) Fed a commercial dry food kibble diet.
3) Fed a dry food kibble diet and offered a dental chew every day.
4) Fed a 'raw food diet'.
5) Ideally a fifth group fed a dry food diet and whose teeth would be brushed every day.

This would have been a very expensive study because of the life-long duration keeping the dogs in a very controlled environment to ensure that the dietary limitations and tooth brushing were followed, and the need for periodic dental scoring under sedation and CBC/chemscreen testing periodically.

I was not really surprised by my inability to obtain funding because of the expense (far higher than the typical veterinary research foundation maximum grant) and because the hypothesis was that there would be a difference in longevity between groups, as a result of development of distant organ conditions such as renal and hepatic diseases in one or more groups—the major pet-food companies, which would be the obvious potential source of funding for a project such as this study, would likely not participate because the result would be that the study would cause significant distant organ diseases and reduced life-span, and they are unwilling to support any study that results in harm to any of their research colony dogs.

I am aware that there does seem to at least a perception of a cultural difference between Australian dog owners, who may be more likely to house and feed their dogs outside, and US dog owners who are less likely to house and fed their dogs outside.

The 1993 project you mentioned pre-dated the availability of 'dental diets' and development work that has resulted in increased efficacy of dental treats. The study should include a group fed a dental diet only (the latter already included as group 3).

You are welcome to include my points of view in your book provided that I am allowed to read and revise if necessary, any comments ascribed to me.

Colin

On November 13, 2021, Tom Lonsdale wrote
Subject: RE: Hello again

Hi Colin,

Not surprisingly lots has changed these 28 years past.

I applaud the increased scope of your proposed project. No matter the cost, the junk pet-food companies ought to have done the work and published the results themselves. They claim their products are suitable and safe—the best available, they say. The onus of proof is on them. Making them accountable is the problem.

Back in 1993 your draft project[7] focused on the: 'Effect of the Form of the Diet on the Development of Periodontal Disease in the Dog—A Long-Term Clinical Trial'.

Purpose: To compare the effects in dogs of food presented in three forms over a long period. Specific questions to be addressed:

1) Can a 'natural diet' keep the mouth healthy (absence of periodontal inflammation)?
2) Is dry food really more effective than canned food in preventing accumulation of plaque and calculus?
3) Is there a difference between processed foods (dry or canned materials) and the 'natural' diet?

At our clinic we found that it takes little time or money to demonstrate early adverse effects of junk 'food'. We took four raw meaty bones fed dogs with healthy mouths and switched them to a diet of Hill's Science Death. Within a week the accumulation of tartar was easily seen in the video we made.[8] We felt bad about harming our pets but, in the interests of scientific progress, I think they would have understood the need for short term pain in the interests of long-term gain.

How about you doing a simple little study over a few months? Does the University of Pennsylvania still feed its research dogs Hill's products? You could offer to feed some of the dogs raw meaty bones and chart the difference.

Back in 1993 you cited[1] my Preventative Dentistry [Appendix D] chapter in support of your Clinical Trial proposal. Are Pennsylvania vet students made aware of the preventative and therapeutic benefits of Nature's remedy—raw meaty bones—or are they taught to put their faith in industrial products and tooth brushing?

Your points of view appreciated and of course will only be quoted accurately and in context.

Best wishes,
Tom

ENDNOTES

Chapter 1

Some background, some context

1. Adam Smith, *The wealth of nations*, Penguin, 1999 (1776).
2. Larry Vogelnest, Taronga Zoo vet, speaking on *The Investigators*, ABC, 1993. http://www.rawmeatybones.com/pdf/ABC_The_Investigators.pdf
3. Rachel Carson, *Silent spring*, Penguin, 2001 (1962).
4. Margaret Thatcher, Speech at 2nd World Climate Conference, 1990. https://www.margaretthatcher.org/document/108237

Chapter 2

Eruption of dissent

1. Tom Lonsdale, 'Oral disease in cats and dogs', *Control & Therapy*, no. 3128, Post Graduate Committee in Veterinary Science, University of Sydney, December 1991.
2. Breck Muir, 'Canned pet food not the healthiest', *Australian Veterinary Association News*, December 1991, p. 28.
3. John Wingate, 'Far fetched claims', *Australian Veterinary Association News*, December 1991, p. 28.
4. Duncan Hall, 'Canine dental decay—many causes', *Australian Veterinary Association News*, March 1992, p. 24.
5. *Australian Veterinary Association News*, March 1993, p. 23.
6. The full text is in Appendix D.
7. This may be a version of Honoré de Balzac's line 'The secret of a great success for which you are at a loss to account is a crime that has never been found out, because it was properly executed', from a serialization of *Le Père Goriot* published in *Revue de Paris* in 1834. (Honoré de Balzac, 'Old Goriot', trans. Ellen Marriage, J. M. Dent & Co., 1896, p. 124.)
8. 'Dogs—food for, and rational treatment of', Agriculturist's Notebook no. 12, *Quarterly Journal of Agriculture*, vol. 11, 1841, pp. 239–45. Available from Google Books.
9. 'Spratt's', *Wikipedia*, accessed 15 March 2022. https://en.wikipedia.org/wiki/Spratt%27s
10. *Rockford: the pet food story, 1923–1987*, Rockford Pet Foods Division, Quaker Oats Company, 1987. Available from Google Books. See also https://history.rockfordpubliclibrary.org/localhistory/?p=36608
11. Tim Philips, 'Learn from the past'. https://www.petfoodindustry.com/articles/401-learn-from-the-past
12. Robin Kaiser-Schatzlein, 'This is how America's richest families stay that way', *New York Times*, 24 September 2021. https://www.nytimes.com/2021/09/24/opinion/biden-tax-loophole.html

13. Jan Pottker, 'From the archives: sweet secrets: opening doors on the very private lives of the billionaire Mars family', *Washingtonian*, 29 April 2008. https://www.washingtonian.com/2008/04/29/from-the-archives-sweet-secrets-opening-doors-on-the-very-private-lives-of-the-billionaire-mars-fami/
14. 'Purina international sites', Purina, accessed 5 May 2022. https://www.purina.com/international-sites
15. Tim Phillips, '8 episodes offer insights for the future', *Learn from the past*, Pet Food Industry, 24 October 2007. https://www.petfoodindustry.com/articles/401-learn-from-the-past

Chapter 3

Food and medicine

1. FDA Consumer Health Information, *No bones about it: bones are unsafe for your dog*, US Food and Drug Administration, April 2010. (Later advice can be seen at https://www.fda.gov/consumers/consumer-updates/no-bones-or-bone-treats-about-it-reasons-not-give-your-dog-bones.)
2. 'BluePearl, Banfield now part of same company', American Veterinary Medical Association, 17 November 2015. https://www.avma.org/javma-news/2015-12-01/bluepearl-banfield-now-part-same-company
3. 'Mars Petcare marks strategic entry into European veterinary care sector as Anicura to join the business', media release, Mars Petcare, 11 June 2018. https://www.mars.com/news-and-stories/press-releases/mars-petcare-strategic-entry-european-veterinary-care-sector
4. Jasdip Sensi, 'Linnaeus expands amid continued investment', *Pet Gazette*, 10 August 2020. https://www.petgazette.biz/27696-linnaeus-expands-amid-continued-investment/
5. Patrick Hatch, 'Vet and pet store giant Greencross set for private equity takeover', *Sydney Morning Herald*, 5 November 2018. https://www.smh.com.au/business/companies/vet-and-pet-store-giant-greencross-set-for-private-equity-takeover-20181105-p50e2j.html
6. Tom Lonsdale, 'Pandemic of periodontal disease: a malodorous condition', presentation to Sydney Metropolitan Practitioners Branch, Australian Veterinary Association, August 1992. http://rawmeatybones.com/pdf/popdamc.pdf
7. Tom Lonsdale, 'Raw meaty bones essentials', *Control & Therapy Series*, no. 291, Centre for Veterinary Education, University of Sydney, June 2018.
8. 'Small animal nutrition TimeOnline, 20 September – 17 October 2021', notice of online course, Centre for Veterinary Education, University of Sydney, 2021. https://www.cve.edu.au/EventDetail?EventKey=CSTOSAN21
9. Dog Food Commercial for Supercoat with Dr Harry. https://www.youtube.com/watch?v=7SY1MVwVm7o
10. Tom Lonsdale, Nestlé Purina assault on pets part 1. https://www.youtube.com/watch?v=t9JTkQC4lJw&t=8s
11. Tom Lonsdale, Nestlé Purina assault on pets part 2. https://www.youtube.com/watch?v=2fTiIjBEhZo

Chapter 4

Protecting your pets

1. 'Get a dental checkup for your dog', undated poster from 1990s, Upjohn, Animal health Operations, Sydney.
2. 'Major health problems can start with gum disease', wraparound advertising feature, *Veterinary Times*, vol. 32, no. 27, 15 July 2002.
3. Cover of *Time*, 23 February 2004. http://content.time.com/time/covers/0,16641,20040223,00.html
4. Tom Lonsdale, 'Maine Coon cats'. https://youtu.be/0l895uWOEiI
5. Rolf Hauptmann, Submission no. 72 to Regulatory approaches to ensure the safety of pet food, *Parliament of Australia*, 2018. https://www.aph.gov.au/Parliamentary_Business/Committees/Senate/Rural_and_Regional_Affairs_and_Transport/SafetyofPetFood/Submissions
6. Jane Hansen, 'Pet vet bills give paws for thought', *Sunday Telegraph*, 2 September 2012. https://www.dailytelegraph.com.au/pet-vet-bills-give-paws-for-thought/news-story/34cc1b416dd221add8bf3d804c2edd60
7. Tom Lonsdale, 'New scientific thought, persistent vet school madness', *RMB Newsletter*, vol. 4, no. 2, 2004. http://www.rawmeatybones.com/newsletters/archive/4-2%20April%202004%20-%20New%20scientific%20thought,%20persistent%20vet%20school%20madness.pdf

Chapter 5

Prescription for health

1. Blaire Van Valkenburgh, 'Incidence of tooth breakage among large, predatory mammals', *American Naturalist*, vol. 131, no. 2, 1988, pp. 291–302.
2. Yue Ma, Risheka Ratnasabapathy and James Gardiner, 'Carbohydrate craving: not everything is sweet', *Current Opinion in Clinical Nutrition and Metabolic Care*, vol. 20, no. 4, 2017, pp. 261–5.
3. Anthony Mills and Antoni Milewski, 'Geophagy and nutrient supplementation in the Ngorongoro Conservation Area, Tanzania, with particular reference to selenium, cobalt and molybdenum', *Journal of Zoology*, vol. 271, no. 1, 2007, pp. 110–18.
4. Albert-László Barabási, Giulia Menichetti and Joseph Loscalzo, 'The unmapped chemical complexity of our diet', *Nature Food*, vol. 1, 2020, pp. 33–7. https://doi.org/10.1038/s43016-019-0005-1
5. The Royal Canin Weight Management Clinic, Small Animal Teaching Hospital, University of Liverpool, accessed 26 March 2022. https://www.liverpool.ac.uk/sath/services/weight-management/
6. Laura McGuire, 'Hill's Pet Nutrition launches new campaign to tackle pet obesity', *Pet Gazette*, 1 April 2021. https://www.petgazette.biz/194561-hills-pet-nutrition-launches-new-campaign-to-tackle-pet-obesity/?omhide=true&cmid=a378df96-5ddc-4466-bebe-fd5ea55ab969
7. 'Pawfect guests at the House of Commons', *PFMA Archive News*, Pet Food Manufacturers' Association, 9 August 2019. https://www.pfma.org.uk/news/pawfect-guests-at-the-house-of-commons-

Chapter 6

Veterinary schools

1. Patrick K. House, Ajai Vyas and Robert Sapolsky, 'Predator cat odors activate sexual arousal pathways in brains of *Toxoplasma gondii* infected rats', *PLoS One*, vol. 6, no. 8, 2011, e23277. https://doi.org/10.1371/journal.pone.0023277
2. Tim Rettig, 'Cultural innovation: growing beyond the constraints of your cultural conditioning', *Intercultural Mindset*, 21 November 2017. https://medium.com/intercultural-mindset/cultural-innovation-growing-beyond-the-constraints-of-your-cultural-conditioning-c36b0ae193aa
3. Ignaz Semmelweis, 'The etiology, concept, and prophylaxis of childbed fever', in C. Buck, A. Lopis, E. Nájera and Terris, M., eds, *The challenge of epidemiology: issues and selected readings*, Pan American Health Organization, 1988, Table 1, p. 47. (Excerpted from Ignaz Semmelweis, *The etiology, concept, and prophylaxis of childbed fever*, trans. K. Codell Carter, University of Wisconsin Press, 1983.)
4. K. Codell Carter and Barbara R. Carter, *Childbed fever: a scientific biography of Ignaz Semmelweis*, Transaction Publishers, 2005.
5. 'Louis Pasteur', *Historical biographies*, Science History Institute, 14 December 2017. https://www.sciencehistory.org/historical-profile/louis-pasteur
6. Frederick F. Cartwright, 'Joseph Lister: British surgeon and medical scientist', *Britannica*, 6 February 2022. https://www.britannica.com/biography/Joseph-Lister-Baron-Lister-of-Lyme-Regis
7. Stefan Riedel, 'Edward Jenner and the history of smallpox and vaccination', *Baylor University Medical Center Proceedings*, vol. 18, no. 1, 2005, pp. 21–5. https://doi.org/10.1080/08998280.2005.11928028
8. 'Alexander Fleming', *Historical biographies*, Science History Institute, 5 December 2017. https://www.sciencehistory.org/historical-profile/alexander-fleming
9. 'Dr Tom Hungerford', *Our story*, Centre for Veterinary Education, University of Sydney. https://www.cve.edu.au/Web/About/Our_Story.aspx?hkey=1d413213-1cbe-4d73-8d83-a06809acf42e
10. Richard Malik, Nomination of Tom Lonsdale for the College Prize of the Australian College of Veterinary Scientists for 2004. http://rawmeatybones.com/vetsay/malik.pdf Douglas Bryden, Nomination of Dr Tom Lonsdale for the College Prize in 2004. http://rawmeatybones.com/vetsay/Doug%20Bryden%20Nomination.pdf
11. Tom Lonsdale, 'Sefi's ear discharge'. http://www.rawmeatybones.com/pdf/C+T%20cat's%20ear%20IIaa.pdf
12. Tom Lonsdale, Letter of complaint to each member of Senate, July 2010. http://rawmeatybones.com/pdf/SU%20Senate%202010.pdf
13. Rosanne Taylor, Response to complaint, 20 July 2010. http://rawmeatybones.com/pdf/Dean%20Syd%20Vet%20School%20July%2010.pdf
14. Freedom of Information, Junk Pet Food Involvement, Australian Vet Schools. http://rawmeatybones.com/foi.php
15. FOI Enquiries United Kingdom Raw Meaty Bones Support & Action Group. https://www.ukrmb.co.uk/showcontent.toy?contentnid=162360

16. Hill's Pet Nutrition Australia, Multi-Project Funding Program. http://rawmeatybones.com/pdf/3.100A%20Prop%20Hill's%20Revised%202013-15(2)%20(2)_Redacted.pdf
17. Murdoch University College of Veterinary Medicine, Proposal for Partnership Opportunities for Royal Canin. http://rawmeatybones.com/pdf/3.195A%20Prop%20Royal%20Canin%202014eh%20IR1%20(2).pdf
18. Sponsorship agreement between Murdoch University and Hill's Pet Nutrition Pty Ltd. http://rawmeatybones.com/pdf/3.212%20Final%20Signed%20Contract%20Hill's%20Australia%202013_Redacted%20not%20released.pdf
19. Royal Veterinary College voted world's leading vet school. https://www.rvc.ac.uk/news-and-events/rvc-news/royal-veterinary-college-voted-world-s-leading-vet-school
20. Tom Lonsdale, Manifesto for RCVS elections 1998. http://rawmeatybones.com/RCVS/RCVS1998.html
21. Royal Veterinary College correspondence. https://www.ukrmb.co.uk/images/RoyalVetCollFOI.pdf
22. Tom Lonsdale, RCVS election statement 2014. http://rawmeatybones.com/RCVS/RCVS2014.php
23. Tara Parker-Pope, 'Colgate gives doctors treats for plugging its food brands', *Wall Street Journal*, 3 November 1997. https://www.wsj.com/articles/SB878509979865406000
24. Royal Dick School of Veterinary Studies and Pedigree Master Foods, Crown Petfoods and Ralston Purina International (UK) Ltd. https://www.ukrmb.co.uk/images/RoyalDickCorres.pdf
25. Dale Hancock, email to CVM Faculty Distribution List re Public Records Request, Washington State College of Veterinary Medicine, Washington State University, 25 June 2009. http://rawmeatybones.com/pdf/Washington%20State%20CVM.pdf
26. Colin Harvey, 'The relationship between periodontal infection and systemic and distant organ disease in dogs', *Veterinary Clinics of North America: Small Animal Practice*, vol. 52, no. 1, 2022, pp. 121–37. https://doi.org/10.1016/j.cvsm.2021.09.004
27. Tom Lonsdale, 'New scientific thought, persistent vet school madness', *RMB Newsletter*, vol. 4, no. 2, April 2004. http://rawmeatybones.com/newsletters/archive/4-2%20April%202004%20-%20New%20scientific%20thought,%20persistent%20vet%20school%20madness.pdf
28. Tom Lonsdale, 'Pet foods' insidious consequences: a modern veterinary snafu', presentation to staff and students, Faculty of Veterinary Science, Massey University, Palmerston North, New Zealand, 9 September 1993. http://www.rawmeatybones.com/PFIC.html

Chapter 7

White-collar criminal collaboration

1. Lonsdale, 'Self-regulation and self-determination for a better future', AVA election manifesto, 1995. http://www.rawmeatybones.com/AVArevised/election.html
2. Breck Muir and Tom Lonsdale, 'Manifesto of Drs Lonsdale and Muir'; AVA elections, 1998. http://www.rawmeatybones.com/AVArevised/election1998.html
3. Tom Lonsdale, Election manifesto, AVA elections, 2003. http://www.rawmeatybones.com/AVArevised/election2003.html

4. Tom Lonsdale, 'Excuses and falsehoods', AVA election manifesto, 2003. http://www.rawmeatybones.com/pdf/Excuses_and_falsehoods.pdf
5. Paul Lynch, 'Mr Tom Lonsdale and the Australian Veterinary Association', *Legislative Assembly Hansard*, 13 May 2004. https://www.parliament.nsw.gov.au/Hansard/Pages/HansardResult.aspx#/docid/HANSARD-1323879322-83464
6. https://en.wikipedia.org/wiki/Regulatory_capture
7. Barbara Fougere, Letter of complaint, 21 March 1994. http://www.rawmeatybones.com/pdf/Master.pdf
8. 'BluePearl, Banfield now part of same company', *JAVMA News*, American Medical Veterinary Association, 17 November 2015. https://www.avma.org/javma-news/2015-12-01/bluepearl-banfield-now-part-same-company
9. Sonia McGill, 'Canine urolithiasis', Small Animal Specialist Hospital (SASH), Tuggerah, 20 November 2020. https://youtu.be/2kIb0yoxZLQ
10. The Board, Veterinary Practitioners Board of New South Wales. https://www.vpb.nsw.gov.au/board
11. Tom Lonsdale, 'Feline gingivostomatitis: nature's best medicine—raw meaty bones—to the rescue', 17 May 2018. https://www.youtube.com/watch?v=W1H-XTSAr_o
12. Royal College of Veterinary Surgeons, *Supplemental Royal Charter 2015*, 17 February 2015. https://www.rcvs.org.uk/document-library/supplemental-royal-charter-2015/
13. Henry Carter, Fax to Tom Lonsdale commenting on Mars Inc. influence on the veterinary profession, 14 March 1995. http://www.rawmeatybones.com/pdf/Henry%20Carter%201995.pdf
14. Tom Lonsdale, Record of meeting with Professor Richard Halliwell, president of the RCVS, 17 June 2004. http://www.rawmeatybones.com/pdf/Halliwell.pdf
15. *The Provet dental solutions catalogue*, Small animal, Provet, July 2021. https://provet-catalogues-au.partica.online/catalogues/the-provet-dental-solutions-catalogue-june-2021/flipbook/1/
16. 'NEW VeggieDent FR3SH dental chews for dogs', email promotional message, Virbac Australia, 23 July 2021.
17. 'Pet legacies', RSPCA, accessed 29 March 2022. https://www.rspca.org.au/support-us/pet-legacies
18. Heather Sandlin, 'Royal Canin warns of rescue centre struggles post-lockdown', *Pet Gazette*, 14 July 2021. https://www.petgazette.biz/196135-royal-canin-warns-of-rescue-centre-struggles-post-lockdown/
19. L McGuire, 'Mars Petcare launches £1.3m TV campaign', *Pet Gazette*, 21 July 2021. https://www.petgazette.biz/196182-mars-petcare-launches-1-3m-tv-campaign/

Chapter 8

Fallacies in the alternative

1. Ian Billinghurst, 'A more natural diet for your dog', client handout, *Control & Therapy*, no. 2275, Post Graduate Committee in Veterinary Science, University of Sydney, August 1986.
   Richard H. Pitcairn and Susan Hubble Pitcairn, *Dr Pitcairn's Complete Guide to Natural Health for Dogs & Cats*, 4th edn, Rodale Books, 2017.

Juliette de Baïracli Levy, *The Complete Herbal Handbook for the Dog and Cat*, Faber, 2005.

2. Ian Billinghurst, 'Canine nutrition: a point of view', presentation at Nutrition Conference, University of Sydney, 1988.
3. Ian Billinghurst, *Give your dog a bone*, Billinghurst, 1993, p. 126. https://drianbillinghurst.com/product/give-your-dog-a-bone/
4. Billinghurst, *Give your dog a bone*, p. 177.
5. Alan Bennet, Ian Billinghurst, Tom Lonsdale, and Breck Muir (Raw Meaty Bone Lobby of Concerned Veterinarians), 'ABC review', media release, 13 September 1996. http://rawmeatybones.com/ABCReview.html
6. Alan Bennet, Ian Billinghurst, Tom Lonsdale and Breck Muir, (Raw Meaty Bone Lobby of Concerned Veterinarians), 'Pet food front', media release, 5 March 1997. http://rawmeatybones.com/ABCReview.html
7. Ian Billinghurst, Resignation letter, 24 March 1997. http://www.rawmeatybones.com/pdf/Resignation%2024%203%2097%20pdf.pdf
8. BARF Hong Kong. http://www.barf.com.hk/en/index.html
9. Nick Thompson, ukbarfclub discussion forum, March 2003. http://rawmeatybones.com/vetsay/Thompson.pdf
10. Raw Feeding Veterinary Society. https://v2h.924.myftpupload.com/rfvs-position-statement-2021/
11. Lotka–Volterra Model, Science Direct. https://www.sciencedirect.com/topics/earth-and-planetary-sciences/lotka-volterra-model
12. Marty Goldstein. https://drmartypets.com/about/
13. Volhard Dog Nutrition. https://www.volharddognutrition.com/

Chapter 9

The media: good, bad and ugly

1. Robin Kaiser-Schatzlein, 'This is how America's richest families stay that way', *New York Times*, 24 September 2021.
2. Hans Christian Andersen, *The emperor's new clothes* (Danish: *Kejserens nye klæder*), C. A. Reitzel, 1837.
3. Michelle Graham, 'Diet debate opens more than just a can of worms', *Veterinarian*, vol. 1, August 1993. http://www.rawmeatybones.com/pdf/TheVeterinarian_Aug93.PDF
4. Australian Broadcasting Corporation, *The Investigators*, 27 April 1993. https://www.youtube.com/watch?v=o2WfMcvrb7k&t=311s
5. Elizabeth Farrelly, 'Within a whisker of being stigmatised', *Sydney Morning Herald*, 11 July 2013. https://www.smh.com.au/opinion/within-a-whisker-of-being-stigmatised-20130710-2pqc1.html
6. John Swinton, circa 1880. http://www.blatantpropaganda.org/propaganda/articles/journalists-are-intellectual-prostitutes-says-John-Swinton-of-the-New-York-Times.html
7. Katrina Warren, 'Avoiding dental problems', *Reader's Digest Australia*, vol. 201, no. 1194, July 2021, pp. 16–17.
8. Correspondence with the *Veterinarian* and NSW Veterinary Practitioners Board, 2003. http://www.rawmeatybones.com/pdf/Excuses_and_falsehoods.pdf

9. Sotheby's Australia, 'The David Newby collection consigned to Sotheby's Australia', press release, 7 March 2017. https://www.smithandsinger.com.au/files//press/AU0813_ART_David_Newby_Collection_20170503.pdf
10. Stuart Littlemore, *Media Watch* transcript, ABC TV, 3 March 1997. http://rawmeatybones.com/MediaWatch.html
11. Crikey Whistleblower Archive, 'ABC's *Catalyst* ignores whistleblower', *Crikey*, 2003. http://rawmeatybones.com/crikey2.html
12. 'We call out a lack of disclosure by the *Science Show* in its "Climate grief" series on ABC Radio National', *Media Watch*, ABC TV, 1 June 2020. https://www.abc.net.au/mediawatch/episodes/climate/12309158
13. Response from an ABC spokesperson, ABC TV, 1 June 2020. https://www.abc.net.au/cm/lb/12309244/data/abc-response-data.pdf
14. Simon Webster, 'What the experts want you to know about your pet's diet', *Sydney Morning Herald*, 27 May 2021. https://www.smh.com.au/lifestyle/health-and-wellness/what-the-experts-want-you-to-know-about-your-pet-s-diet-20210518-p57sza.html
15. Tom Lonsdale, 'Three-part test', *RMB Newsletter*, vol. 6, no. 5. http://rawmeatybones.com/newsletters/archive/6-5%20Dec%202006%20-%20Three%20Part%20Test.pdf

Chapter 10

Politicians and regulators: let dog food companies lie

1. Miranda Combs, 'Raw pet food: veterinarians warn about trendy diet for dogs and cats', *WKYT Investigates*, 25 April 2019. https://www.wkyt.com/content/news/Raw-Pet-Food-Veterinarians-warn-about-trendy-diet-for-dogs-and-cats-509016631.html
2. Poppy Noor, 'AOC finds her perfect puppy—which other politicians have found theirs?', *Guardian*, 8 January 2020. https://www.theguardian.com/us-news/2020/jan/07/aoc-finds-perfect-puppy-which-other-politicians-found-theirs
3. Shane Goldmacher, 'How Alvin the beagle helped usher in a Democratic senate', *New York Times*, 23 January 2021. https://www.nytimes.com/2021/01/23/us/politics/raphael-warnock-puppy.html
4. 'What are early day motions?', *UK Parliament*. https://www.parliament.uk/about/how/business/edms/
5. 'Processed pet foods and vets', *Early Day Motions*, EDM 335, UK Parliament, tabled on 7 December 2004. https://edm.parliament.uk/early-day-motion/26858
6. 'Raw Meaty Bones group', *Early Day Motions*, EDM 1003, UK Parliament, tabled on 11 November 2005. https://edm.parliament.uk/early-day-motion/29343
7. Paul Lynch, 'Mr Tom Lonsdale and the Australian Veterinary Association', *Legislative Assembly Hansard*, 13 May 2004. https://www.parliament.nsw.gov.au/Hansard/Pages/HansardResult.aspx#/docid/HANSARD-1323879322-83464
8. Kevin Conolly, 'Animal welfare', *Legislative Assembly Hansard*, 14 August 2018. https://www.parliament.nsw.gov.au/Hansard/Pages/HansardResult.aspx#/docid/HANSARD-1323879322-103187/link/56
9. Sterling Griff, 'Senate to inquire into problem-plagued pet food industry', Centre Alliance, 20 June 2018. https://centrealliance.org.au/media/media/senate-to-inquire-into-problem-plagued-pet-food-industry/

10. Regulatory approaches to ensure the safety of pet food, Parliament of Australia, 2018. https://www.aph.gov.au/Parliamentary_Business/Committees/Senate/Rural_and_Regional_Affairs_and_Transport/SafetyofPetFood
11. Regulatory approaches to ensure the safety of pet food, Submissions received by the Committee, Parliament of Australia, 2018. https://www.aph.gov.au/Parliamentary_Business/Committees/Senate/Rural_and_Regional_Affairs_and_Transport/SafetyofPetFood/Submissions
12. Published submissions, 2018. http://www.rawmeatybones.com/pdf/SenateSubs151.pdf
13. Barry O'Sullivan, Address to Public Hearing, Senate Rural and Regional Affairs and Transport Reference Committee, Parliament of Australia, 29 August 2018. https://parlinfo.aph.gov.au/parlInfo/search/search.w3p
14. Sterling Griff, Address to Public Hearing, Senate Rural and Regional Affairs and Transport Reference Committee, Parliament of Australia, 29 August 2018. https://parlinfo.aph.gov.au/parlInfo/search/search.w3p
15. Melanie Christie, Regulatory approaches to ensure the safety of pet food, Submission 62, 2018. https://www.aph.gov.au/DocumentStore.ashx?id=6f637452-9ad9-4469-8083-2defba3de722&subId=613406
16. Regulatory approaches to ensure the safety of pet food, Report, Parliament of Australia, 16 October 2018. https://www.aph.gov.au/Parliamentary_Business/Committees/Senate/Rural_and_Regional_Affairs_and_Transport/SafetyofPetFood/Report
17. Christine Lewis, Regulatory approaches to ensure the safety of pet food, Submission 61, 2018. https://www.aph.gov.au/DocumentStore.ashx?id=bd22a34d-a817-4c52-9ca7-77888b2f2524&subId=613532
18. Tom Lonsdale, Correspondence with officers of the Department of Agriculture commencing 5 November 2019. http://www.rawmeatybones.com/pdf/Petfood_review_emails.pdf
19. David Littleproud, Correspondence on file, 2020.

Chapter 11

The art of war

1. Sun Tzu, *Quotable Quote*. https://www.goodreads.com/quotes/17976-if-you-know-the-enemy-and-know-yourself-you-need
2. The 'wh—' questions echo Rudyard Kipling's version of the journalist's maxim: 'I keep six honest serving-men / (They taught me all I knew); / Their names are What and Why and When / And How and Where and Who', in *Just so stories for little children*, Macmillan, 1902.
3. Australian Veterinary Association, *Veterinary Workforce Survey 2021: analysis report*, December 2021, p. 4. https://www.ava.com.au/siteassets/news/ava-workforce-survey-analysis-2021-final.pdf
   Frédéric Michas, 'Number of veterinarians in the United Kingdom (UK) 2010–2021', *Statista*, 16 December 2021. https://www.statista.com/statistics/318888/numbers-of-veterinarians-in-the-uk/

U.S. Veterinarians 2020, *Reports*, American Veterinary Medical Assocation, updated January 2021. https://www.avma.org/resources-tools/reports-statistics/market-research-statistics-us-veterinarians

4. Tom Lonsdale, RMB Campaign & Elections. http://rawmeatybones.com/elections.php
5. Royal College of Veterinary Surgeons, Code of professional conduct for veterinary surgeons. https://www.rcvs.org.uk/setting-standards/advice-and-guidance/code-of-professional-conduct-for-veterinary-surgeons/#responsibilities
6. American Veterinary Medical Association, Veterinarian's oath. https://www.avma.org/resources-tools/avma-policies/veterinarians-oath
7. Veterinary Practitioners Board of New South Wales, Oath for veterinary graduates in NSW. https://www.vpb.nsw.gov.au/sites/default/files/images/GR03%20Oath%20for%20Veterinary%20Graduates%20in%20NSW.pdf
8. 'Scopes trial', *Wikipedia*, accessed 11 April 2022. https://en.wikipedia.org/wiki/Scopes_Trial
9. Katie Pfaff, 'Fortune Business Insights: pet food market to reach nearly $128B worldwide by 2027', *Veterinary33*, 9 July 2021. https://www.veterinary33.com/action/www.veterinary33.com/veterinary-today/the-veterinary33-debates/74/fortune-business-insights-pet-food-market-to-reach-nearly-128b-worldwide-by-2027.html?mc_cid=9922475ffb&mc_eid=aeb9e9784d/?comment=ok
10. *Pet food market: global industry trends, share, size, growth, opportunity and forecast 2021–2026*, IMARC Group, ID:5330937, May 2021. https://www.imarcgroup.com/pet-food-market/
11. Nils-Gerrit Wunsch, 'Global sales of the Nestlé Group 2005–2021', *Statista*, 16 March 2022. https://www.statista.com/statistics/268892/nestle-groups-global-sales/
12. Jill Krasny, 'Every parent should know the scandalous history of infant formula', *Business Insider Australia*, 26 June 2012. https://www.businessinsider.com.au/nestles-infant-formula-scandal-2012-6?r=US&IR=T
13. Andrew Jacobs and Matt Richtel, 'How big business got Brazil hooked on junk food, *New York Times*, 16 September 2017. https://www.nytimes.com/interactive/2017/09/16/health/brazil-obesity-nestle.html
14. All About Mars. https://www.mars.com/about
15. Robin Kaiser-Schatzlein, 'This is how America's richest families stay that way', *New York Times*, 24 September 2021.
16. Susan Thixton, 'A day to never forget', *Truth about Pet Food*, 16 March 2019. https://truthaboutpetfood.com/a-day-to-never-forget/
17. Jennifer Fiala, 'Hill's aims to settle vitamin D case for $12.5 million', *VIN News Service*, 2 February 2021. https://news.vin.com/default.aspx?pid=210&Id=10055228
18. 'Update: FDA says Hill's failed to follow own procedures', *JAVMA News*, 29 January 2020. https://www.avma.org/javma-news/2020-02-15/update-fda-says-hills-failed-follow-own-procedures
19. 'Racketeer influenced and corrupt organizations (RICO) law', *JUSTIA*, reviewed October 2021. https://www.justia.com/criminal/docs/rico/

20. 'PrimeSafe and Agriculture Victoria statement—pet meat investigation', Agriculture Victoria, 17 August 2021. https://www.primesafe.vic.gov.au/news/primesafe-and-agriculture-victoria-statement-17-august-2021
21. ' "Act now to prevent future tragedy": RSPCA says lack of pet food safety regulation is putting Australian pets at risk', media release, *RSPCA*, 18 August 2021. https://www.rspca.org.au/media-centre/news/2021/%E2%80%98act-now-prevent-future-tragedy%E2%80%99-rspca-says-lack-pet-food-safety-regulation-0
22. Code of Professional Conduct, Australian Veterinary Association. https://www.ava.com.au/about-us/code-of-professional-conduct/
23. 'About us', RSPCA. https://www.rspca.org.au/about-us

Chapter 12

Sparking the revolution

1. 'The next evolution in feline hydration', *Provet Group Marketing Newsletter*, 9 September 2021. https://mailchi.mp/provet/nestle-purina-pro-plan-veterinary-hydracare-10-september-2021?e=c38915290b
2. Tony Johnson, 'The nightmare that is blocked cats', *VetzInsight*, 24 February 2014. https://www.vin.com/vetzinsight/default.aspx?pId=756&id=6133546
3. 'Facts & figures about dog attacks', UPMC Children's Hospital of Pittsburgh. https://www.chp.edu/injury-prevention/safety/home-and-yard/dog-bites/facts-and-figures
4. C. O'Herlihy and T. O'Herlihy, Regulatory approaches to ensure the safety of pet food, Submission 69, 2018. https://www.aph.gov.au/DocumentStore.ashx?id=a90f90d8-3e08-4791-9a86-adcea7fcc11e&subId=613488
5. R.A. Mugford, 'The influence of nutrition on canine behaviour', *Journal of Small Animal Practice*, vol. 28, no. 11, 1987, pp. 1046–55. https://onlinelibrary.wiley.com/doi/10.1111/j.1748-5827.1987.tb01328.x
6. 'Tackling the mental health crisis in the veterinary profession', *Vet Practice*, 16 August 2021. https://vetpracticemag.com.au/tackling-the-mental-health-crisis-in-the-veterinary-industry/
7. Maurizio Pompili, 'Critical appraisal of major depression with suicidal ideation', *Annals of General Psychiatry*, vol. 18, 2019. https://doi.org/10.1186/s12991-019-0232-8
8. L. Myers, 'Predilection to dental calculus formation in a group of dogs: influence of calculus on the sense of smell', paper presented to International Working Dog Breeding Conference, 2003. Reported in *RMB Newsletter*, vol. 4, no. 2. www.rawmeatybones.com
9. Gregory S. Okin, 'Environmental impacts of food consumption by dogs and cats', *PloS One*, vol. 12, no. 8, 2017, e0181301. https://doi.org/10.1371/journal.pone.0181301
10. Dylan Byers, 'How Facebook and Twitter decided to take down Trump's accounts', *News*, NBC Universal, 15 January 2021. https://www.nbcnews.com/tech/tech-news/how-facebook-twitter-decided-take-down-trump-s-accounts-n1254317
11. Latika Bourke, ' "Boiled alive": new footage shows full scale of live exports horror', *Sydney Morning Herald*, 5 May 2018. https://www.smh.com.au/politics/federal/boiled-alive-new-footage-shows-full-scale-of-live-exports-horror-20180503-p4zd9q.html

12. 'Vatican admits Galileo was right', *New Scientist*, no. 1846, 7 November 1992. https://www.newscientist.com/article/mg13618460-600-vatican-admits-galileo-was-right/
13. 'Plate tectonics', Wikipedia, accessed 30 March 2022. https://en.wikipedia.org/wiki/Plate_tectonics
14. Fred C. Kelly, 'A study in human incredulity', *Harper's Magazine*, August 1955, pp. 286–300. Available from: https://www.wright-brothers.org/History_Wing/Aviations_Attic/They_Wouldnt_Believe/They_Wouldnt_Believe_the_Wrights_Had_Flown.htm#top
15. Tara Parker-Pope, 'Colgate gives doctors treats for plugging its food brands', *Wall Street Journal*, 3 November 1977. https://www.wsj.com/articles/SB878509979865406000
16. Frederick Kaufman, 'They eat what we are', *New York Times Magazine*, 2 September 2007. http://rawmeatybones.com/pdf/NYT2007.pdf
17. 'The Kennel Club announce Purina PRO Plan as their new partner in pet nutrition', Kennel Club, 20 February 2018. https://www.thekennelclub.org.uk/media-centre/2018/february/the-kennel-club-announce-purina-pro-plan-as-their-new-partner-in-pet-nutrition/
18. Fred Southwick, 'Opinion: Academia suppresses creativity: by discouraging change, universities are stunting scientific innovation, leadership, and growth. *Scientist*, 9 May 2012. https://www.the-scientist.com/news-opinion/opinion-academia-suppresses-creativity-41016
19. Mark Lawrence, 'Ultraprocessed foods and cardiovascular health: it's not just about the nutrients', *American Journal of Clinical Nutrition*, vol. 113, no. 2, 2021, pp. 257–8. https://doi.org/10.1093/ajcn/nqaa333
20. Marion Nestle, 'Should dogs eat pea and lentil proteins?', *Food Politics*, Marion Nestle blog, 20 November 2019. https://www.foodpolitics.com/2019/11/should-dogs-eat-pea-and-lentil-proteins/
21. George Hajishengallis, Interconnection of periodontal disease and comorbidities: Evidence, mechanisms, and implications, *Periodontology 2000,* vol. 89, no.1, June 2022, pp. 9–18.
22. Anthony R. Pratkanis and Elliot Aronson, *Age of propaganda: the everyday use and abuse of persuasion*, W.H. Freeman & Company, 1992.
23. Colin Harvey, Correspondence, 1993. http://rawmeatybones.com/pdf/Colin%20Harvey%2020-7-93.pdf
24. Tom Lonsdale, 'There's a cuckoo in the nest: a deceptive bird', *Raw meaty bones: promote health* (ch. 12), Rivetco Pty Ltd, 2001, p. 266.
25. Louise Delagran, 'What is spirituality?', *Taking Charge of Your Health & Wellbeing*, Earl E. Bakken Center for Spirituality & Healing, University of Minnesota, no date. https://www.takingcharge.csh.umn.edu/what-spirituality
26. Tom Lonsdale, 'Cybernetic hypothesis of periodontal disease in mammalian carnivores', *Journal of Veterinary Dentistry*, vol. 11, no. 1, 1994, pp. 5–8.
27. Desmond Tutu, 'Truth and Reconciliation Commission, South Africa', *Encyclopedia Britannica*. https://www.britannica.com/topic/Truth-and-Reconciliation-Commission-South-Africa

28. Desmond Tutu, 'Truth and reconciliation', *Greater Good Magazine*, 1 September 2004. https://greatergood.berkeley.edu/article/item/truth_and_reconciliation
29. https://www.youtube.com/channel/UCzZmYoLjxA8bFUepVvHmv_A
30. 'No bones (or bone treats) about it: reasons not to give your dog bones', *Consumer Updates*, US Food and Drug Administration, 21 November 2017. https://www.fda.gov/consumers/consumer-updates/no-bones-or-bone-treats-about-it-reasons-not-give-your-dog-bones
31. Sonia McGill, 'Canine urolithiasis', Small Animal Specialist Hospital (SASH) Tuggerah, 20 November 2020. https://youtu.be/2kIb0yoxZLQ
32. Caroline Mansfield and Lina Maria Martinez Lopez, *Report on regulation and safety of pet food in Australia to the Department of Agriculture and Water resources*, Melbourne Veterinary School, University of Melbourne, 2019. http://rawmeatybones.com/pdf/Pet%20Food%20Health%20and%20Safety%20Report.pdf
33. Caroline Mansfield, 'Save the puppies: contact your MP'. www.aph.gov.au. https://www.youtube.com/watch?v=XwgfVEAHpG0&t=250s

Appendix A

1. James Thomas and Alison McClymont, 'Cat food study leads to ethics overhaul at University of Sydney veterinary faculty', *ABC News*, 24 March 2016. https://www.abc.net.au/news/2016-03-24/cat-food-study-leads-to-ethics-overhaul-at-university/7272488
2. Sarah Whyte and Lesley Robinson, 'Vet industry compromised by influence of pet food and pharmaceutical companies, expert says', *ABC News*, 12 November 2015, updated 22 January 2016. https://www.abc.net.au/news/2015-11-12/vet-profession-compromised-by-commercialisation-of-industry/6936732
3. James Thomas and Alison McClymont, 'Some supermarket cat food brands may cause "severe illness", study finds', *ABC News*, 21 March 2016. https://www.abc.net.au/news/2016-03-21/some-supermarket-cat-food-brands-may-cause-severe-illness-study/7263634
4. RSPCA, 'Pet Food Hills Science Diet', *RSPCA Word for Pets*. https://www.rspcaworldforpets.com.au/categories/Dog-Merchandise/Dog-Food/Pet-Food-Hills-Science-Diet
5. Feline Greenies Dental Treats. https://www.greenies.com.au/
6. Hill's Science Diet, Adult Oral Care Chicken Recipe Cat Food. https://www.hillspet.com.au/cat-food/sd-feline-adult-oral-care-dry
7. Tom Lonsdale, 'Raw meaty bones essentials', *Control & Therapy Series*, no. 291, Centre for Veterinary Education, University of Sydney, June 2018. http://www.rawmeatybones.com
8. http://www.rawmeatybones.com/foi.php
9. 'AS 5812:2017: Manufacturing and marketing of pet food', *Standards Australia*. https://infostore.saiglobal.com/en-au/standards/as-5812-2017-99333_SAIG_AS_AS_208845/
10. 'Pet food standards: Cat and dog food ingredients', Pet Food Industry Association Australia. https://pfiaa.com.au/pet-food-standards/

11. 'PetFAST reporting', Australian Veterinary Association. https://www.ava.com.au/library-resources/other-resources/petfast/
12. https://www.ava.com.au/veterinarians/technical-information/petfast
13. 'Senate to inquire into problem-plagued pet food industry', media release, Centre Alliance, 20 June 2018. https://centrealliance.org.au/media/media/senate-to-inquire-into-problem-plagued-pet-food-industry/
14. Kelly Burke, 'Cat-food irradiation banned as pet theory proved', *Sydney Morning Herald*, 30 May 2009.
15. Susan Thixton, 'Pet food regulations: how the "system" works against pet food consumers', Truth about Pet Food, 26 April 2018. https://truthaboutpetfood.com/how-the-system-works-against-pet-food-consumers/
16. https://petleadershipcouncil.org/pet-industry-news/mars-petcare-announces-support-of-australian-pet-food-regulation

Appendix F

1. Small Animal Specialist Hospital. www.sashvets.com
2. The Board, Veterinary Practitioners Board. www.vpb.nsw.gov.au/board
3. AVA Corporate Supporters, Australian Veterinary Association. https://www.ava.com.au/sponsorship-advertising/
4. Feline gingivostomatitis: Nature's best medicine—raw meaty bones—to the rescue, 17 May 2018. https://www.youtube.com/watch?v=W1H-XTSAr_o
5. Diabetes with Dr Darcy, SASH Vets, 28 Oct 2020. https://www.youtube.com/watch?v=-We52Tw-_KQ
6. Nestlé assault on pets, Part I, 14 May 2021. https://www.youtube.com/watch?v=t9JTkQC4lJw
7. Nestlé assault on pets, Part II, 14 May 2021. https://www.youtube.com/watch?v=2fTiIjBEhZo
8. Maine Coon cats. https://www.youtube.com/watch?v=0l895uWOEiI&t=346s
9. R. Hauptman, Submission 72 to Regulatory approaches to ensure the safety of pet food. https://www.aph.gov.au/DocumentStore.ashx?id=0dfe6f3c-8f29-4209-9895-df563f3e015c&subId=613355
10. Stop the mass poisoning of pets by vets, 19 August 2015. https://www.youtube.com/watch?v=20EjO8mmk7A&t=400s
11. Canine Urolithiasis, SASH Vets, 20 November 2020. https://www.youtube.com/watch?v=2kIb0yoxZLQ
12. Avenging Kitty, 25 September 2019. https://www.youtube.com/watch?v=deyz0-G-jyg&t=80s
13. J. Vale, Submission 134 to Regulatory approaches to ensure the safety of pet food. https://www.aph.gov.au/DocumentStore.ashx?id=1c3bbf91-3b7c-444a-850c-3703bc252233&subId=613667

Appendix G

1. Nestlé assault on pets, Part I, 14 May 2021. https://www.youtube.com/watch?v=t9JTkQC4lJw
2. RMB Campaign & Elections. http://www.rawmeatybones.com/elections.php
3. Stop the mass poisoning of pets by vets, 19 August 2015. https://www.youtube.com/watch?v=20EjO8mmk7A&t=400s
4. Feline gingivostomatitis: Nature's best medicine—raw meaty bones—to the rescue, 17 May 2018. https://www.youtube.com/watch?v=W1H-XTSAr_o
5. R. Hauptman, Submission 72 to Regulatory approaches to ensure the safety of pet food. https://www.aph.gov.au/DocumentStore.ashx?id=0dfe6f3c-8f29-4209-9895-df563f3e015c&subId=613355
6. Maine Coon cats, 25 June 2020. https://www.youtube.com/watch?v=0l895uWOEiI
7. C.E. Harvey, Correspondence, 1993. http://rawmeatybones.com/pdf/Colin%20Harvey%2020-7-93.pdf
8. Science Death Experiment, 21 February 2015. https://www.youtube.com/watch?v=nr7TLXg-vd4&t=93s

ACKNOWLEDGEMENTS

Many people have helped me understand and communicate the raw meaty bones message. Chance remarks, random comments and examples from a wide circle of people have found their way into the inner recesses of my brain and helped me list the facts and opinions expressed in these pages. Dr Breck Muir, from our first meeting in 1982 until today, has been a source of knowledge, inspiration and support. Bill Bowes arrived with impeccable timing in 2000 to help me with the sprawling IT needs of research and publishing *Raw Meaty Bones: Promote Health* and then *Work Wonders: Feed your dog raw meaty bones*. Bill is the perfect ally and friend who ensured the publication of *Multi-Billion-Dollar Pet Food Fraud.* Many clients and staff have supported the campaign. Some names appear in the text. However, there are many whose names are not included. I extend my thanks to all.

Many books, periodicals and films have provided important information. I acknowledge all sources referenced in the Endnotes section and the many more that came across my desk this past fifty years.

Dr Laurel Cohn and Helen Williams wrestled with the early *Multi-Billion-Dollar Pet Food Fraud* manuscript and provided excellent structural advice. Dr Juliet Richters provided vital guidance, copy-editing, proofreading and indexing. Simon Goodway provided inspiration and created the illustrations. My admiration and thanks go to Joy Lankshear of Lankshear Design for book design and typesetting of the final product, and to book PR agency Palamedes for designing the book jacket.

Over the 50 plus years of my veterinary career many thousands of animals have taught me about stoicism and the silent endurance of suffering. I hope that this book provides some acknowledgement and provides the animals with a voice. Lastly, I acknowledge you, the reader, for your interest in our unfinished work. Thank you.

INDEX

Q

R

S

Made in the USA
Middletown, DE
21 May 2023

31018683R00249